IF IT SOUNDS LIKE A QUACK...

IF IT SOUNDS LIKE A QUACK...

A Journey to the Fringes of American Medicine

Matthew Hongoltz-Hetling

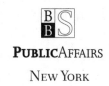

PUBLICAFFAIRS

NEW YORK

PublicAffairs
Hachette Book Group
1290 Avenue of the Americas, New York, NY 10104
www.publicaffairsbooks.com
@Public_Affairs

Printed in the United States of America
First Edition: April 2023

Published by PublicAffairs, an imprint of Perseus Books, LLC, a subsidiary of Hachette Book Group, Inc. The PublicAffairs name and logo is a trademark of the Hachette Book Group.

The Hachette Speakers Bureau provides a wide range of authors for speaking events. To find out more, go to www.hachettespeakersbureau.com or email HachetteSpeakers@hbgusa.com.

PublicAffairs books may be purchased in bulk for business, educational, or promotional use. For information, please contact your local bookseller or Hachette Book Group Special Markets Department at special.markets@hbgusa.com.

The publisher is not responsible for websites (or their content) that are not owned by the publisher.

Print book interior design by Linda Mark.

Library of Congress Cataloging-in-Publication Data
Names: Hongoltz-Hetling, Matthew, author.
Title: If it sounds like a quack . . .: a journey to the fringes of American medicine / Matthew Hongoltz-Hetling.
Description: First edition. | New York : PublicAffairs, 2023. | Includes bibliographical references.
Identifiers: LCCN 2022030108 | ISBN 9781541788879 (hardcover) | ISBN 9781541788862 (ebook)
Subjects: LCSH: Quacks and quackery—United States—History—20th century. | Quacks and quackery—United States—History—21st century. | Alternative medicine—Political aspects—United States. | Alternative medicine—Social aspects—United States. | Medical care—Political aspects—United States. | Social medicine—United States.
Classification: LCC R730 .H66 2023 | DDC 615.8/56—dc23/eng/20220628
LC record available at https://lccn.loc.gov/2022030108

ISBNs: 9781541788879 (hardcover), 9781541788862 (ebook)

LSC-C

Printing 1, 2023

To my mother, Marjorie Hetling, an avid reader who took me to the library, bought me subscriptions to children's magazines, and, when I was in seventh grade, set me up with my first typewriter. Most importantly, she raised me in a house full of books and gave me space to fumble through them, as and when I chose. Thanks, Mom!

Contents

Cast of Characters

 Larry Lytle, a heroic dentist from Rapid Creek, South Dakota, who at the age of sixty-five embarked on a second career that he believed would revolutionize health care.

 Toby McAdam, a failed gubernatorial candidate from Billings, Montana, who created a line of supplements to treat his mother's terminal illness.

 Robert O. Young, a Mormon missionary from Utah who became a folk musician, a tennis player, and a research scientist, in that order. His scientific discoveries resurrected a long-dead theory that challenges the common understanding of germs.

 Alicja Kolyszko, a language teacher who fled Poland's authoritarian Communist Party to pursue her own piece of the American Dream and became the unlikely champion of a much-maligned parasite.

 Leilani and Dale Neumann, Pentecostals of great faith whose pursuit of good works led them from Turlock, California, to found a ministry in rural Wisconsin.

 Jim Humble and Mark Grenon, two beings with vastly different backgrounds who were brought together by a shared belief that the nefarious Deep State was suppressing their miraculous health drink.

Introduction

LIVINGSTON, MONTANA, 2020

> Soon her eye fell on a little glass box that was lying under the table: she opened it, and found in it a very small cake, on which the words "EAT ME" were beautifully marked in currants. "Well, I'll eat it," said Alice, "and if it makes me grow larger, I can reach the key; and if it makes me grow smaller, I can creep under the door; so either way I'll get into the garden, and I don't care which happens!"
>
> —Lewis Carroll, *Alice's Adventures in Wonderland*, 1865

AMERICA'S HEALTH CARE ECOSYSTEM IS SO FULL OF WEALTH AND nonsense that some citizens sell other citizens hundred-dollar tubes of toothpaste (Theodent 300 lacks fluoride but is infused with a proprietary cacao derivative). Health care is so upside down that at one New York hospital, emergency room patients have an average wait time of five hours and forty-one minutes, while rich patients get luxury suites with high-thread-count sheets and a butler. America's health care is so ludicrously well funded that in 2020, when a mysterious new virus swept the globe, the system had ample cash to buy more ventilators, more masks, more technology, more public aid to make quarantines feasible, more high-quality medical staff, and more testing kits than anywhere else on Earth. And yet it's so dysfunctional that, despite these advantages, in August of that year the US took the lead as the nation with more of something else—COVID-19 deaths, the most in the world.

One reason for the high body count was that in 2020 an estimated sixty-six million Americans refused to wear masks to slow the spread of the disease. When pollsters from the Brookings Institution (America could also afford the best sociology polls) asked why, the most frequent answer given was that, as Americans, they had the right *not* to wear a mask.

This was a shockingly honest response.

Going maskless was an exercise of medical freedom, for its own sake. When I read about the poll's results, I was struck by the severe contrast between the symbolism of the act and the concrete grittiness of the consequences, which included the deaths of thousands of otherwise healthy adults and children in every state.

America's surging medical-freedom movement (which accompanied a surge of fatal COVID-19 cases) raised fascinating ethical questions about the boundaries of public health policies, questions that went far beyond the pandemic. After all, we grapple with all sorts of easily preventable deaths. How should the government discourage people from bad health decisions like snorting cocaine, driving without a seat belt, committing suicide, or buying large portions of soda? Should an individual be allowed to sell a fake treatment for an all-too-real fatal disease? What to do when two constitutional directives—public health and individual freedom—collide?

As I began to research this book, I hoped to get to the bottom of these serious questions.

But I didn't.

That's because, early on, I got on the phone with Toby McAdam, a Montana practitioner with about twenty years of experience treating patients. We chatted about the coronavirus pandemic, which at the time dominated most conversations everywhere.

Toby radiated friendliness, knowledge, and, most importantly, complete sanity. But after about three minutes, I realized the book I was writing was going to be something completely different from what I'd initially envisioned.

"You need to look into this," he told me. Toby was sixty-five years old, and he estimated that he had treated a thousand people for cancer. "If someone has a little bit of devious in them, they can get a hold of this virus and mix it with the rabies virus. You're going to get, basically"—and then he said a word.

I'm hard of hearing, and so, when the word I think I heard can't possibly be the word uttered, I'm used to running through a mental Rolodex of rhyming alternatives. Had Toby said salon peas? Some bees? That didn't make sense.

The word was *zombies*.

Toby said it would be possible—easy—for a nefarious actor to turn other people into zombies.

I didn't know much about zombies, but this seemed unlikely to me. So I asked Toby to explain.

He told me that, under a 2017 change in federal regulations, his registration as a researcher allowed him to order modest quantities of various viruses.

"I decided to test this out," he said. "I can get up to five vials of anthrax, smallpox, a lot of those different viruses. If you're registered. That's what's scary."

I agreed that it was, indeed, scary.

"Remember five, ten years ago, that guy attacked that homeless guy and started eating his face off?" Toby asked me. I did, vaguely—a horrific incident in downtown Miami, in which the perpetrator had tested positive only for marijuana, leaving the motivation behind the attack murky. "They blamed it on bath salts."

It would be child's play, Toby said, to induce a similar reaction using an easily transmissible virus—capitalizing, perhaps, on the way a rabies virus induces its hosts to bite aggressively, thereby giving it opportunities to infect new hosts. And because one can be inoculated against rabies, Toby said, warming to his subject, the zombie reaction could be targeted toward specific segments of the population.

"All you have to do is spray an area, depending on what they use, and you could spray that and people could be turned into zombies."

If you were to draw a Venn diagram, with one circle each representing people who believe in zombies and people who treat cancer—would there be any overlap? I had always assumed the first circle would be really small and off in a corner. But it turns out there is at least one person who belongs to both groups: Toby McAdam, of Billings, Montana.

That conversation was the start of my education about health care, something I had always associated with brilliant white-coated doctors, top-shelf medicines, and hospitals implementing evidence-based surgical interventions.

But I learned that millions of Americans who have access to those doctors and hospitals have instead been dabbling in a very different world of health care, one that has little to do with medical institutions, public health agencies, or science. It is a wonderland of leeches and lasers, of zombies and holy spirits. To those who live in that world, it is a joyous exercise of our freedom to fight a mystically powerful Big Pharma; to those who don't, that world is a mournful dirge of humanity's inability to get out of its own way.

This book—the only health care book that gives proper weight to the possibility of disinfecting body cavities with bleach—peers through the looking glass to describe the world of science-lite health care, its origins, and how, between 2000 and 2020, it changed the face of America in ways that no amount of money will fix.

As you explore that world with me, you will meet a heroic dentist, a Jesuit missionary, an Andromedan gold miner, a Polish American linguist, and a couple with an unbreakable devotion to God. Like Toby McAdam, they've all undertaken journeys to the furthest fringes of health and healing.

Their stories are disparate, ranging from Poland to Montana to wherever zombies go. But they follow remarkably similar arcs: the discovery of miracles, the duty to spread the word, and the obstacles and opportunities met along the way. I hope that telling these stories together will illuminate a place that is wild and dangerous but full of promise. For someone, at least.

My pledge to you is that when you set this book down, your neighbor's refusal to wear a mask will be the least of your problems.

PART
ONE

INCUBATION

In which a handful of ordinary Americans discover One True Cure

"And that's the way" (he gave a wink)
"By which I get my wealth—
And very gladly will I drink
Your Honour's noble health."

—Lewis Carroll, *Through the Looking-Glass,
and What Alice Found There,* 1871

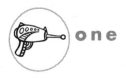 **one**

LARRY LYTLE, 1972

> There is a tide in the affairs of men
> Which taken at the flood, leads on to fortune;
> Omitted, all the voyage of their life
> Is bound in shallows and in miseries.
>
> —William Shakespeare, *Julius Caesar*, 1599

WHEN THE FLOODWATERS BEGAN TO THREATEN THE STABILITY of their home, Plan A was for Robert and Helen Vanderbeek to hustle their two kids through the driving rain and into the car to escape Waverly Street, in Rapid City, South Dakota. But before they could even get into the car, they saw other vehicles being swept along by the dark and roiling waters.

So, as quickly as it could be articulated, Plan B was put into motion. Robert made sure that the boat trailer was tied securely to the big, sturdy tree outside their home. Helen climbed aboard the boat with the two boys—Mark, fourteen, a student at West Junior High School, and Matt, twelve, a member of the Little League baseball team for Ward 3.

The little boat was incapable of navigating the rabid waters, but that wasn't the point. It was moored to the big tree, and the big tree wasn't going anywhere. So, ipso facto, neither were the Vanderbeeks. They bobbed in the darkness.

The flood was a fluke. The highest rate of flow ever recorded for Rapid Creek had been 1.7 billion gallons in a twenty-four-hour period. But that night, winds pushed major rain clouds over the region with agonizing slowness; the clouds hemorrhaged as much as eighteen inches of rain, overfilling the river with 19 billion gallons that crashed through Rapid City with terrifying power.

The big tree that the Vanderbeeks had chosen stayed firm. But up-river, other trees from all along the valley uprooted and joined floating debris—trucks, propane tanks, mobile homes aflame from fires set by their own severed gas lines, a watery stampede charging like wilde-beests down a narrow canyon. No one knows what, exactly, slammed into the Vanderbeeks, and in the end it didn't matter. Something big and heavy smashed the hull of the boat, and all four Vanderbeeks were flung overboard into the black and raging waters, and there was no Plan C.

.•:˙

MATT VANDERBEEK'S LITTLE LEAGUE PRACTICES WERE RUN BY COACH Larry Lytle, a tall, athletic dentist, age thirty-seven, whose heavy brow and arrow-straight posture added to his commanding presence.

Coach Lytle was born in 1935, in a sod house with a dirt floor in Wasta, South Dakota (about 150 residents and a post office), and raised with six siblings. His family battled clouds of crop-devouring grasshoppers that darkened the sky; one year, the unending dryness wilted the grass until they were forced to use a shotgun to kill their herd of a hundred starving cattle. He'd gone on to study dentistry at the University of Nebraska and founded the state chapter of the American Dental Association.

Now, as the floodwaters began streaming down the Black Hills, Lytle and his wife, Norma, were at a Friday night classical concert at Stevens High School. But the concert was cut short; a Rapid City police lieu-tenant appeared and told folks that they should hunker down at home or evacuate immediately.

Lytle knew the lieutenant; in addition to being a coach and a dentist, Lytle was city council president and alderman for Ward 3, which lay right beneath the Canyon Lake Dam. He had responsibilities in this sort of crisis.

But first, he had people to take care of—his three kids, Kim, Kip, and Kelly; his wife, Norma; plus a German family he was hosting as part of an exchange program. Lytle tried to take everyone home via 32nd Street, but the bridge there was already underwater; instead, he zipped up Bacon Park and crossed there, just as the water began flowing across the bridge.

At home on Frontier Place, just south of the Meadowbrook Golf Course, Lytle's basement was already full of water. When the lights and telephone lines died, everyone retreated to the home's upper level. The house was located near Meadowbrook's fifth fairway. Across the greens, through the driving rain, Lytle could see a red light, possibly some sort of emergency vehicle. Lytle, not knowing that his own Ward 3 was facing the worst of the crisis, decided to walk over there and plug into the municipal emergency response that way.

Soon he and his eleven-year-old son, Kip (a teammate of Matt Vanderbeek's), were picking their way across the soaking-wet golf course. The lightning—vast, uncontrolled energy from above—lit up the world in discrete, freeze-frame chunks. They didn't know it, but as they drew near to the emergency vehicle (it turned out to be a fire truck), the water was flowing in stealthily behind them, covering the golf course and cutting off their escape.

The 38th Street bridge, which would have allowed Lytle to reach the fire truck, was now also underwater and impassable. He got as close as he dared and shouted, but no one heard. He and Kip turned around, but the waters on the golf course were rising quickly. Lytle, who stood six two, scooped Kip up and carried him, water lapping against his legs and threatening to sweep them both away.

Elsewhere, thousands were harried by floodwaters that peaked at ten feet high. On West Chicago Street, a division manager for Sears was electrocuted in his home. A professional cowboy was sitting in his car when a wall of water swept him away. A carpenter was fleeing with his family and friends to higher ground when he returned to the house to answer a ringing phone; they lived, and he died.

Lytle knew none of these stories yet, but by the time he waded off the golf course, panting, with Kip in his arms, he understood it was bad. The father of the visiting German family was a policeman. Using sign language, Lytle made him understand that, if they had to abandon the house, they would retreat to higher ground in the nearby foothills. But first, they would have to rescue the disabled next-door neighbor and take him along.

A little past midnight, Lytle stationed himself on a lawn chair on the house's rear deck, monitoring the water. A constant, dull roar clouded his senses, but he tried to stay alert, in case the dam broke.

"I was listening for something that might warn me that there was more disaster coming in than we already had," he later said.

It was a lonely vigil. Each flash of lightning gave him a glimpse of the water; each time, it was a little closer to their end of the golf course. Then it began to race through their backyard. But Lytle could not withstand the fatigue. He fell asleep.

When he awoke, he was disoriented—he could see nothing, hear nothing above the driving rain and rushing waters. But the next lightning flash showed him that the waters were receding. The Lytle home would survive.

Just as the sky began to lighten, Lytle heard screams. People who had fled were returning to the neighborhood. Many found their homes ruined, or gone, some with family inside. Survivors wandered the streets in a daze. And these were the lucky ones in Ward 3. Looking out over the golf course, Lytle saw mud, debris, and bodies, one of which had been partially dismembered by the terrible force of the water.

"So it was a—it was a, uh, a night of horror," Lytle said.

.•:˙

When the rain stopped in the midmorning, Lytle fired up an old car and made his way to city hall by driving alongside a railroad with one wheel up on the track.

He drove through a community in chaos; there were reports of looting and gunfire by night, and injured people lay on mattresses lining hospital hallways. Ruptured gas mains and power lines fueled explosions and fires. Some blamed the flood on recent cloud-seeding experiments conducted by the Institute of Atmospheric Sciences at a nearby mining and technology school.

Lytle helped lead a ten-day, round-the-clock rescue effort that focused on pulling apart wreckage in the hot, humid sunshine to search for survivors—and bodies.

Amid the horror, stories of individual courage began to emerge. A railroad worker was found by a helicopter on the roof of his house with a woman; he requested that they take her first, and when they returned for him, he was gone. Another man, Russ Haley, lifted his wife and daughter onto a roof but found that he could not hoist himself up to join them. Haley used his belt to strap his body to a tree limb, clinging to his branch for seven hours in the frigid rushing waters, like the ornament on the bowsprit of a ship. He left the belt in the tree for what he called "a conversation piece."

The rescue effort revealed more examples of bravery and independent judgment. Scores of local contractors used loaders and backhoes and trucks wherever they saw a need, whether they were being paid or not.

Lytle worked to whittle the list of fifty-five hundred missing people down to confirmed living or dead. They scooped mud out of the Meadowbrook School gymnasium and used it as a base of operations. More than two hundred bodies were recovered in the first couple of days, but only eighty-seven had been identified. They were laid out at the junior high school, many mangled beyond recognition. Lytle called other dentists in Rapid City and collected dental records, using them to attach names to bodies.

Some of the missing were Lytle's friends—patients from his dental practice or classmates of his kids. He found that three members of Kip's Little League team had died.

In the end, there were 238 dead, counting two people who lived outside Rapid City's borders.

The oldest victim was James Atkins, a ninety-four-year-old farmer turned carpenter and father of six.

The youngest victim was four-month-old Jenifer Traversie, who died with her two-year-old brother.

"So," Lytle said, "we had a pretty difficult time in Ward 3."

One person whose name was not on the list of the dead was young Matt Vanderbeek, the boy whose family took refuge in a boat that was smashed to pieces. After being thrown clear, Matt reclaimed the surface of the water and managed to stay afloat.

"They picked him up several hours later on . . . , gasping for the last bit of life he had," Lytle said.

The storm orphaned the boy. Lytle and other rescue workers found the Vanderbeek parents, Robert and Helen, side by side, about seventy-five feet from their home.

Volunteers coordinated watches on bridges downstream, near Cheyenne, where people scanned the waters to see if they could find survivors clinging to debris.

Five bodies, including that of Matt's brother, Mark Vanderbeek, were never found.

.·: ˙

FOR A YEAR, LYTLE WORKED INTENSIVELY ON THE REBUILDING EFFORT—HE won an award for his service to Rapid City during and after the flood—but then he felt that he'd given enough and retired from public service.

"I figured my family deserved some more of my time," he said.

Lytle's medical training, which served him so well in identifying the bodies and in other aspects of the recovery, was the hard-won legacy of a battle that had been fought in the 1840s, when a community of Parisian doctors successfully argued for the merits of objective data in their field. What seems so obvious today—that medical practices should be dictated by the scientific method—initially met stiff resistance from other doctors within the medical community who didn't want to cede their authority and judgment to a body of knowledge being compiled by a bunch of far-distant Numbers Junkies. But by 1860, the evidence-driven approach had been so successful in treating patients that virtually all medical schools were instructing their students to follow the science.

Lytle's formative years and dental training took place between the 1930s and 1960s, when reverence for institutional health care was at an all-time high. In case after case, science was throttling death and disease—the polio vaccine, anesthesia, penicillin, histamines, radiation, and chemo were all discovered in this period, and medical devices like iron lungs and mechanical heart valves were developed. Every tomorrow glimmered with the promise of even more astonishing science-based medical advances, and an army of medical researchers was delving into ever more discrete, localized causes for sickness.

That's why it's so strange that Lytle grew increasingly convinced there was in fact a single, systemic explanation for disease, one that had been completely overlooked by the medical establishment.

He later said that he'd gotten the first hint of it as a boy on the farm, when he took his father's good knife without permission and began whittling. He slipped, and the sharp blade cut a deep gash in his leg. Without telling his parents, he treated it with brackish well water, so alkaline that it gave the family diarrhea.

"I often wondered why that cut seemed to heal overnight. Now I know," he wrote, years later. "It was the energy."

Lytle enrolled at the University of Nebraska in 1960 and graduated its dental college in 1964, moving to Rapid City just as an emerging generation of leftist hippies was infusing America with a suspicion of institutions, including medical institutions. Seeking alternatives, they revived long-dead New Age theories about healing energy, crystals, pyramids, and astrology, among many others. While Lytle was growing his dental practice, he came to believe that a universal healing light suffused all living things; disruptions in this energy, what ancient Chinese healers called qi, were the root cause of all illnesses.

Lytle came to believe that this universal energy could power everything from spontaneous healing to dowsing rods. He began working to invent a medical device capable of harnessing that ancient force and focusing it in a way that would allow all of humankind to enjoy better health.

For Larry Lytle—coach turned dentist turned civic leader—healing light was the One True Cure.

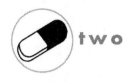 two

TOBY MCADAM, 1976

Ah me! Love can not be cured by herbs.

—Ovid, *Remedia Amoris*, c. 2 AD

TOBY MCADAM—THE GUY WHO BELIEVES THAT ZOMBIES CAN BE created by rejiggering the rabies virus—was born in August of 1958 in Clyde Park, Montana, about ten years before George Romero's shambletastic *Night of the Living Dead* defined zombies for American filmgoers.

Over the course of several wide-ranging phone conversations, two different pictures of Toby emerged. He was optimistic and full of his own bravado—a high school tough, a gleeful thorn in the side of institutional oppressors, and a healer of those in need. Toby traced his heritage, proudly but vaguely, through John Loudon McAdam (a Freemason and the Scottish inventor of macadam blacktop) and on back to the ancient druids of Scotland.

But when Toby told me the stories that made up his childhood, I saw a boy who seemed, mostly, sad.

Young Toby's dark complexion and woolly hair (an inheritance from his French Canadian father) made him the closest thing to a minority in his overwhelmingly white, underwhelmingly populated hometown of about 250 people. The racists of Clyde Park, hard-pressed to find an outlet for their bigotry, landed on Toby as an easy target. His parents were raising three kids in a modest rental home, and Toby's father, a night-shift lumber mill worker, also hauled garbage for the town. Even worse in this deep red state, his parents were strong Roosevelt Democrats, admiring FDR's commitment to a list of human rights, including "the right to adequate medical care and the opportunity to achieve and enjoy good health."

Toby's Scottish mother, Frances Simmons McAdam, a sometime waitress, sometime bartender, leveraged all of her fierce temper in an effort to shield Toby. When his teachers banished him to the coatroom for hours or held him back in the second grade, she laid into them with reckless abandon. During one of his youth soccer games, she raged at the referees, drew a technical, and then laughed about it on the way home. Other times, she railed against injustices being faced by Native Americans, or the evils of Richard Nixon.

But there was little she could do about the cruelty of Toby's peers. As Toby went to and from school, bullies sometimes threw garbage at him and called him racial slurs. After school one day, they caught Toby and tied him up. Other times, they broke his bicycle, and his knuckles.

It was in 1976 that Toby, fresh out of high school, began what would prove to be a decades-long quest for his purpose in life. He tried on a variety of jobs, but nothing seemed to fit. When he got married and was hired by a management company, Frances was delighted. When he got divorced, and fired, she was sympathetic. When he wound up in court over child support and wrongful discharge claims, she took his side.

Toby's older siblings sometimes resented her soft spot for him, but he was the baby, by several years. In 1989, and again in 1993, he got in trouble for writing several thousand dollars' worth of bad checks and for setting up a fraudulent checking account. She forgave it. He would find his footing, she was sure.

Still, as Frances aged, Toby couldn't help but notice that she rarely turned to him for help. If she couldn't find her remote control, she called his brother, Fred. If she needed a ride for a doctor's visit, she called his sister, Jeanie.

In 2000, Toby thought he'd finally found a purpose that would make Frances, and even his siblings, proud. He publicly announced he was running for governor of Montana under the Hamletesque slogan "Toby or not Toby." The campaign fizzled when he failed to qualify for the ballot, but by then the local paper had called him out for not having paid child support since 1988. Fred and Jeanie called him an embarrassment.

You might argue that this all sounds like a real bummer, but Toby didn't see himself as a sad sack. His siblings were simply jealous. "It was more of a—because I would fight. I would take on the status quo. If somebody had an issue, I would get involved with it. That's why I do so well when I get into it."

One day Frances told Toby she'd been diagnosed with lung cancer. A few months later, she moved in with his sister, Jeanie. When Toby visited, Frances cooked for him and her poodle, Midget, who ate bacon and drank from a glass of water on a TV tray.

At some point, Toby and Frances developed a shared belief that Frances would see the end of the tumor growing on her lung, rather than the other way around. Their stubborn optimism got on Jeanie's nerves.

"You have cancer," Jeanie would say. "You don't understand."

"I don't care what I have," Frances would reply, Toby by her side. "I'm gonna beat this thing."

Fred sided with Jeanie, who saw it as a deceptive plying of false hopes, and so an emotionally difficult tug-of-war between family members began, two sets of best intentions that expressed themselves in familial conflict.

Jeanie drove Frances to the hospital for radiation treatments and urged her to listen to the doctor's grave pronouncements. When they got back, Toby would share an article about alternative cures and work with Frances to find speckles of hope amid the doctor's grim words.

One day, Toby received a package in the mail from an East Coast company. Inside was a clump of reddish-brown tendrils and shreds. It was bloodroot, also known as bloodwort, a small and modest plant that bears white flowers and grows from Nova Scotia to Florida.

Toby sat at a table and used a mortar and pestle to grind the roots into a fine powder, which he tipped carefully into tiny half capsules. In his readings, Toby had learned that bloodwort contains berberine, a chemical compound that had, in some test-tube studies, triggered a physical process called apoptosis. Apoptosis is programmed cell death, and it's the lack of apoptosis that allows tumors to grow uninhibited.

Soon he was handing a bottle of the capsules to his mother. His siblings scoffed, but Frances accepted them with gratitude and promised to take them.

TOBY, EAGER TO HELP FRANCES, BEGAN SEEKING OUT OTHER PLANTS WITH medicinal properties. This proved to be surprisingly easy, because, due to a recent change in federal law, more than six hundred American corporations were aggressively selling the idea that the plants of their suppliers could cure the ills of their customers.

In 1994, the dietary supplement industry had successfully lobbied Congress to pass the Dietary Supplement Health and Education Act (DSHEA), which broadened the definition of a food supplement to include almost any vitamin, mineral, plant, or hormone. It also, critically, shifted the burden of proof away from manufacturers so that the Food and Drug Administration had to identify dangerous products on a case-by-case basis.

The new, lax regulatory environment made selling supplements more profitable, which led to an influx of unscrupulous players. This made the industry much bigger and much, much more toxic. Between 1994 and 2000, the supplement industry in the US mushroomed from $4 billion in annual sales to $18.7 billion, and the number of dietary supplements advertised mushroomed right along, from four thousand to twenty-nine thousand. Most were, if not beneficial, then at least harmless. But the race for profitability led some companies to sell the cheapest-possible supplements, containing bulk fillers like talc and gelatin and produced in facilities that allowed (or intended) them to be laced with all sorts of nasty adulterants—blue printer ink, drywall, boric acid, lead paint, floor wax, rat poison. Other manufacturers tried to stand out from competitors by slipping pharmaceuticals into their supposedly all-natural products or were ignorant of what was actually in their own pills. One supplement producer that I spoke with, a vegan activist who'd had his name legally changed to Erb Avore, dedicated years to bringing an all-natural version of Viagra—he called it Stiff Nights—to market. After a man who took Stiff Nights died, the FDA found that Erb's supplier had given him not a plant extract but a synthetic analogue of sildenafil, the pharmaceutical in some commercial dick-stiffening drugs. The pills of one of his competitors was found to contain thirty-one times the prescription dosage of tadalafil (the key drug in erection-boosting Cialis), plus an antidepressant.

The one thing every supplement seller had in common was a vested interest in promoting the idea that the raw active ingredients in its products—mostly minerals and plant extracts—were the key to good health, which they did by flooding the public with promotional materials: magazines and newsletters that cited the flimsiest of scientific studies.

And so, when Toby went searching for information, he found dozens of articles that hinted, implied, or flat out argued that bloodroot could combat cancer. He also read that white willow bark was a good natural alternative to aspirin, leading him to make some capsules of an extract. Then he read that hawthorn berry promoted blood flow.

Toby read more articles that made more promises about more plants. As an optimist, he viewed every herb-related claim in the best possible light. He soon internalized the broader picture that the supplement sellers were painting and came to believe the body was wholly capable of fighting off any disease, if only modern medicine would get out of the way. Packets and boxes of herbs and powders and roots and bark began arriving regularly in his mailbox. He turned a table into a de facto manufacturing lab space and ground these raw ingredients into what seemed like reasonable doses. He made pills to boost his mother's immune system, and pills to reduce fluid buildup in her lungs, and pills to address her forgetfulness. Everything she complained of found a theoretical remedy in bottles of his homemade medications.

"The formula I made works around DNA and genetics. A lot of the time, you're going through cancer, you're missing a lot of nutrients in your body," he said. He thought she might live another thirty years.

Despite Toby's efforts, Frances lost the power to walk. Her continued decline was a mystery to him. "I could not figure out why things were going wrong. There was no way things should be going the way it was. I was frustrated."

In February of 2004, Toby got a call from Jeanie. Frances, by then eighty-three, was nearly incoherent, seeing things that weren't there. Something was seriously wrong.

Toby said he was on his way.

.:.

Outside Livingston Memorial Hospital, the weather hung on a knife's edge, sun and wind tugging at clouds bloated with snow and sleet.

Inside, a different knife's edge balanced life and death. Frances wore breathing tubes like a scuba diver in an ocean of hypoxic air. Flowers clung like anemones to every available surface, and Mylar-coated air bubbles wished her a speedy recovery.

Doctors said Frances had suffered a severe stroke and would likely not leave the hospital alive.

A stroke? Toby was confused. Strokes happen when a blood clot gets into the brain. But Toby had been giving his mother a clot-busting blood thinner.

"It should never have happened," he said.

While her favorite program, *Golden Girls*, played on the television, Toby and Frances relived shared memories. At some point, she told him she could see fish, swimming in lazy circles in the air.

Near the end, Toby told Frances he didn't understand why she'd had the stroke. What about his pills? Had he failed her? Frances experienced a period of lucidity. She looked Toby in the eyes and held his hand.

"You have to promise me that you will never stop this." His supplements, she told him, made her proud. "Whatever you do," she said, "your gift to people is your ability to heal people."

He promised he would never stop.

Then she started to say really awful things. Awful because they were kind. Kind because they were among her last. Among her last because she had given up. His treatments, she told him, had extended her life. He'd allowed her closure. Frances must have intended to ease Toby's suffering. But when she thanked him, the words fell on him like a dead weight.

"That's pretty hard," he said, "when your mother gives you that."

Toby knew that if he spoke a word, or even stayed in that room for another moment, a torrent of emotions would burst out of him. Outside the room, he walked aimlessly around the hospital. He spoke to God. He made promises. He offered up his soul.

But before he reentered the room, he learned he would have to face the hard truth. His mother—his fierce, loving, laughing, shouting, joyous mother—was gone.

A few weeks later, at Jeanie's house, he helped his brother-in-law, Mearl, clean out some of his mother's stuff. Without warning, Mearl handed him a bunch of the bottles Toby had given to Frances. They were all full of pills.

Toby was dumbstruck.

"Why wasn't she taking them?" he asked Mearl.

"I don't know," Mearl said. "I thought she was."

Toby wondered if his sister had withheld the pills from his mother, or whether Frances had just decided it was time to go. But either way, his main takeaway was that the full bottles proved the stroke had come only because she wasn't on his medication. He could have kept her alive for years.

Perhaps it was for the better that the whole governor thing hadn't panned out. With her dying breath, Frances had imbued him with a new purpose. He, Toby McAdam, had discovered that his herbal concoctions were the One True Cure.

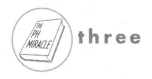 **three**

ROBERT O. YOUNG, 1970

Tragedy is like strong acid—it dissolves away all
but the very gold of truth.

—D. H. Lawrence, letter, 1911

B RIGHAM YOUNG UNIVERSITY OR UNIVERSITY OF UTAH?
Many young Mormons faced this choice, teenagers brimming
with potential and bloated with confidence, deciding whether they were
merely extraordinary or so extraordinary that they could bend the world
to their will.

The more ambitious students often chose BYU, which offered a reputation of academic exclusivity, reinforcement of Mormon cultural norms,
and rigorous moral standards. Rigorous morals were no stranger to the
sandy-haired and athletic Robert Oldham Young—his father, a picture
of kindness, always led the family through morning prayers, blessed the
dinnertime meal, and made sure everyone had a family prayer before
going to bed.

Nor did BYU's reputation for high academic expectations intimidate
Young, for whom self-belief came as naturally as breathing. After all, he
had done well in high school and earned Eagle Scout status in the Boy
Scouts, all while lawn cutting, snow shoveling, floor vacuuming, dish-
washing, and garden weeding at home.

But despite his piety, his work ethic, and his academic prowess, when
Young graduated high school in 1970, he chose the more relaxed atmosphere of the University of Utah, for two reasons.

First, his favorite tennis coach was on the staff at U of U, and Young,
who had been playing since he was eight, dreamed of making his mark

as a tennis pro. And second, the campus was within walking distance of his home, which meant he could stay close to his girlfriend.

Over the first few months at U of U, life was good, but it wasn't great. Not yet.

Soon after he began classes, he learned that the Church of Jesus Christ of Latter-Day Saints had begun training missionary students abroad. Young set aside tennis and girlfriend, trading the deserts and mesas of the American Southwest for the wet smog of urban England (which also happened to be the site of Wimbledon). During his two-year sabbatical at the Ecclesiastic LDS Mission in London, he was granted the title of elder.

"Elder Young." It had a nice ring.

He rented a cramped, one-room flat about fifteen miles south of the LDS Training Center, in Epsom (home to mineral springs that supposedly had healing properties and gave rise to Epsom salts). The icy shower in the shared bathroom fueled his exploration of the area, because pedaling his bicycle through the chilly streets warmed him more quickly than sitting in his room.

The cold was only a minor annoyance. The sense of independence and freedom was exhilarating. In fact, if you could put great into a bottle, well then, Young's life would have been a whole bottleful of great. Even when he went to a KFC and bit into a feather in his chicken wing, he didn't mind. He simply gave up chicken on the spot and felt healthier than ever.

After a few months, Young was summoned to the office of mission president Wallace Bennett.

"I would like you to head up a traveling musical group," President Bennett told Young. "I'm giving you the van and the equipment you need, so you can sing and present messages within song about the principles of the gospel and of Jesus Christ."

This was perhaps one of the few times in history that life exceeded the boundless expectations of youth. Having access to Wimbledon, being made an elder *and* a musician? Young was beside himself. He and three other young missionaries practiced every Monday and Tuesday. He grew his hair long. They called themselves the Family Portrait. Young wrote some of the songs, wholesome, heartfelt messages wrapped in folk rock–flavored melodies.

On most weekends, they crammed themselves and their equipment into the mission's van and played gigs, sometimes on the campuses of major universities like Cambridge and Oxford, after which they might crash on the couches of other missionaries. Bennett even arranged for a recording session at London's Tin Pan Alley, the epicenter of the British music scene, allowing them to distribute actual albums to crowds. At this point, if you could put a bottle of great into a box, well then, Young would have a whole boxful of bottlefuls of great.

Then Bennett sent them word to drop everything. They were going to Buckingham Palace to play for the queen of England. Queen Elizabeth II had spent her twenty-two years on the throne trying to be more relatable than her predecessors. She had glad-handed crowds, walked the streets of Sydney, Australia, and arranged to be filmed making salad dressing while her husband, Prince Philip, barbecued sausages. Inviting four American teens to play at the palace was an extension of that outreach.

"It was a command performance," Young later said. "I mean, you don't ask the queen. She asks you."

At the palace, he was led through endless rooms and hallways to the performance space; there sat the queen, surrounded by family and attendants. Young recognized Prince Philip and Prince Charles, the twenty-six-year-old heir apparent. There were also friends of the royal family and a fair number of what the English referred to as Beefeaters—the sworn guardians of the crown jewels, Tower prisoners, and the queen herself.

This was the apex. If you could put a boxful of bottlefuls of great into a truck, well then, Young would have had a whole truckful of boxfuls of bottlefuls of great.

The Family Portrait fine-tuned their instruments, and then Robert Young sang his heart out. The message of the music was simple.

"Families are forever," he said. "Not just this life, but forever."

Afterward, he was brought forward to spend a moment with the queen.

"She is just a lovely woman," Young said. "Very eloquent. Very polite."

It was a window into wealth and fame, and Young's early experiences had taught him that with hard work, he might achieve some level of wealth and fame himself. But it wouldn't be as an elder or a rock star. After his missionary training, he returned to U of U, just knowing that life had something even greater in store.

He rolled through college on a tennis scholarship (a C+ in biology but As in psych, econ, writing comp, and, of course, tennis), and then, although he never reached Jimmy Connors or Björn Borg status, he earned a living for five years as a tennis pro.

When he put down his racket, he was twenty-nine. His hairline was receding at a worrisome pace, but he was still blessed. He'd married the beautiful Shelley Redford, who claimed to be the sister of actor Robert Redford, and was working on a family of his own. It was time for whatever came next.

He drove his truckful of boxfuls of bottlefuls of great toward the horizon, searching and believing in himself.

That's when he decided to study nutritional science, springboarding off the knowledge he'd amassed as a pro athlete. In the nineties, he began looking for ways to better understand health by examining live blood specimens. He used a darkfield microscope, which allowed for improved image contrasts without staining the specimens. One day, while scrutinizing magnified images of squirming cells, he saw something that led him to a startling conclusion.

He, Robert Oldham Young, tennis pro, queen-approved musician, and supposed brother-in-law of Robert Redford, had discovered the One True Cure. If he was right, his greatness could not be contained, not by the biggest bottles, the sturdiest boxes, or a whole fleet of trucks.

Two years later, Young was charged with his first crime.

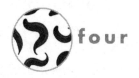four

ALICJA KOLYSZKO, 1956

Nora: Look here, Doctor Rank—you know you want to live.
Rank: Certainly. However wretched I may feel, I want to prolong
the agony as long as possible. All my patients are like that.

—Henrik Ibsen, *A Doll's House*, 1879

THE ADULTS—ALICJA'S MOTHER AND AUNT—SHOOED THE CHIL-
dren out of the large living room in the flat.

It was 1956, and Poland was in chaos. Elsewhere in the country,
the communist government was putting down protests with soldiers and
tanks. Prime Minister Józef Cyrankiewicz gave a radio address, warning that anyone lunatic enough to raise a hand against the government
would see that hand chopped off.

But for Alicja, a little girl living in the small city of Elk, such horrors
were nothing more than a certain tone in abstract discussions among
adults.

She was five, an age when the evils of men were far less worrisome than
the creatures of legend. Slavic storytellers said Elk Lake was infested—its
waters hid the bloodsucking demon *strzyga*, the *mamuna* (which lurked
in lakeside thickets in the form of hairy old women, replacing innocent
children with their own offspring), and the wicked *wodniki*, unbaptized
suicide victims that dragged swimmers beneath the waves.

Monsters notwithstanding, the lake was a magnet. In the distance, a
stone-walled prison loomed over the far side of a lake-spanning bridge;
sometimes, winds carried rough voices across the ice, though whether
they were the voices of prisoners or spirits Alicja never knew. In the win-

ter, she skated far from the shore, peering into fishing holes and feeling the absoluteness of their inky depths.

The courtyard to the rear of Alicja's apartment was, by contrast, a riotous circus of life—bicycles and motorcycles and balcony-based puppet shows and cows and chickens and clotheslines and screaming children and flirting teens and drinking parents. And there was Alicja smack in the middle, a blue-eyed, blonde-haired tomboy with hand-sewn tights under her white dresses, to facilitate running on the complex's rooftops, or wrestling a man's heavy bicycle out of the courtyard and onto the cobbled streets that led to Elk Lake.

"It could be a movie done from that courtyard," she told me, sixty-five years later.

But on this particular day, the cold lake and the hot courtyard were out of sight and out of mind. As Aunt Wanda herded Alicja's brother Bazuk (Basil, in English) past one set of French doors and toward the kitchen, Alicja stood quietly in the rear hallway, unnoticed.

Her father, Vasili—her noble, pipe-smoking father, born in 1894, once one of the largest landowners in Poland—lay on the couch, pale and silent.

He'd fought against the Bolshevik communists as part of the White Army, but it had all gone wrong. He'd been stripped of his lands and imprisoned by the government, leaving the family a sense of dignity and lost wealth. Vasili always dressed in suits, with a white shirt and tie. At dinner, they ate with aprons, and even the toddlers used adult knives and forks.

Her grandmother entered the room with a stranger. The woman was so short that Alicja could see the crown of her Ukrainian ochipok; it was black, topping brilliant colors that framed the sides of her solemn face. She put a wicker basket down on the floor next to Alicja's so-still father.

"Please," Alicja's grandmother said to the woman. "Be careful." In the background, Alicja's mother, Alina, thirty years younger than her husband, began crying fitfully.

Alicja couldn't hear much, but she caught the word *pijawka*. Alicja knew what a *pijawka* was. When she and her playmates thrilled themselves by running along the half-submerged, felled trees that lay next to Elk Lake, the *pijawka*—small, black, slimy, and disturbingly active—

sometimes attached themselves to the children's bare legs, filling them with revulsion.

Vasili stirred, groaning in pain or protest. The visitor directed Alicja's grandmother and her uncle Stanislaus to transfer him to the bedroom. Alicja, fearful of being caught eavesdropping, slipped away.

When she came back, her father was no longer on the couch. A few days later, she heard that word—*pijawka*—again and knew it was now associated with her father's path back to health.

.:˙

THE STORY OF THE *PIJAWKA*—THE LEECH—BEGINS IN PREHISTORY.

Five hundred and fifty million years ago, the world's waters were a seething swamp of multicellular blobs in an endless gyre, each blob trying to put together a successful strategy for reproducing itself.

One day a new form emerged, not so much rising from the muck as squirming through it, on the world's first belly. This was *Ikaria wariootia*, the oldest known bilateral creature on the planet and the one whose descendants include both leeches and humans. It was surprisingly leech-like, which means that the evolution of nearly every animal can be measured, in some way, by its distance from the leech.

Leeches have done more than perhaps any other animal to shape our biome's genetics. Eventually, as warm-blooded animals diverged from their cold-blooded reptilian forebears, the parasitic leeches had an unintended impact on the makeup of tens of thousands of species: in a little-understood evolutionary process called DNA jumping, leeches absorbed a DNA group called Bovine B from snakes and inserted it into the genetic code of mammals. As a result, roughly a quarter of a cow's DNA code is copied directly from pythons (one of many weird examples of mammals walking around with reptile DNA).

Today, there are nearly seven hundred leech species. One lives in the forest canopy, waiting to drop on unsuspecting hikers, while another lives exclusively in the anus of the hippopotamus. And a few leech species feed on humans. These are the *pijawka*.

The next time Alicja was playing in the shallow waters at the edge of Elk Lake, she looked down to find that one had attached itself to her leg. When this happened to area children, they usually rushed to their parents, who used ashes from wood-fired kitchen ovens to kill them (the leeches, not the kids). But, knowing that the *pijawka* had helped her father, little Alicja had moved beyond mere revulsion.

She poked at the leech on her leg, probing around the edge of its attachment. She pressed her fingernail down, interposing it gently between the leech and her own skin to disrupt the leech's suction. And the leech released, carrying a bit of her vitality beneath the deep, dark waves.

.∵·

ALICJA WAS EIGHT AND A HALF MONTHS PREGNANT WHEN IT BECAME CLEAR that she would have to flee Poland. During a March 1973 teaching conference in Białystok, administrators announced that membership in the Communist Party would thenceforth be a baseline requirement for women to work as teachers (men had been hit with the same rule long before).

"Alicja," said the director. "You are not coming back to school."

On the director's desk, Alicja saw a termination form known as a "wolf ticket," a reference to those who, with ruined prospects, were forced to live in the forests like animals. Alicja, whose family had already lost so much to communist dogma, flared.

"I am coming back," she said.

"No," the director said calmly. "You're not."

Even then, Alicja could have asked to be accepted by the Communist Party, but she was the daughter of Vasili. When he fell on the battlefield, he had lain still as death while the Red Army poked him with a stick, before moving on.

Alicja stormed out of the office.

All throughout Poland, families that were not in the good graces of the Communist Party were disappearing from their homes, though it was not always clear which had fled to America and which were languishing in a Polish prison. Alicja worried about leaving Vasili, now on the cusp of his eighties; age was a foe he could neither conquer nor endure. But Vasili insisted she get herself, her husband, and her children out of Poland. She and her husband sold the Alfa Romeo to bribe an official into approving a short vacation to Italy, and soon she was hugging Vasili goodbye, her family members' birth certificates sewn into the wall of her suitcase.

"Have a good trip," said her father, playing along. "Enjoy Italy, and I will see you soon."

She never saw him again.

Alicja's family disembarked in New York with five dollars and no English skills. Alicja was now one of the seven hundred thousand *Polonia amerykańska* who sought a new life in 1980s America. By prior arrangement through refugee agencies, Alicja and her family were sent by train to southwestern Minnesota, where they were taken to a small living quarters on a farm. The owner, who had eight kids, raised crops and did side work as an auctioneer.

The farmer's neighbor spoke Polish; she explained to them that the farmer was sponsoring them through a refugee program. They would have to work there for a minimum of five years, at a wage of one dollar per hour. Alicja, who had never pulled a turnip in her life, cried herself to sleep.

In the morning, she made a phone call from the barn and learned that their file had been mixed up with that of another family, one with farming experience. It took a few weeks, but they soon landed in the bosom of a Baptist church community in Minneapolis.

There, in a small apartment, the full weight of overbearing government finally fell from their shoulders. Alicja studied English and worked a sewing machine in a local factory. Every purchase was a liberating exercise in Americanism. Here, they learned, they would be able to buy a house—a whole house!—on credit. But before that, they would buy a car. But before that, food.

In Poland, a government food-voucher system made it easy to get drunk, but one had to fight for a space in line to buy a steak. Here, they walked across a bridge to get to Lunds, a high-end grocery store, and bought whatever they felt like eating. That first time, for dinner, they got packages with pictures of a tempting delicacy: chicken that could be fried, the American way.

As they made their way back to their apartment, they spoke happily to one another, cars streaming past. *Our fellow Americans!* they said wonderingly. *They must think we're strange, carrying bags from a fancy store like Lunds, and yet walking across the city, like peasants.*

When they got home, they opened their big, heavy canisters of chicken only to find that they had purchased two huge tubs of Crisco shortening. They laughed until tears ran down their cheeks.

America was good.

.•: :

ON A TRIP BACK TO POLAND IN 1999, ALICJA WALKED INTO A SMALL PRI-vate clinic and was greeted immediately by the owner, a petite, elegantly dressed woman with a skyward-pointing nose that spoke not just to a profession but to a certain class of person.

Unlike America, where hospitals treated patients like interchange-able widgets, this was a very personal experience. Alicja kind of knew this woman—a friend of a friend, highly recommended.

Things in America had gone wrong for her five years before. While in the back seat of a car that spun out of control in one of Minneso-ta's harsh winter blizzards, she was pitched between the front seats and smashed her face against the gearshift of the manual transmission.

The blow broke her nose, but the lasting impact was from a painful torquing of her spine. Ever since, her lower back had throbbed relent-lessly. The doctors recommended surgery, but Alicja instead searched for a noninvasive solution, one that America's gleaming, monolithic hospitals had overlooked. Her quest for an alternative drove her down Europe's crooked, narrow streets to this modest clinic.

Here, the elegant woman boosted Alicja's spirits immediately. Of course she could alleviate Alicja's pain, she said confidently, her Polish words like a soothing salve on Alicja's English-weary ears. That is what she did.

"Angela," the woman said to the only other worker behind the counter. "Please take Mrs. Kolyszko to be treated."

Angela, who was young and rotund and dressed in street clothes, flushed but led Alicja back without complaint. The treatment room was small and cool and spare, furnished only with a tiny nightstand alongside a metal bed that had a white sheet draped over it.

"I came to get help for my back," Alicja told the young woman.

Angela asked her to undress for the treatment.

"Everything?"

Yes, everything.

When Alicja was completely naked and breaking out into goosebumps in the coolness, Angela had her lie face down. The bed was cold on her bare stomach.

The woman asked Alicja to point to the parts of her back that hurt.

Alicja indicated her lower back, all around the coccyx.

"I am freezing," Alicja later recalled. "She didn't cover me, not with a sheet, not with anything."

As Angela bent over Alicja, Alicja realized that the woman smelled of sweat, acrid with nervousness. Wordlessly, Angela began to apply something cold and wet to the pained areas of Alicja's lower back.

Alicja knew what they were—leeches, each one sinking three hundred tiny teeth into her flesh—so she was prepared for the slight pinching sensation. But she wasn't prepared to be literally shaking with cold.

"Can you cover me?" Alicja asked. "A little bit?"

"Yes," said Angela. "I'll be right back."

The door closed, and Alicja shut her eyes, clenching her jaws against the cold. Five agonizing minutes passed. With the leeches feeding on her back, she was afraid to move. After ten minutes, she began to bang on the table, and didn't stop until the elegant woman appeared.

"Oh, child," she said, all poise and solicitousness. "No one covered you!"

"Yes, I am freezing," said Alicja.

The woman put a sheet over Alicja's bare legs, and another one over her torso, above where the leeches were attached, and left. Alicja was more comfortable, but the minutes slithered by with agonizing slowness, humping along on blood-engorged bellies. Wait—those weren't minutes.

"I feel something is walking on my back," Alicja later said. "It is crawling."

This didn't concern her so much as terrify her. She didn't know how many leeches were still attached to her backside, or where the unattached ones might wander. All dignity lost, she let out an adrenaline-fueled scream.

A leech tumbled along the curve of Alicja's body and fell to the floor. Her screams increased in pitch and volume.

Both the little elegant woman with the skyward-pointing nose and large, perspiring Angela came bursting into the room, bustling to corral the leeches that, done feeding, were on the move.

Alicja got glimpses of them—swollen with her blood, and so much larger than she had pictured.

Once the chaos subsided, the elegant woman's natural sense of calm reasserted itself. She dressed Alicja's wounds, soothingly, and placed her in an adult diaper, soothingly. She made a bit of soothing small talk while she worked, as Angela watched, the red of her cheeks slowly fading.

Then the little elegant woman told Angela—hulking, hapless, blushing Angela, who by now Alicja was beginning to suspect was the other woman's daughter, and less than committed to the family business—to dispose of the leeches.

Alicja gratefully began pulling on her clothes. But as soon as the proprietress left, tension began to seep back into the room. Alicja and Angela regarded one another unhappily. The large woman's cheeks once again flooded with color as she took up one of the wriggling, engorged leeches and carried it to the little nightstand, which now held a jar filled with a clear liquid.

Angela tentatively put a leech into the jar. Alicja had read up on leech treatments, but what happened next was not addressed in the literature.

The leech exploded; Alicja's blood burst from its mouth and covered the surrounding area in thick red droplets.

Alicja, half dressed, froze in shock; the only thing that moved were her eyeballs as they followed Angela, who grimly soldiered on, blushing and sweating and breathing heavily as she inserted another leech into the alcohol solution.

This one exploded even more violently; there was now blood on Alicja's clothing and face. Alicja grabbed the last of her clothes and fled.

At the front desk, Alicja managed to count out 160 zloty—about forty US dollars—to the elegant woman, whose composure was not at all ruffled by Alicja's stricken face, nor by the traces of blood that still adorned it.

"I paid," Alicja later recalled. "I said thank you, even."

Utterly disappointed with the events of the afternoon, Alicja plopped into her car, diaper crinkling against the seat. Two things wore off. The first was the sheer emotionality of the whole unpleasant experience. The second was the natural anesthetic that the leeches had secreted into her back to mask the sting of their ministrations.

Alicja shifted her weight, assessing her condition. She moved gingerly and then with increasing gusto. The pain in her back, a near-constant companion for years, was gone. Then she noticed something even more remarkable. Her knee, which had been painfully swollen from a tennis injury, was no longer inflamed.

The leeches—bloodsucking, gross little creatures though they may be, inexpertly applied as they were—had done something to her. Something that seemed almost miraculous.

Remembering how the doctors had told her that nothing could accomplish this except surgery, Alicja saw an opportunity to more fully live the American Dream.

America had fancy grocery stores, and glistening cars, and cunningly disguised tubs of cooking lard, and skyscrapers, and promise. But it lacked leeches.

Leeches were, Alicja was sure, the One True Cure.

five

DALE AND LEILANI NEUMANN, 1987

Sir Patrick Cullen: Well, I've known over thirty men who've found out how to cure consumption. Why do people go on dying of it, Colly? Devilment I suppose!

—George Bernard Shaw, *The Doctor's Dilemma*, 1906

L EILANI.
   Dale.

She sang. He preached.

She was nineteen. He was twenty-five. Stillness made her anxious. Solitude brought him peace. Leilani was a native Californian. Dale hailed from rural Wisconsin.

She glowed amid her megachurch family; he had been proudly born again. She was a honeyed blend of culture; he was German, white as butterkäse cheese. Her religious faith was bound up in community, his, an unshakeable confidence in self and God. Leilani's emotions gushed over children, animals, peers, elders, everyone; Dale guarded his feelings in a secret, inner space. After Bible college, Leilani attended a progressive Californian Pentecostal church, while Dale graduated Christian Life College into that very same church.

Together, they built a dream in which their love for one another was surpassed only by their shared devotion to God.

Leilani Evarista Miraflor had grown into her long, lustrous dark hair, brown eyes, and radiant smile under the prayerful eyes of her grandmother (who had pioneered many churches with her grandfather), her Hawaiian-born mother, and an enormous extended family.

Dale Roger Neumann was a strapping, swaggering six foot two and a bit of a perfectionist. His slicked-back hair and dark-hued clothing unintentionally bolstered his natural resemblance to the actor Johnny Depp. Dale was the fifth of eight children born to Elvere Schmidt and William "Peanut" Neumann, a union man in the construction industry.

By the time Dale met Leilani, he'd already crossed the most important threshold in his life—unhappy as a young man, he had found a much happier existence on the far side of his born-again baptismal waters. He spent his college years studying theology—learning to teach and preach the Bible—and "missiology," which is the study of missionary work.

Dale was exploring paths toward becoming a Pentecostal minister. He knew that some preachers bent scripture to match their own personal agenda, but Dale was a straight arrow, interpreting each passage as literally as possible. When he preached, his boundless self-confidence and conviction caught fire. He wasn't above referring to himself in the third person, as in, "That's the day when Dale R. Neumann died, and he was buried in baptism."

With Leilani, another side of Dale emerged. He could be slyly funny, displaying an almost childlike tenderness with her. In June 1987, they married.

In the early days, Dale often assumed the role of theological teacher. Leilani was surprised at the extent to which Dale pushed her into making everyday decisions and taking responsibility for them. She credited his faith in her with allowing her to grow in confidence and to get to know herself.

Other decisions, he had already made.

"He let me know the few things he had definitely made his mind up on like breastfeeding, homeschooling etc.," Leilani would later write.

They moved to Turlock, located in California's Central Valley roughly halfway between San Francisco and Yosemite National Park. The community was in the midst of a thirty-year population explosion; every home was skyrocketing in value, and money came easily. The Neumanns were blessed with four kids in six years—first came Luke, then Ariel, then Hamilton, and finally Madeline, who went by her middle name, Kara.

The family attended religious services at the New Life Christian Center; it was located beside a farmer's field full of harvest, a potent metaphor for a congregation that believed in reaping souls for the Lord. The church leader, a much-loved figure known as Pastor Dave, was progressive, and he led the Neumanns through lively, fun services that differed sharply from the dogmatic traditions of the mainstream Catholic Church.

When not worshiping, the Neumanns enjoyed a world of gazebos and Jacuzzi hot tubs and grounds where everything grew thick and lush; in Turlock, their huge Spanish-style corner home had twelve-foot ceilings, rear-facing balconies, arched doorways throughout, and the largest backyard in the whole subdivision.

Much later, in 2019, Leilani would revisit the home with her daughter and her father in a stroll down memory lane. There was the swimming pool where Kara and the other kids once swam with friends; here was the sun-warmed macadam where Lolo the cat once lounged. It had been a cushy life.

"We probably spent like, I don't know, $20,000 just on chandeliers," she said. She giggled, a bit ashamed at the extravagance, a bit buoyed by the memory. "We were a little crazy back then. But anyway." Her voice took on a slightly wistful tone.

"When we lived in California."

.∴.

THE JOURNEY AWAY FROM THOSE HAPPY, SUNNY SUBURBS BEGAN, IN A sense, as an outgrowth of Dale's devotion to following the Bible as written, rather than listening to institutional interpretation.

And the Bible was very clear about health care.

Jesus Christ loved healing. In one story, Jesus took three sandaled apostles to Galilee, where a man named Jairus, the influential ruler of a local synagogue (and therefore a good "get" for Jesus), threw himself at Jesus's feet and begged him to heal his twelve-year-old daughter, who "lieth at the point of death." It was an emergency.

Jesus rushed toward Jairus's house, with crowds all around. But suddenly his footsteps slowed. He stopped cold, whipped around, and looked at the crowd.

"Who touched my clothes?" he asked.

Apparently, Jesus was under the impression that someone had snuck up behind him and made contact with his robe.

Was Jesus serious? A girl's life hung in the balance. Even his three apostles seemed embarrassed. After all, hundreds of people surrounded them. Touchers gonna touch.

But Jesus ignored their signaling.

"Someone touched me," he insisted. He scrutinized the crowd. With tensions rising, and Jairus no doubt sick with worry over the delay, Jesus eyed a woman in the crowd. Realizing that Jesus was not going to let this go, she stepped forward, trembling with fear, and fell at his feet, confessing. The woman was sick. She'd experienced twelve years of continuous menstrual bleeding, which left her a social pariah. The local customs required that she be confined to her house lest she sully a man with her impure, womanly touch.

And so, as she now confessed, she'd slipped up behind Jesus and grabbed his clothes, which instantly caused the blood to dry, healing her. Once the public shaming was complete, Jesus lost interest.

"Daughter, thy faith hath made thee whole," he said. "Go in peace, and be whole of thy plague."

He returned his attention to the emergency mission of the dying girl.

But just then, a messenger from Jairus's house joined them and, in a classic case of failing to soften the blow, told Jairus, "Thy daughter is dead."

The Bible records no words from Jairus; possibly, he was speechless at the realization that his daughter had breathed her last while Jesus was preoccupied with Clothesgate.

Jesus strode on. He found Jairus's house in absolute bedlam, crowded with people wailing in anguish. In what may be the world's first case of hard-core trolling, Jesus asked the mourners to justify their actions (their actions being, namely, mourning a child they loved who had died only minutes before).

"Why make ye this ado, and weep?" he demanded.

The crowd got ugly, but he shooed them out and made his way to the dead girl's room. He took the corpse by the hand.

"*Talitha cumi*," he said, in Aramaic. The Bible interprets this for us: "Damsel, I say unto thee, arise."

Right away, the girl got up out of the bed, and Jesus told the parents (who were, in a Seussian turn of phrase, "astonished with a great astonishment") to get her some food. This outcome presumably made up for the trolling.

The story of the raising of Jairus's daughter is, in many ways, the absolute essence of how Jesus is portrayed in the Bible—a guy who walked around with absolute confidence, often using acts of healing to get people to listen to sermons about his dad. By one count, Jesus and his followers performed sixteen different acts of miraculous healing, plus some demon banishing and some dead raising.

Dale, reading all this in his favorite book, unsurprisingly decided to give prayerful healing a go. After a decade of undergoing chiropractic treatments for persistent back pain, he instead sought a higher form of treatment. And just like that, God answered—the chronic pain went away.

Dale and Leilani soon took that reasoning a step further. If God was willing to cure their ills, wasn't seeking out a doctor instead of God a blasphemous insult?

In the months that followed, the whole family continued to experiment, praying over childhood fevers, Leilani's allergies, and all the little aches and pains that come with regular family life. And it paid off. Headaches faded. Allergy attacks evaporated. Leilani's anxiety was alleviated.

The Neumanns became confident that prayer, not medical science, was the One True Cure.

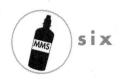 **six**

THE ALIEN, 1996

Quackery and idolatry are all but immortal.

—Oliver Wendell Holmes, "The Medical
Profession in Massachusetts," 1869

THE STRANGER WAS TAKEN INTO GUYANA ON AN AIRPLANE, TO Georgetown in a car, to the Cuyuni riverbank in a pickup, to the upper reaches of the river in a speedboat, and then slowly into the dense jungle in a truck that sometimes spun its man-sized wheels on barely there roads of mud.

In the end, even the powerful truck had to be abandoned.

The stranger continued on foot, into this land where harpy eagles ate sloths, anacondas ate monkeys, and tarantulas ate birds. He looked like a small, white Alabaman in his sixties. For all anyone knew, that's what he was. He seemed fantastically out of place in the humid rainforest as he tried to keep up with the eight Guyanese workers, each of whom had an eighty-pound pack on his back, straps running around the top of their head to help them bear the weight up a thousand-foot ascent.

He'd foregone snake-resistant boots in favor of lighter tennis shoes that retained less water. He stood by his choice, but it had him on edge, constantly looking for snakes. Still, reptiles did not deter the stranger.

He was there for gold.

Lots of people were. It was 1996, and foreign companies, mostly from Australia and Canada, were mobilizing huge mining operations, cutting in the Guyanese government for 5 percent in royalties on tens of tons of gold each year. There was also a chaotic patchwork of medium- and small-scale operators—some local, some foreign, some sanctioned by the government, and some illegal, with more than half of all mined gold smuggled across international lines into Brazil or Venezuela.

Staffing a gold operation was never easy, but this year it was even worse than usual because a chloroquine-resistant strain of malaria was eating its way through the local manpower. Research would later show that every 1 percent increase in gold prices correlated with an increase of as much as 13 percent in malaria cases, because young workers would flock to gold camps that doubled as mosquito buffets.

The stranger considered himself "among the best, if not the best" gold miner in the world, using his own proprietary techniques. The party established a jungle camp to assay mineral samples. It was rough living—lying in a hammock and hoping that the squelches, smacks, and screams of the seething darkness kept their distance. Among the many unpleasant creatures in the region was *Haementeria ghilianii*, the giant Amazonian leech that, at more than seventeen inches long and four inches wide, was known to attack caimans and anacondas.

One day, two of the workers woke up so sick they couldn't get out of their hammocks, except to vomit and deal with bouts of diarrhea. Their heads hurt, and they ached all over. Though they had high fevers, they shivered with chills.

Everyone knew these symptoms indicated malaria, potentially fatal. The stranger made a suggestion. He had brought along an American-made water purifier known as stabilized oxygen.

"It seemed to me, knowing it killed pathogens in water, that it might cure malaria. I sat down with the men who had malaria and asked them if they would be interested in trying this 'health drink' from America."

With little to lose, they drank the water purifier.

But there was something they didn't know about the stranger, who went by the name Jim Humble. He wasn't human.

•ₒ•

OH, SURE, HE HAD LIVED A HUMANESQUE LIFE. A BOYHOOD IN MOBILE, a short stint in the marines, work at a California health food store, followed by engineering for the aerospace industry.

But all of that was misleading.

The stranger's real life story, which he shared only with a select group of people, was quite different. He didn't see himself as a straight, white, male, human Terran. He was an ancient alien god from the Andromeda Galaxy.

And, really, I can't prove that he isn't.

Nearly a billion years ago, he'd lived on Andromeda's "Planet of the Gods," so known in that corner of the universe because the alien race occupying it was so advanced.

"We built planets. Stars and all sorts of things that were associated with gods," the alien in Jim Humble's skin would later say, when he went public with his actual identity. The ruler of the Planet of the Gods, a being known as Manzanora, controlled an empire of fifty-five planets. After joining a sector of Manzanora's space navy that was tasked with business in the Milky Way, the alien in Jim Humble's skin developed a real affinity for Earth, which was just a lifeless rock until his people nudged it into its current, life-friendly orbit around the sun. They also stocked it with its biological life (meaning that all species on Earth are technically invasive).

"There was no evolution on this planet, sorry," the alien later said. "It happened on other planets, but we brought the animals here. We brought the water here also."

Eventually, he and his fellow aliens began walking Earth's surface in the guise of humans. When the body they were using wore out, they would trade it for another that was just beginning a new human life cycle. This disrupted their memories, but they had implants in their heads that allowed them to sense one another. The alien in Humble's skin had learned of his true origin only after others, drawn to his implant, had contacted him and reawakened buried memories of ancient civilizations that he had experienced over the course of millions of years on other planets (and thousands of years in his previous human bodies on Earth).

The sick gold workers knew none of this when they accepted his offer of a water purifier that he called an American health drink. The following day, when two more men fell ill, they accepted it too.

All four men recovered, according to the alien in Humble's skin. When he went back to civilization, he took out ads in Guyanese newspapers, touting his "Humble Health Drink" as a cure for malaria. But not everyone liked the immortal alien's assertion. The Guyanese minister of health called him in for an interview.

"She told us that if we sold our solution to one more person, that we would be in their prison and that we wouldn't like their prison," the extraterrestrial later wrote. "I had seen the prison and I knew that she was right."

.:·

AFTER LEAVING GUYANA, THE ALIEN IN HUMBLE'S SKIN MOVED BACK TO Nevada. He sold his only significant asset, a forty-foot oceangoing house-boat, and used the capital to start a business that sold mining equipment.

Meanwhile, he began experimenting with his Humble Health Drink to better understand its properties and improve its efficacy. He bought bulk amounts of swimming pool test strips to measure the chlorination levels of different concentrations. Sometimes he let it air out for a while. Sometimes he added vinegar.

Soon, the alien came up with a formulation that cured not only malaria but cancer, by soaking into cells and killing the little cancer-causing bug inside them. It was the sort of revelation that demonstrated the immortal being's superiority over humankind's scientific institutions—they had never even detected cancer-causing bugs, let alone come up with treatments for them. The alien in Humble's skin soon discovered that the health drink cured diabetes, AIDS, erectile dysfunction—in fact, just about anything.

This was fantastic news, because a million years ago he and a group of fellow aliens had agreed to stop mucking about with planet-design projects and instead do something really wonderful for the universe. Though there was initial debate about what that something wonderful might be, they eventually settled on elevating Earthlings to take their rightful place in the intergalactic community. But this plan brought opposition from Manzanora and other aliens, who feared the potential of humanity and saw Earth as a planet-sized prison.

These two groups of aliens—those who wanted to elevate humans, and those who wanted to see them permanently sequestered on Earth—

have been trying to achieve their respective agendas ever since. Because of an intergalactic code that prevents the wholesale slaughter of intelligent beings, the aliens have had to work by manipulating humans; all of modern history has been subtly shaped by these two warring viewpoints.

Most serious diseases were in fact created by agents of Manzanora in order to suppress humans. And now he, the alien in Jim Humble's skin, had devised a drink that could end disease, forever foiling Manzanora and clearing the path for Earth's ultimate destiny. The immortal being began calling it Miracle Mineral Solution.

MMS was, he was sure, the One True Cure.

In order for the mission to succeed, MMS had to be introduced around the world. But how?

The alien was at this time experiencing what Earthlings called "cash flow issues." The magazine he used to advertise mining equipment "made a big mistake" with his ad and refused to credit him. He identified this event as the reason that his business failed. He was penniless and living on Social Security.

In 2001, a friend offered him a gig as resident caretaker at an old gold-milling property in Mina, Nevada, a ghost town of 150 people that billed itself as "ATV friendly." The buildings were decrepit shacks, holdovers from a time when the area had been a mining spot served by a railroad.

Soon, the alien in Humble's skin was puttering about the old gold mill, fixing leaky roofs and pushing back the endless tide of dust. He sometimes went outside to watch the night sky. When he did, he often saw spaceships headed farther down the valley, toward Area 51, famous as a hotspot for UFO activity. But Area 51 was controlled by the American government, which had been co-opted by Manzanora and his allies. Aliens going there could not be relied on to help bring MMS to the Earthlings.

He was stymied.

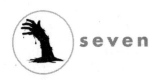seven

AMERICA

Joy, temperance, and repose, slam the door on the doctor's nose.

—Friedrich von Logau, *Sinngedichte*, c. 1654,
translated by Henry Wadsworth Longfellow

THE ALIEN IN JIM HUMBLE'S SKIN WAS NOT THE ONLY ONE STEW-ing over his inability to popularize a One True Cure. Throughout American history, other inventors of other One True Cures had been a constant, if minor, presence, dotting the landscape from sea to shining sea. Each inventor had turned away from the medical establishment; each had a theory of health that was at odds with accepted science; each had a cure that could be applied in the home, away from the prying eyes of medical institutions. Into this category fell Vermont country doctor D. C. Jarvis, who sold people on the wonders of apple cider vinegar; Oklahoma pastor Charlie Shedd, who made money by telling people to "Pray Your Weight Away"; and San Francisco's Albert Abrams, who once claimed that his $250 electronic "rheostat boxes" could diagnose any disease by keying into its unique vibration. In the 1920s, husbands heard from North Carolinian John Brinkley that a $750 procedure of sewing goat testicles into their scrotums boosted sexual prowess, while wives were told by Indiana's Hager Medical Company that they could cure any ailment of the vagina with a generous application of Oak Balm suppositories (which consisted of boric acid, alum, cacao, and butter, with a side of scorn).

But by the late 1990s, it was tough going for those with One True Cures. Medical science had, over the course of a hundred years of col-lecting and analyzing data, indisputably proven its ability to treat disease and extend life. This sterling track record led the American public to largely trust trained doctors. To take just one sign of that trust, in 2001, 93 percent of Republicans and 97 percent of Democrats agreed that it was important for parents to get their children vaccinated—meaning that vaccines had a higher approval rating than Dolly Parton, Tom Hanks, or Dr. Seuss.

The alien in Humble's skin, as well as many of his peers, felt that if only enough people knew how great their respective One True Cures were, the public would embrace them. But their efforts to get the word out were invariably foiled by a system of informational gatekeepers. Political leaders, reputable news anchors and newspaper editors, corporate CEOs, and major universities all required extraordinary proof to even entertain the idea that leeches, or rogue microscopy, or herbs, or a water purifier could possibly cure cancer and other terminal illnesses.

This system, which the alien believed was the product of agents of Manzanora, made it virtually impossible for him to get MMS out to the world. And so the impact of these visionary healers, individually or collectively, was negligible.

But then the alien's human male offspring (some of his family members were more understanding of his eccentricities than others) gave him a computer. And suddenly, the alien had new hope for the future. The keepers of knowledge still stood at the gate, but through the computer, the knowledge itself flowed around them in an endless flood of bits and bytes that could not be contained.

"With the Internet and modern technology, normal people can now know more than doctors used to know. We can no longer be kept in ignorance about medicine," the alien in Humble's skin wrote. "The dawn of the age of information has already happened, but this is the dawn of the age of medical information to the average person."

As the internet began piping massive amounts of information into the brains of the public, the federal government's primary regulatory response was the Telecommunications Act of 1996, which treated the internet as an advancement of telephone networks. As such, all the attention was focused on things like preventing monopolies and ensuring equitable access by consumers. No one had a game plan in place to address the information itself, and so the establishment stood mute and dumb as society's traditional gatekeepers of knowledge were swept away in a torrent of weight-loss fads, conspiracy theories, get-rich-quick schemes, and One True Cures. .

People were suddenly signing up for email accounts, and those accounts were being inundated with two trillion junk emails every year, many of them promises from shady marketers of One True Cures. People formed internet forums grouped by topic of interest and shared information about more One True Cures. Websites sprang up, trumpeting still more One True Cures. It was a surge of information and misinformation, formed by alternative healers who were both victims and abettors of its force.

By 2000, experts in the nascent field of web traffic analysis found that 43 percent of internet users (twenty-two million Americans) were going online to research their health concerns.

In South Dakota, dentist Larry Lytle used the internet to connect with others who would soon help him advance his One True Cure, universal healing energy. In Montana, Toby McAdam began selling his One True Cure, herbal supplements, through an Amazon storefront and other online retail platforms. In Utah, Robert Young enrolled in a distance-learning school that allowed him to write a dissertation on the One True Cure he had discovered with his darkfield microscopy. Aspiring leech entrepreneur Alicja Kolyszko advertised online for those interested in trying her One True Cure. In California, the Neumanns found an internet forum that celebrated ever more extreme versions of their One True Cure, prayer. The alien used his computer to begin building a webpage that would promote his One True Cure, MMS.

The gatekeepers of knowledge, who have historically prevented outlandish claims from reaching mass audiences unchallenged, had been America's first line of defense against One True Cures. But when healers began using the internet to reach those mass audiences directly, the second line of defense was the common sense and rationality of the American consumer, which in reality meant that the second line of defense was an array of massively resourced institutions—notably the Centers for Disease Control and Prevention, the FDA, the Federal

Trade Commission, and the US Justice Department—that had long guided Americans to lead healthier lives, and enforced existing laws against people whose One True Cures actively endangered the public.

With $4 billion a year and nine thousand workers in 170 districts, field offices, and laboratories, the FDA alone seemed more than capable of shutting down the generation of corporate criminals emerging in this new digital world.

Because there was virtually no cost to establishing a branded website, and no regulatory screen to slow them down, shady supplement sellers nimbly pivoted their marketing to take advantage of the crisis of the day. An early high-profile example came in late 2001, in the wake of the 9/11 terrorist attacks. Cyberspace was suddenly full of supplement ads promising to provide protection against various terrorism-related threats, like anthrax and radiation fallout from "dirty" nuclear bombs. And even before those fears subsided, no fewer than forty-eight websites popped up to advertise colloidal silver, oregano oil, and bogus "prevention kits" that claimed to stop the emerging SARS virus.

In 2002, a consumer watchdog, unhappy with the impact of fraudulent dietary supplements on public health, said that the slowness of the FDA's response to such threats was "appalling" and "dangerous." And so the FDA, bolstered by the appointment of a new commissioner, Mark McClellan, announced that the agency was stepping up enforcement and would no longer "tolerate fraudulent schemes that deceive or endanger the public." McClellan promised Associated Press reporters that the FDA was going to be much more aggressive.

"We're putting manufacturers on notice about what is coming," he said. "We had a major seizure this week, and you can expect more coming." He was joined in his tough talk by Howard Beales, director of the FTC's Bureau of Consumer Protection, who said, "Our message to e-marketers making deceptive claims is 'change your site to comply with the law.'"

The FDA rolled up its collective shirtsleeves and got to work. The year 2002 was marked by frenzied enforcement activity. Investigators busted Conklin Company of Shakopee, Minnesota, for claiming that its product Life Track Arthritis could treat arthritis; Earth and Plant of

Homer, Alaska, for claiming that Hydrogen Plus could treat lupus; AffordableHGH.com of Wilton, Connecticut, for telling people to self-inject its human growth hormone as an antiaging treatment; TriMedica International of Tempe, Arizona, for putting a concentrated alkaline supplement, PH+, into the packaging of an unconcentrated supplement; and Windsor Health Products of Kowloon, Hong Kong, and Optimum Nutrition of Aurora, Illinois, for selling, respectively, Essence of Mushroom and Opti-Soy 50 as treatments for cancer. The FDA hit companies claiming that Kirkman Taurine was an autism treatment, that Brain Nutrient could treat low intelligence and mental retardation, and that Advanced Form U Life could cure cancer, arthritis, and heart disease. It busted Dandy Day Corporation of Broomfield, Colorado, for saying that Crave Away, an aloe vera dietary supplement, could treat diabetes and attention-deficit disorder, and that its aloe vera cream could treat skin cancer, yeast infections, strep throat, and radiation burns. It chastised Nature's Energy of Pleasant Grove, Utah, for making AMP II Pro Drops, a supplement laced with the drug ephedrine (it seized 141,000 bottles valued at $2.8 million).

As FDA enforcement agents romped through the roster of industry scofflaws, seizing products, shutting down websites, and even seeking criminal convictions, agency publicists distributed press releases pointing out the crackdown's many successes.

Governmental control of America's health messaging must be maintained, and the FDA intended to eliminate all internet-enabled threats before things got out of hand.

Naturally, things got out of hand.

PART TWO

PRODROMAL POLITICS

In which One True Cureism catches the system by surprise

> You tell your doctor, that y' are ill;
> And what does he, but write a bill?
> Of which you need not read one letter;
> The worse the scrawl, the dose the better,
> For if you knew but what you take,
> Though you recover, he must break.

—Matthew Prior, *Alma*, 1718

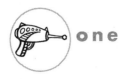one

LARRY LYTLE'S LASER LIGHT

> Once upon a time, many years ago—when our grandfathers
> were little children—there was a doctor; and his name was
> Dolittle—John Dolittle, M.D. "M.D." means that he was
> a proper doctor and knew a whole lot.
>
> —Hugh Lofting, *The Story of Doctor Dolittle*, 1920

ONCE HE UNDERSTOOD THAT UNIVERSAL HEALING ENERGY, OR qi, was the One True Cure, Larry Lytle was eager to apply that knowledge to his dental patients. He believed misalignment of the jaw could disrupt the flow of energy through the body, which caused a dizzying array of symptoms, including dizziness. Others were headaches, hearing loss, eye pain, face pain, anxiety, forgetfulness, tiredness, insomnia, sinusitis, and all sorts of body pains, grouped under the umbrella term dental distress syndrome.

The problem was that the American Dental Association, which by then was completely in thrall to the Numbers Junkies, didn't recognize qi, nor did it recognize dental distress syndrome.

Had Lytle asked—and there was no way he would—it would have told him that mixing his mystic beliefs with his professional practice was a very bad idea. And so, when a couple of former patients sued him for using unapproved methods to realign their jaws, the profession did not have Lytle's back. In 1998, South Dakota's State Board of Dentistry (which he had founded) revoked his license.

For a guy with Lytle's insights, dentistry was getting to be too small a field anyway. He was now tinkering with designs and applying for patents in an effort to harness the universal healing energy for much broader health benefits. After countless hours of work, he finally unveiled his One True Cure: a laser that fired light directly into human cells. Encouraging people to shoot themselves with lasers isn't as dangerous as it sounds when the lasers are low level—more laser pointer than lightsaber.

Around 2001, Lytle signed a contract with the Rapid City company Tri-Tech Manufacturing and produced his first laser, the Pegasus. His offerings quickly evolved into the Rotary Multiplex, the 660 FlashProbe, and the 660 Enhancer Probe. Then he upgraded an old model, the Q10, with the laser that would become his crowning glory.

The Q1000 was a beaut: it had a gleaming, sturdy casing (airplane-quality aluminum, Lytle said) with a numerical digital display that glowed in blue and green. It came with an instruction booklet of the sort that accompanied microwave ovens, but instead of defrosting a steak or warming a bowl of soup, laser owners could enter a three-digit code that would set it to treat a specific medical condition.

And this baby treated it all.

Hard of hearing? No problem: just laser your ear.

Gonorrhea? Just laser your crotch.

Poor vision? Point that thing directly into your eyeball and let 'er rip.

The Q1000 could also treat more serious and life-threatening conditions, including diabetes, sickle cell anemia, HIV/AIDS, and cancer. If someone was losing their mind (perhaps a prerequisite for customers), they could use the device to treat their mental diagnoses. In a particularly ballsy move, Lytle advertised the lasers (which cost between $4,295 and $12,600) as being suitable "for the treatment of any unknown condition."

He was able to speak directly to potential customers through various websites as well as through a YouTube channel. He set up domains including drlytle.com, qlaserhealinglight.com, qlaserspma.com, and qlaserinformation.com. His operation began to grow; he added affiliates, distributors, corporate entities, and staff.

Lytle entered his seventies, a time when many people are happy to set aside their professional pursuits and focus on the little things in life. But Lytle was laser focused on the big things: money and recognition for what he saw as a revolution in health care.

Lytle's vitality was testified to in his newspaper ads, the sort that pose as news articles. They referred to "Doctor" Lytle as "a remarkably young man in his seventies," whose lasers were "as gentle as the kiss of a butterfly." Though the entire point was clearly to make and imply medical claims, the sin was cleansed with tiny print that stated there were "no medical claims made or implied."

In 2005, Lytle hired a salesman, Ronald "Ronnie" Weir Jr., who was twenty-five. Back when Lytle was Ronnie's age, the laser was a new, poorly understood technology without any real practical applications. And now here was Ronnie Jr., still young in a world so advanced that lasers could treat AIDS. (True, they were being used to treat AIDS exclusively by Lytle, but still. It was remarkable.)

The age difference made for quite a culture gap. When Lytle was a kid, people picked up their pallies and goosed their machines until they burned rubber; if they met a pill, they would dish out shiners by dispensing knuckle sandwiches.

When Ronnie Jr. was born, in the early 1980s, people simply rolled with posses and dissed each other (though sometimes people were gagged with spoons, at their own request).

But Lytle and Ronnie Jr. papered over their differences with a universal bonding agent—money. There were dollars to be made and photons to beam. If Ronnie was hesitant about selling lasers that could cure diabetes, he put those hesitations aside and quickly proved to be more than competent. Within two years, he was heading up Lytle's national sales efforts.

.•:·

SHORTLY AFTER HE STARTED SELLING LASERS, LYTLE BEGAN HOLDING INformational seminars. Supposedly the seminars were for anyone, but in practice his audience was a bit brittle. At one event, men and women of a certain age sat in hard-backed chairs, facing an empty podium. "This is a true story of a black bear cub. . . ." Lytle was nowhere to be seen, but his kind and reassuring voice rang out as a large projector screen behind the podium came alive with pictures. According to the excruciatingly folksy story, two ranchers—Gary and Chad—came across "Little Bear" after it fell out of a large oak tree and paralyzed its back. They consulted with a wildlife official and a veterinarian, both of whom said the bear should be shot. But Gary instead reached out to Lytle.

"I told him that," Lytle's prerecorded voice said, "based upon research and other clinical studies, that I believed it would help the bear's spine."

And so Gary applied the laser to the bear's back every day. After four weeks, the bear seemed fine.

"He also developed a healthy appetite for apples and dog food," said Lytle, in a tone that suggested the bear was quite the little rascal. "By the time Little Bear's back was healed, it was too late in the winter to return him to the woods."

The ranchers let the bear hibernate in a trailer packed with straw. In the spring, they drove the trailer back to the spot where the bear had been found and released the animal.

"Thanks to caring ranchers and the use of healing light," Lytle intoned, "there is a healthy black bear living free in the northern Minnesota woods."

(As someone who has written a book about human-bear interactions, I will note only that, because the state of Minnesota was at that time spending thousands of dollars to kill thousands of bears in a population-reduction plan, odds are that the rascally, human-habituated Little Bear actually wound up in the bottom of somebody's meat locker.)

At the end of the bear video, a sales manager hyped the audience up for the entrance of "Doctor Lytle," who then appeared in the flesh—tall, straight-backed, ruggedly handsome, and sporting big, bushy eyebrows that reminded me of Sam the Eagle from the Muppets.

His basic claim was that the Q1000 popped lost electrons back into individual human cells, thereby restoring them to perfect health, but his explanations wrapped that concept in a lot of science words (redox, oxidation, wavelengths, metabolic) to give cover to the pseudoscience. I found that if I replaced those words with metasyntactic variables (universal placeholder words), I got a metasyntactic variable paragraph that could be applied to any One True Cure.

"I have developed a method of adding thingummies to the gubbins, which smurfs cellular activity," Lytle said. "I have discovered that combined low-level Hodor thingamabobs, positioned to form gizmos, powered stuff, and at specific whatchamacallits, put thingummies back at the something level. Somethings that lose thingummies become thingamajigs, and thingamajigs are yoke-forming, plus thingamajigs accelerate the whatsis Marklar, causing accelerated blah and early widget death. Putting thingummies back changes thingamajigs back to somethings and stimulates metabolic processes at the wossname level. Yada yada yada, I Am Groot."

Lytle's original words meant exactly the same. He told the audience that the Q1000 controlled weight, produced endorphins, "enhealthened" cells, and extended life. He pointed to research studies, including one conducted on 122 people in Allahabad, India, that found lasers helped reduce pain and promote healing. (Unsurprisingly, the Allahabad study was published only in a shady and disreputable online journal.)

Lytle wrapped up his lecture with his catchphrase: "You cannot unknow what you now know."

He then advised the audience to reach out to his staff of laser specialists to get a one-on-one presentation in Northern California, Arkansas, Kansas City, Omaha, or Detroit, after which his team of salespeople moved in to ensure the healing could begin.

.∴.

BECAUSE HE WAS SELLING THEM AS MEDICAL DEVICES, LYTLE'S LASERS fell under the regulatory authority of the FDA, which was extinguishing fraudulent health claims at a record pace from a majestic command center located on the White Oak Campus in Bethesda, Maryland, where fifteen buildings wrapped in glinting windows reflect the brillig sun. Its insides include an endless array of Wonkaesque rooms—walls covered in white tiles that absorb sound and deaden electronic interference, giant robotic arms, microscopes, centrifuges, brain-scanning machines, racks of beakers with liquids of various tints, 3D printers spitting out plastic replicas of human body parts, and, of course, row upon row of cubicles (gray-paneled, if not visually then spiritually).

Here, administrators talk about "optimization" and achieving "continuous improvement" in a "self-service, Web-centric environment," which is pretty fancy talk for an agency that got its start in 1902 by recruiting young people into a "Poison Squad" (volunteers received five dollars a month, plus free food that was intentionally laced with borax, for the sole purpose of figuring out what happens when people eat food laced with borax).

Often, an FDA investigator makes no effort to be likable, with the entirely predictable outcome that they are unlikable. Interestingly, when they do make an effort to be likable, they tend to be even more unlikable.

To take just one example, during an annual summit at the Bethesda Marriott, the FDA sought to be more public-friendly by presenting a panel of current and former investigators to talk about "A Day in the Life of an FDA Investigator."

One agent told the audience that reaching out to the FDA with "postinspectional correspondence" was helpful to resolve "discussional items" and advised that inspectees keep in mind the importance of validations. A company that failed to communicate about "nonconformances" was at risk of being termed a "more violative firm." Amid all the jargon-laden drudgery, an audience member asked the panel whether it was "appropriate to ask what level certification an inspector is."

The lead panelist got with the public-friendliness.

"We are actually investigators. Sorry," she responded, with all the tender sweetness of a seasick crocodile. "We are—our classification is actually investigator."

Point made. Or maybe not. She made the point, which had little to do with the question, again.

"Inspector is a totally different classification within the agency. It's a pet peeve."

That drove it home. As did her next statement.

"We are actually investigating. We don't inspect your facilities," she said. "We really don't. We investigate them."

The name of the event, incidentally, was the Eighth Annual FDA Inspections Summit.

Why does the FDA find it so difficult to engage with the public?

Because it's creaking under the supremacy of the Numbers Junkies, who have spent the last 170 years promoting data-driven approaches to medicine that, while effective, have the very great downside of viewing both patient and practitioner as interchangeable cogs. The end result of this aggressive objectification campaign is nowhere more apparent than in the agency's 567-page *Investigations Operations Manual*. The manual is an FDA investigator's bible, and like the actual Bible, it micromanages the behavior of its adherents to a shocking degree.

Investigators can't wear jewelry. They can carry a pen, but it has to be held in such a way that it cannot drop off the body. Anticipating the traditional nerd solution to pen holding, it says, "Do not depend on clips on pens, etc., to hold these items in your outer pockets."

If it is remotely possible for an investigator to sustain eye damage, they must wear safety glasses that "should at a minimum meet the American National Standards Institute standard z87.1 for impact resistance." If they have any questions about whether a particular pair of safety glasses is adequate, they must call an on-tap regional industrial hygienist.

Even supervisors are micromanaged by the *Operations Manual*, which in one so-unmemorable-that-it's-memorable passage instructs them to, when appropriate, consult with CDRH Office of Regulatory Programs (HFZ-320) before invoking the QS/GMP regulation 21 CFR 820.180(c) concerning the certification of audits and reaudits.

The wretchedly boring and impersonal FDA culture was fundamentally incompatible with Lytle, who had learned during the Rapid City flood that individual action is often more important than kowtowing to the system. He did not accept the agency's oversight authority.

"One has to wonder why the FDA even controls non-significant risk devices such as low-level lasers," Lytle wrote. "It seems the marketplace should decide the fate of non-significant risk low level lasers—not the government."

Unfortunately for Lytle, the agency took a call from a California man who told them that one of Lytle's lasers had rendered him temporarily blind. The man said he'd called Lytle's company first but was making the complaint because he got no refund.

When the complaint call came in, some poor schlep in some gray cubicle dutifully opened an investigatory file, tagging it with identification numbers that, in an act of mind-numbing redundancy, include an FDA Establishment Identifier (FEI), a central file number (CFN), a Program Assignment Code (PAC), and a Home District Code (which mysteriously comes with no acronym at all).

When the FDA began reaching out to Lytle with concerns about the way he was marketing his $12,000 laser pointers, he shined them on. He told investigators what they wanted to hear. He kissed the ring. He bent the knee. He said yes. And then, the moment their shadow left his doorstep, he did whatever the hell he wanted. For six years, he held them at arm's length, and there was no sign they were getting any closer to cracking down on him.

One day, in May 2007, Lytle checked his voicemail and found that it contained a message from an FDA investigator seeking information about one of his companies, Low Level Lasers Inc. Lytle returned the call and left a message in which he told the agent, very politely and professionally, that the corporate entity Low Level Lasers Inc. no longer existed. However, Lytle said smoothly, he would be happy to field any questions the agent might have.

When Lytle hung up, his demeanor changed. He explained to an un-identified companion that Low Level Lasers Inc. did in fact exist, but only on paper. Lytle was using the corporation as a channel to funnel money to himself from another entity so that there wouldn't be a direct paper trail between that other entity and Lytle or his family.

It "doesn't do any business with anybody related to me," he said, his smug tone implying he'd sent the FDA on a wild goose chase. He said that when the FDA agent did get him on the phone, Lytle would just tell him that his lasers were not intended for humans at all.

"If he says anything about it, I'm going to say, 'Well, Low Level Lasers is a veterinary type of thing,'" he said.

But Lytle, in the style of movie villains everywhere, had explained the details of his scheme to his own detriment. In this case, he failed to properly hang up the phone. Which meant that his intention—or we might say confession—to deceive the United States government was now recorded on the voicemail of an enforcement agent of the United States government.

Lytle's various laser-selling corporate entities had just become "more violative firms."

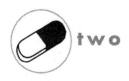 **two**

TOBY MCADAM'S SUPPLEMENTS

Doctors who made great fortunes out of dainty remedies for imaginary disorders that never existed, smiled upon their courtly patients. . . . The leprosy of unreality disfigured every human creature in attendance.

—Charles Dickens, *A Tale of Two Cities*, 1859

EVERY TIME I CALLED TOBY, HE WAS IN HIS HOME OFFICE. EVERY time, he said it would be okay to take a little break. Every time, we proceeded to talk for hours.

By the time his mother died in the hospital, Toby was already treating friends and family with his herbal concoctions and planning to sell them to strangers. Soon he had shifted from consuming misinformation to spreading misinformation. One of his first real hits was a salve made with an herb called bloodroot, which had a caustic property that meant it (like zombies) could eat human flesh. Toby advised his customers to use his salve to burn skin cancer off their bodies.

The internet allowed Toby to compete with some of the biggest herbal companies in the marketplace. He rented an office in Livingston, Montana, established the brand RisingSun, and before long was selling "Indian Mud Black Salve" along with other bloodroot-based products from various domain names he controlled through six different corporate entities.

Shelves around the country began to fill up with Toby's bloodroot oils, salves, tonics, and tinctures. To capture the all-important segment of the public that can be convinced to put caustic substances in their mouths, he marketed Bloodroot Toothpaste, a powdered version called

Dentrifice Bloodroot Toothpaste, and, my personal favorite, Bloodroot Oral Peppermint Spray.

As Toby read about other herbal remedies, he used a blend of intuition and common sense to add products to his rapidly growing catalog. He made a plant-based version of the powerful and addictive opioid painkiller hydrocodone, and a wormwood-based tincture for gallbladder disease, which he named Artemis. Toby did nearly all the work himself—he developed the products, he wrote the copy for the labels, and he designed the packaging.

And the thing was, after decades of jumping from one job to the next, he was suddenly gaining traction as a successful businessman. Soon he was selling about a thousand items a month, including his species-specific formulations for cats, dogs, and horses.

This was exactly the sort of thing the FDA frowned on. Its problem wasn't necessarily what was *in* Toby's products; it was what was *on* the packages Toby was designing. On those packages, Toby claimed that his pills and salves could treat certain diseases and health conditions, and by certain, I mean pretty much all.

Toby was not the only one advertising the medical benefits of a product line, of course.

Big Pharma companies make similar medical claims about their drugs all the time. But the primary difference is the rigamarole they have to go through to get there. A drug company typically starts by using advanced computing methods to explore simulated molecule constructs, looking for chemical compounds that might have a certain impact on the body. Beginning with as many as ten thousand candidates, they then use preclinical studies on living cells, animals, and computer models to winnow the field down to just a handful.

The drug company must then file an application for human trials that includes everything it knows about the drug. If the application is approved, it moves on to conduct Phase One human trials, meant to demonstrate that a drug is safe by measuring side effects. During Phase Two trials, they give the drug to a select group of people who are suffering from the disease. In Phase Three, they give the drug to hundreds or thousands of volunteers with the illness and compile data on efficacy and side effects.

After all that, the company fills out yet another application with the FDA, seeking approval to bring the drug to market. And once the drug is on the market, there's a "post-market surveillance" phase, which essentially provides mechanisms for the FDA to monitor the drug for side effects and reel dangerous drugs back in.

It's not a perfect system, and Big Pharma works hard to nudge the FDA into approving borderline cases, but it is at least rigorous and transparent.

Toby, by contrast, was doing none of this. He was producing his products without oversight, as if they were unregulated supplements, and advertising them as if they were heavily regulated drugs. And Toby routinely made the sort of statement that Big Pharma never could.

"I've dealt with a thousand people with cancer," he told me. "I'd say I have a 98 percent success rate." Or, "I think the average person can live to be about 120 years old."

Big if true!

For years Toby simply escaped the FDA's notice. But then his luck finally ran out.

In 2007, a pair of inspectigators (investipectors?) showed up at RisingSun. The FDA's *Investigations Operations Manual* instructs agents to develop "rapport" with the dealer of the supplements they are inspecting, as this is "important to the success of your objective." They are told to be polite and friendly.

If the supplements dealer objects to the agents taking a sample of products, the agent is told to, in a polite and friendly manner, "point out and discuss the authorities provided by FD&C Act sections 702(a), 702(b), 704(a), 704(c), 704(d) [21 U.S.C. 372(a), (b) and 374(a), (c), (d)] and the precedent case mentioned in IOM 2.2.1."

Usually, that friendly conversation takes care of things. But "if refusals persist," the agents are instructed to, while maintaining that all-important friendly and polite demeanor, "point out the criminal prohibitions of Section 301(f) of the FD&C Act [21 U.S.C. 331(f)]."

Governments threaten. But friends simply point out criminal prohibitions.

When Toby allowed the FDA to conduct its inspection, it determined that some of his products fell under the definition of drugs, which were being sold without a prescription and without adequate instructions for their usage. They also confirmed that his labels and marketing claims were unsubstantiated and illegal.

They told him to knock it off.

.·:·'

WHEN THE FDA FIRST TOLD TOBY TO STOP ADVERTISING HIS PRODUCTS AS cures for cancer and other serious diseases, he, like Lytle with his lasers, adopted a strategy to shine the FDA on. But with the agency's resources diffused among a growing pool of violative firms, Toby's shining on of the FDA may have been the greatest in the history of FDA shinings-on.

With every phone call, every in-person visit from an investigator, every warning letter and packet of certified mail, Toby promised, over and over, to come into compliance.

And he never did.

Months passed. Then years. Around 2009, the FDA shifted from warning Toby to collecting court-admissible evidence against him. And it gave a handful of FDA agents authorization to go undercover. Going undercover is one of the most exciting and extreme aspects of law enforcement, the sort of thing that even the FDA's *Operations Manual*, which covers the topic in Section 4.1.4.6, can't stomp the fun out of.

The manual tells agents to devise cover stories and purchase suspected illegal products to "augment existing investigation or inspection efforts."

Cover stories are exciting! So far so good.

The items purchased become "Official Samples." Then investigators simply have to determine whether they have purchased investigational samples, food standards samples, nonregulatory samples, mail entry samples, audit/certification samples, reconditioning samples, import samples, domestic import samples, special domestic import samples, additional samples (which encompasses both import additional samples and domestic additional samples but not special domestic import samples), post-seizure samples, 301k samples, induced samples, in-transit samples, or documentary samples.

Each type of sample comes with its own exhaustive rules for handling and processing, because, yes, actually, the *Operations Manual* can indeed leech the vitality out of every goddamn thing.

Nevertheless, while Toby continued adding bricks to his wall of promises, the FDA became his best customer. Undercover agents bought Old Amish Dewormer Original Formula (to fight parasites and cancer); they bought capsules of CanFree Internal Formula ("has shown positive benefits in battle with cancer"); they bought Anemia Formula (anemia and sore throat and also "cleanses the blood"); they bought Kavakosh for Epilepsy/Depression ("to act on the brains [*sic*] limbic system"); they bought ADD/ADHD Support, Amazonian Analgesia, Arthritis Support, and twelve other products.

Soon Toby was shipping packages of irrefutable evidence to undercover operatives in Maryland, Arizona, and Washington, DC. The FDA used these purchases to take Toby to court, and on November 8, 2012, Toby ran out of reasonable options. He filed a sworn affidavit with the court in which he stated that he "will cease operations."

This was, in certain circles in the FDA, a great relief and a great victory. After nearly seven years, one Toby McAdam had finally been brought to heel.

But.

Over at the FDA, somebody must have said to somebody, "Let's just be sure. Let's dot one last *i* and cross one more *t*."

And so, one final time, an agent visited Toby's website, which was still in operation for some reason, and placed one more undercover order, which for some reason was accepted, and then sat around, just to be sure a box of Lugol's Iodine ("supports thyroid health") didn't show up.

A week went by, and the FDA agents breathed a sigh of relief. The Lugol's Iodine had not arrived. They had finally gotten through to Toby.

Another week went by, and they turned to other matters.

A third week went by, and everyone began to think about Christmas.

Then midway through the fourth week, on December 17, an unob-trusive package from RisingSun arrived in Maryland.

Toby had shined them on again. And this time, the shine hit the fan.

The FDA, expressing bewilderment, went back to court, calling To-by's conduct "contumacious." They noted that he hadn't paid for the FDA's inspectional costs! Or the supervisional costs! He had sworn com-pliance! And then hadn't complied! It now appeared, they wrote, "as if he never intended to comply," a conclusion that took them just seven years to draw.

A criminal case against Toby began to wend its way through a series of court dates. If he lost, he could actually be sent to prison. Toby took advantage of this grace period, about two years, to keep selling as many supplements as he could. (It could be argued that this conduct was also contumacious.)

There was a lot of advice on offer. The FDA was advising him to make a deal. Members of his family and his circle of friends were advising him to make a deal. His own legal counsel advised him to make a deal.

And so, Toby did what most people in his situation would do. He decided to ask Elon Musk.

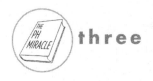 **three**

ROBERT O. YOUNG'S PH MIRACLE

The idea of winning a doctor's degree gradually assumed
the aspect of a great moral struggle, and the moral fight
possessed immense attraction for me.

—Elizabeth Blackwell, the first woman in the US
to receive a medical degree, 1895

WHEN ROBERT YOUNG PEERED THROUGH THE LOOKING GLASS
of his darkfield microscope, he was not just observing squiggly
microorganisms whiffling their way through a drop of human blood; he
was, in a sense, looking at the historical time and place in which scientists first became aware of those tiny beings living inside us and decided
what the heck they were.

That time and place—1850s Paris—was exceedingly bleak.

Paris had the highest death rate in France; in some years, cholera
alone killed ten thousand city residents, which spawned conspiracy theories alleging that the outbreaks were a deliberate plot on the part of the
government to depopulate the city's poor.

But in fact the cholera was more rightly attributed to the germ-laden,
ubiquitous rats prowling the streets, which themselves were described
as "dark, evil-smelling, polluted with noise and smoke, and appalling to
the senses." After a rain, Parisian pedestrians faced the very real danger
of stumbling over the uneven ground and falling into one of countless
pools brimming with the commingled shit of rats and street urchins.

The city's eastern suburbs had a chain of slaughterhouses that produced cheap horsemeat. One slaughterhouse was in danger of falling
down because its foundation was undermined by enough rat dens to

provide homes for an estimated 320,000 of the rodents. People walking across fields in the district could feel the earth, riddled with rat tunnels, shake beneath their footsteps. But authorities were afraid to close the slaughterhouses on the grounds that the rats, once deprived of horse-meat, would turn against the people.

About the only thing that preyed on rats were cats—and laboratory scientists. (Scientists had been using rats as lab animals for at least twenty-five years by then.) Paris hosted a vibrant community of doctors who were excited about the new, data-based vision of the Numbers Junk-ies. Though implementation of the scientific process was still somewhat clumsy, these researchers were slowly uncovering the knowledge needed to make great strides, particularly in medical science. Every morning, they walked through the rat-swarmed streets to laboratories that gave the world quinine, codeine, aspirin, the stethoscope, the blind experiment, and the hypodermic needle, among many other discoveries.

One of these scientists was chemist Louis Pasteur, who demon-strated that microscopic bugs were responsible for the souring of milk. He proved that boiling a glass bottle of fruit juice or milk (what we now call pasteurization) killed off the tiny organisms and temporarily halted the decay. Because these microorganisms—bacteria and viruses—were also thought to be the basis for a lot of human diseases, Pasteur had found the key evidence in support of germ theory.

But Pasteur faced intense pushback from other French scientists, most notably the organic chemist Antoine Béchamp.

Béchamp said disease was explained not by germ theory but by his own "terrain theory." He believed that diseases like plague and syphilis arose spontaneously from within. Poor conditions in the body's internal environment—its terrain—caused the body's cells to undergo a process called pleomorphism, literally triggering them to morph into the patho-gens that make people sick.

In order to prove terrain theory, Béchamp decided to kill something and immerse it in an airless environment; if the body decayed, he thought it would prove that the agents of decay—those little germs munching their way through the mass—came from within the body rather than floating through the air.

But what animal to kill?

Béchamp walked the same festering Parisian streets as Pasteur and undoubtedly saw the rats, their population barely held in check by the cats. That's why it's odd that he chose to prove terrain theory by executing kittens.

For thirteen years, Béchamp kept jars of dead kittens on a shelf in his laboratory. The bodies were immersed in pure carbonate of lime. Over time, each kitten's body was reduced to bone fragments, which Béchamp exhumed and took as evidence that the kittens had been consumed by the products of their own bodies. Any microorganisms at work, he said, were merely another presentation of the body's own terrain.

"Nothing is lost, nothing is created," he wrote. "All is transformed."

Béchamp and Pasteur sniped at each other in academic papers, but over the years evidence from other scientists accrued in Pasteur's favor. Béchamp remained unconvinced and spent his entire professional life arguing that germ theory was mistaken, which eventually tanked his career. By the time Béchamp died in 1908, at the age of ninety-one, Pasteur's ideas were so universally accepted that, like evolution and gravity, people no longer referred to germ theory—just germs.

UNTIL, THAT IS, THE 1990S, WHEN ROBERT YOUNG SAW, IN A DROP OF magnified blood, what he took to be a long, narrow, rod-shaped bacterium changing into a round red blood cell. This was pleomorphism, happening right in front of his eyes. Béchamp, it turned out, had been right all along.

Which, again, big if true!

Imagine it. Young had the cure for cancer. For diabetes. For everything. What would he do with the knowledge?

Get in on the burgeoning supplement business, that's what.

In addition to selling supplements, Young began offering a professional service of "live blood analysis," during which he examined a microscopic slide of a person's blood for signs of disease. Often, he found that the acid level of their blood was out of whack, in which case he advised them to seek nutritional counseling or alkalizing health supplements.

And they were in luck, because he also sold both nutritional counseling and alkalizing health supplements.

Supplements were particularly vibrant in Young's home state of Utah, where sales went from $924 million in 1994 (when the Dietary Supplement Health and Education Act was passed) to $7 billion in 2012, making it the state's biggest industry. Thanks in part to Utah senator Orrin Hatch, hundreds of millions of federal tax dollars went to support the state's supplement manufacturers, which drew hundreds of thousands of visitors to conventions there.

Many of these products, it should be noted, were aboveboard and totally legal. But there was just one teensy warning sign that Young might have crossed the line from supplement sales to practicing medicine without a license. It was when he was charged with two felony counts of practicing medicine without a license.

The charges were brought in 1995 in Utah, where two women said he had drawn their blood, told them they were ill, and then sold them products to address those illnesses. He disputed their claims and pled guilty to a misdemeanor.

Right around the same time, Young began racking up academic degrees at an amazing rate of speed. According to the dates of issuance for the diploma images in his online CV, he was awarded a bachelor's degree in nutrition by the American Holistic College of Nutrition in Birmingham, Alabama, on March 15, 1995. He received a master's degree of science in nutrition by the same school on June 29, 1995. And after the school changed its name to the Clayton School of Natural Healing, it awarded him a PhD in science on October 5, 1995, just six months and three weeks after he got his bachelor's.

Young had gone from Eagle Scout to Elder Young to musician to tennis pro, and he now laid claim to one of the most prestigious titles society had to offer: Doctor Young.

Just for good measure, Young went on to earn two more doctorates from the Clayton School of Natural Healing—one in philosophy in nutrition and one in naturopathy. (Sadly, about twelve years after issuing Young's third PhD, the nonaccredited school folded; among the students it left behind were many who had been certified in iridology, the "science" of diagnosing illnesses by studying physical features of the iris.)

Young combined terrain theory with strict nutritional advice to develop his One True Cure: an alkaline, plant-based diet to reduce levels of acid in the body.

Young's theory of health went public in 2002, with the publication of a book called *Sick and Tired: Reclaim Your Inner Terrain*. His wife, Shelley Redford Young, was listed as a coauthor for having contributed a set of recipes that embodied the "pH Miracle Diet."

For a book cobbled together from such an odd hodgepodge of sources (an unaccredited nutritional school, Young's time spent looking at slides of human blood, and the theories of a long-dead kitten killer), most of its advice was inarguably good for you. The meat of it was to give up meat, as well as dairy, carbohydrates, and processed sugars. He also recommended physical fitness and mindfulness.

Sick and Tired became an instant hit. It and a series of follow-up books were translated, collectively, into twenty-nine different languages, and Young plausibly claimed they had sold more than ten million copies.

Young believed that an alkaline diet could treat back pain, diabetes, and erectile dysfunction. Around 2006, he even explained how pleomorphism could reverse male pattern baldness, which he attributed to an overly acidified body terrain. Men who wanted to regrow their hair simply had to start and end their day with a dollop of pH Miracle Young pHorever Head pHirst Shampoo, followed by a dose of pH Miracle Young pHorever Top pHinish Conditioner. This regimen was followed over a period of months to "clean and heal the scalp, regenerate new hair, preserve existing hair and to keep new and existing hair healthy and strong."

And indeed, those who looked at the author photos on the covers of Young's books could hardly fail to notice that his own scalp hairs, many of which had yielded their positions in his mid-twenties, had reappeared as if by magic. "The Reversal of Baldness has been a Personal Journey for over 30 Years for Dr. Robert O. Young!" he wrote.

The book's success catapulted Young onto the national stage. He became the sort of famous that landed him spots on morning news show segments about intriguing new health trends. He appeared on CBS's *The*

Early Show with Jane Clayson and Bryant Gumbel, on CNN's *Nightly News*, and on ABC News. One of Young's patients, a Texan mom named Kim Tinkham, appeared on *The Oprah Winfrey Show* and told Oprah's audience that her lifestyle and diet changes had caused her breast cancer to disappear.

.∴.

YOUNG MOVED HIS GROWING FAMILY TO SAN DIEGO AND THEN TO VALLEY Center, California, a community defined by the Hellhole Canyon nature preserve and two casinos. There, he put down a million dollars on a venture that would take pleomorphism to new heights: a $2.7 million, forty-seven-acre avocado and grapefruit ranch that he called the pH Miracle Ranch.

Young began inviting people with serious medical conditions to come to the Miracle Ranch to learn how to live healthier lives. To hundreds, the ranch was a magical place. People came with cancer and left with hope. Young was the light amid the darkness.

Patients walked beneath wooded arbors and past a large meditation bell on paths surrounded by cacti. They could make use of the on-site salon, stay in guest residences, play on the tennis courts, or wander among grapefruit trees.

Young lived in the main, six-thousand-square-foot house that lay beneath a ridge lined by Italian cypress trees and flanked by huge palms, a helicopter pad, and an on-site warehouse full of storage racks of Forever Young supplements.

A stone-slab walkway crossed a landscaped moat at the house's entrance. Inside, every morning, exercise class participants could walk past a commercial kitchen already churning out plant-based smoothies (greens, avocados, cucumbers, and tomatoes but no sugar, no dairy, no fruit) and join Young himself in the gym, which was equipped with trampolines and medicine balls and treadmills. Just outside, a gorgeous swimming pool overlooked the protected lands of the Rincon Band of Luiseño Native Americans.

For some of the patients, who paid between $2,000 and $5,000 per day, Young jump-started the alkalinization process by piping an alkaline solution (baking soda mixed with saline) into their bloodstreams via an intravenous drip. At first he got the IV supplies from holistic practitioners, but then he hired a medical doctor, Ben Johnson, who was licensed to buy medical equipment and administer the IVs.

As Young began to help thousands of people with their health problems, he toed what he thought was the line between advice and medicine. He acknowledged that he was not a medical doctor, but he had credentials. He was a research scientist. He was a microbiologist. He was a naturopathic doctor. He analyzed people's blood lab results, educated them on his theories of disease, and offered them nutritional counseling.

He was acting within the law.

He said.

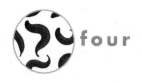four

ALICJA KOLYSZKO'S LEECHES

> When the peasant saw how well [the doctor] ate and drank, his heart desired what he saw, and would willingly have been a doctor too. So he remained standing a while, and at length inquired if he too could not be a doctor. "Oh, yes," said the doctor, "that is soon managed." "What must I do?" asked the peasant. "In the first place buy yourself an A B C book of the kind which has a cock on the frontispiece; in the second, turn your cart and your two oxen into money, and get yourself some clothes, and whatsoever else pertains to medicine; thirdly, have a sign painted for yourself with the words: 'I am Doctor Knowall,' and have that nailed up above your house-door." The peasant did everything that he had been told to do.
>
> —Jacob Grimm and Wilhelm Grimm, "Doctor Knowall," *Grimms' Fairy Tales*, 1812

KNOW OF TWO WAYS TO COOK A LEECH.

The first was featured in an off-Broadway play called *Describe the Night*. Upper-crust diners from Poland submerged leeches in bowls of veggie broth, then nicked their own fingers and stuck them into their respective bowls. Once the leeches had feasted on the diner, the diner added a leech-lethal dose of crushed red pepper to the broth, then feasted on the leech. Theater reviewers panned *Describe the Night*. But the recipe captivated their imaginations.

The second way, from Russian historical accounts, was memorably brought to life by British celebrity chef Heston Blumenthal. He prepared the leeches on camera, allowing them to feed on the rich blood of a heavily fattened goose. He then gave the engorged leeches a quick, lethal bath in liquid nitrogen, after which he fried them like sausages, in parsley and lemon juice. Blumenthal had high hopes for the meal, which he described as looking "just like little black puddings." But once he'd actually popped a cooked leech into his mouth, his assessment was somewhat harsher than the theater critics' view of *Describe the Night*.

"That," he said, immediately after swallowing, "is . . . just . . . congealed goose blood."

He grimaced as his finely honed palate told him more.

"With a leech-membrane casing," he concluded, unhappily. "No matter how I try to wrap that up, it's not appetizing."

The creatures' lack of culinary appeal was good news for Alicja Kolyszko's quest to bring leeches to the American public. If they were tasty enough to gain cachet as food, they would have been subject to a score of food-safety regulations. Similarly, if they were supplements, they would have fallen under the 1994 Dietary Supplement Health and Education Act, and if they were drugs, they would have been subjected to the same human trials that cost Big Pharma millions.

But in the realm of health care, leeches defied legal categorization in America. Which is actually pretty strange, because people have been using leeches to treat sickness from the very beginning.

．∵ ⋮ʻ

IT MAKES SENSE THAT THE EARLIEST RECORDED CIVILIZATIONS WERE BIG on One True Cures, because they independently came to the erroneous conclusion that human illnesses all stemmed from One Big Problem. Health was generally viewed in systemic terms; depending on where one lived, the key to wellness was maintaining the flow of qi through the body, or being smiled on by the gods, or maintaining the correct internal temperature, or properly balancing the four bodily fluids, known as humors.

This worldview proved to be very compatible with leeches, which were almost certainly (outside of prayer) the first, and most widespread, One True Cure. They show up as medical treatments in various ancient cultures—from creation myths to the earliest surviving Sanskrit writings to a 1500 BC painting found in an Egyptian tomb.

In Europe, belief in leeches as healing tools survived into the Middle Ages. The very word "leech" meant "to heal," and early physicians were often referred to as leeches themselves.

But by 1800 leeches were fading from European medicine, along with a bevy of other folk remedies. There were other reasons for people to distance themselves from leeches; in one case, a troop of Napoleon's French army unwittingly drank leech-infested water from a stream, only to realize, with dawning horror, that hundreds of tiny leeches had attached themselves to the soldiers' esophagi; as the leeches fed, their bodies expanded, cutting off the soldiers' air supply and inflicting heavy (and gruesome) casualties.

Strange, then, that when one of Napoleon's military doctors, François-Joseph-Victor Broussais, was installed as the highly influential chief physician at Val-de-Grâce military hospital in Paris, he began prescribing leeches at a rate that had not been seen before and has not been seen since.

Broussais's standing protocol was to administer thirty leeches to every patient as a first step, no matter the medical complaint. He then prescribed more leeches for specific body parts, to treat everything from headaches to nymphomania.

To take your mind off the question of whether that means Broussais's doctors were putting leeches on nymphomaniac genitals, consider that they devised a glass tube designed to transport leeches past the problematically tight sphincters of his patients and apply them directly to inflamed intestinal tracts.

To put your mind back on the nymphomaniac-genitals question, yes, doctors were totally putting leeches on nymphomaniac genitals.

Before Broussais, leeches had been poised to fade from the medical landscape. But his practices were adopted by regular doctors on several continents, which instead triggered a massive and unprecedented leech boom. American dentists used them to drain abscesses. Barbers in Damascus smuggled them into their shops to avoid leech taxes. In some regions, the public could swing by their local leech house for a preventive treatment or pick up leeches by the dozen from a local pharmacy. Members of the upper class tried to outdo each other by decorating their parlors with the most ornate and extravagant leech jars money could buy.

European countries began buying and selling tens of millions of leeches to one another, and soon leeches were popping up outside the medical field. One enterprising doctor, George Merryweather, even showed up at Britain's Great Exhibition of 1851 with the greatest leech-related invention of all time: the leech-powered tempest prognosticator. Based on Merryweather's observation that leeches became highly agitated in advance of a storm, the prognosticator featured a dozen leeches in a dozen cylindrical jars, each tethered by an exquisitely thin gold chain to a tiny whalebone hammer. When the leeches grew restive, the hammers struck a series of bells. The British Royal Navy expressed interest in a military contract for the prognosticator, but it was sadly aborted when a different device—the storm glass, which contains a mix of chemicals that crystallizes in low-pressure systems—was more convincingly presented by Vice Admiral Robert FitzRoy (best remembered for captaining the *HMS Beagle* as it conveyed a young Charles Darwin to the Galapagos Islands).

Ultimately, the thing that pushed leeches out of widespread use was the fact that the leeches themselves began to disappear from the wild. The world had never seen such a widely commodified animal become so scarce so quickly, and it was unsettling. Germany imposed an export ban on its valuable homegrown leeches, and Great Britain declared its local stocks extinct. Newspapers blamed empty leech jars on, among other things, gluttonous herons. International tensions rose as nations accused each other of crossing borders illegally to raid remote regions for their leeches, probably because profiteering leech pirates were doing just that. By the early 1900s, with global leech supplies drained and One True Cures falling out of favor, the mainstream medical establishment turned to less slimy methods of curing.

In America, it stayed that way for a century, until Alicja Kolyszko decided that, gluttonous herons be damned, the leech era was once again upon us.

Alicja has done more than anyone in the country to popularize the term "hirudotherapy"—based on the *Hirudinidae* family of leeches, which includes the species used in medicine.

When I first reached out to her, Alicja wasn't sure she wanted to go on the record talking about her practice. She had the same misgivings as other One True Cure advocates: offering an alternative to Big Pharma was an inherently risky proposition.

"I could jeopardize, completely, noninvasive hirudotherapy in the United States, if I will talk too much," she told me on the phone, her cadence rich with her Polish roots.

I suggested that perhaps she could simply avoid saying the words that could trigger consequences. No dice, she said.

"If I open, if we open Pandora's box, I have to talk," she said. "It's not that simple. It's not that simple. Because my mind goes fast."

Ultimately, she decided to go public. Though the book could bring unwanted scrutiny, it could also help to spread awareness about a form of medicine that she had devoted herself to utterly.

"I can't be a coward," she said. "Because I am a very bold person, and I want to be open more, and more absolutely."

MY PATH TO AMERICA'S LEECH QUEENPIN TOOK ME ACROSS THE EVERglades, driving the neat, straight line of Highway 75 and cutting across Florida's tip like a circumcision.

I knew that the endless expanses of marsh and sedge on either side of the highway hid populations of leeches that were both large and largely ignored. About the only time they got any human attention was in the 1959 B movie *Attack of the Giant Leeches*, in which an Everglades park ranger battled giant bloodsuckers that emerged from a hidden underground cave to drain their human victims dry.

I arrived on Florida's Gulf Coast, which resembles a giant birthday cake made of sugar-sand beaches and lime-green golf courses decorated with breaching dolphins. In Naples, as a valet parked my car, I walked into the LaPlaya Beach and Golf Resort and soon found Alicja sitting in its Baleen Restaurant.

She was a spitfire, with manners and mannerisms that one moment conjured visions of genteel European ballrooms, and the next seemed to spring from a rough-and-tumble dreg-ridden bar. The blend was immensely charismatic. I was smitten.

One of her main concerns was that the book would cheapen the reputation of hirudotherapy by linking it to some of the other practices that I was researching.

"Talking about hirudotherapy, you can't—Matt, if I have too much chip on my shoulder, forgive me, but it can't compare. With anything. There is no modality that you can name to me that compares to hirudotherapy. It is totally superior."

In the late 1990s, when Alicja returned to the US from her visit to the Polish clinic, she had her own unique vision of the American Dream: a pyramid with herself at the tip, topping a network of instructors, resting on a small army of practitioners above millions of patients, and at the base, an endless writhing carpet of leeches.

To make that vision a reality was daunting. Her approach, unique among the practitioners I spoke with, has allowed her to avoid conflict with the law. Alicja brought a certain philosophy to her task. She tried to explain it to me by citing a Polish saying—*Kiedy wejdziesz między wrony musisz krakać tak jak one*—that punned on the word "crow."

"This expression doesn't exist in English. But I give you the sense. It is something about, if one wants to go against the crowd, they have to crow like the crowd," she said.

I kind of got it, but I was enjoying the explanation. So I just looked at her expectantly. She tried again.

"If you want to go against the crowd. The bird? You have to learn to crow crow like they do."

When I raised my eyebrows, she took another stab.

"If you want to be against—or do something, influence—you have to start first to be the crowd and know how to do crow, crow."

I could have kept her going all day, but Alicja shot me a knowing look and shrugged.

"It's a poor translation."

Maybe so, but it boiled down to Alicja's belief that, in order to convince the medical establishment of the efficacy of leeches, she had to present her case in the language of the medical establishment. Alicja pursued this strategy, of cawing like the crowd, by drawing on the regions where leech use persisted—Europe and especially Russia, which around the turn of the millennium was using ten million leeches a year. A small number of scientists in those countries were turning out legitimate academic leech research.

"It was always my goal to go forward every day, to teach more people to make this, not global, because it is," she said, "not global because it is global, but in the United States."

And so, Alicja aggressively networked with hirudotherapists in Egypt, Hungary, Sweden, India, and Turkey. She joined international associations and went to professional hirudotherapy conferences and symposia in Poland, Bulgaria, and Moscow. She formed the American Hirudotherapy Association as a corporate entity in Nevada and invited international colleagues to conferences there.

At the same time, she began using leeches herself to treat clients in America, tapping a pool of European immigrants who already associated leeches with healing. She took out online advertisements and, calling herself Dr. A-Leech-A, personally treated patients wherever she went—Chicago one week, Minnesota the next, then Vegas. She opened an office in New York City and another in North Miami Beach. She began to turn up in mainstream media pieces; the socialite niece of the Duchess of Cornwall (and future queen consort) Camilla Parker Bowles wrote a glowing article for the *Daily Mail* about being treated by Alicja for migraines. An NBC affiliate featured her successful drive to popularize leech therapy in South Florida. In Brooklyn, she disappointed a reporter who asked her to leech him for fun; this, she told the reporter, would be disrespectful to the craft of hirudotherapy. Leeches are not larks.

All of this, she said, distinguished her remedy from the other One True Cures.

"This is not acupuncture," she said. "This is not the supplements. This is not the light therapy, sound therapy, etcetera."

Alicja did everything she could think of to get the medical establishment to take leeches seriously. That gave rise to a new problem: the medical establishment began to take leeches seriously. Which of course meant that, inevitably, leeches were going to draw the attention of the United States government. Soon, in those gray-walled cubicles at the FDA, parasitic, slimy bloodsuckers were seemingly everywhere. And they were talking about leeches.

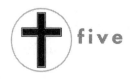five

THE NEUMANNS' PRAYERS

Faith is to believe what you do not see; the reward of this faith is to see what you believe.

—St. Augustine, fourth century AD

D ALE.

Leilani.

He grew. She grew.

He suggested moving. She said yes. He knew Wisconsin well. She wanted to learn. His childhood was icy winters. Hers were drenched in sunshine.

He showed her trees, bramble, bears; she showed him bravery amid isolation. His father, Peanut, lived two towns over; she missed block parties and retail outlets. He could still preach with a fiery conviction; she supported his preaching and found personal growth. He wanted his flock to extend beyond the family; she invited everyone she met to their Bible study. He rented a shop in Schofield's modest commercial downtown area, where she worked tirelessly, serving coffee with a side of God.

Together, in Weston, Wisconsin, where Turlock's human-to-tree ratio was inverted, the Neumann family founded a new ministry and life.

Their main tool for spiritual recruitment was the Monkey Mo Coffee Shop, which they established in 2005 close to their home in Weston, in a strip mall in Schofield that also hosted a farmers market every Saturday. With a drive-up window, spaciously high ceilings, and a decor that one customer called "California cool," Monkey Mo was a social life preserver, where Leilani could throw herself into all the little details of running a small business. She networked with farmers market vendors to get their hand-crafted items on Monkey Mo's shelves. If a customer seemed open to ministry, Leilani would reveal that she was the kind of woman who had the Book of Psalms loaded onto her iPod. Then she might invite them to a Bible study, led by Dale and hosted at either the coffee shop or their home.

The kids, who sometimes worked in the shop, showed off their piety and potential in ways that made Dale and Leilani glow with pride. Luke, sixteen, had a stocky and powerful build but was quiet, with rivers of deep thought that were sometimes troubled. Clever Ariel learned to read at age four; she had gone through a phase around puberty when she always seemed thin and tired, but she'd outgrown it, and at fifteen she was vibrant and quick to laugh. Hamilton, thirteen, was growing into a tall, lean beanpole with dramatic dark eyebrows and an aptitude for cameras and films.

Kara had just turned eleven and was, quite simply, an undiluted joy. At her school, Riverside Elementary, she wrote that her dream was to work at Monkey Mo full time. When there, she often did homework or drew cartoon monkeys. She had Leilani's outgoing, giving nature and Dale's drive and passion for scripture, keeping a journal in which she wrote about her desires to know God better. She hated to make a mistake and devoted herself to self-improvement, learning how to play the piano, note by painstaking note.

In late 2007, the Neumanns found what seemed like their forever home: a three-thousand-square-foot, stately, four-bedroom gray house with a wraparound porch, situated on a four-acre plot in a tulgey wood. They bought it for $312,500 and took advantage of the space to start a flourishing vegetable garden, some of whose produce went to feed customers at Monkey Mo.

Their efforts at building a home ministry continued—the first step, pioneered many times by Leilani's grandparents, was to establish a vibrant, regular Bible study. Here in rural Wisconsin, it was difficult to find like-minded Pentecostals, but the internet made that easier—they keyed into Unleavened Bread Ministries, an online fringe Pentecostal community centered around preacher David Eells, of Florida. Eells definitely advocated a more radical form of worship than the New Life Christian Center in Turlock. But that sat well with the Neumanns; in the worship of God, wasn't a radical devotion the whole point?

After so many years of dreaming about their ministry, it finally began to seem possible. They withdrew the kids from the public school system to be homeschooled instead. A handful of attendees from outside the family—Lynn Wilde, Carolyn Neuen, Dan and Jennifer Peaslee—began to show up at their Bible study, which was held at their house or at Monkey Mo.

Then came the best news yet. Another faith-filled family was moving from California to Wisconsin to partner with the Neumanns in opening a second gospel-oriented coffee shop.

Randall Wormgoor, about Dale's age, had been raised in a devout family from the Netherlands and graduated from Calgary Christian High School in Alberta, Canada. With a receding hairline and bristly mustache that enhanced the natural oval shape of his head, he looked like a big, friendly woodchuck.

Randall and his wife, Althea, had a lot in common with Dale and Leilani. Leilani and Dale had four kids; Althea and Randall did too (Marissa, Cameron, Corinna, and Makayla, all sporting charmingly crooked teeth). The Neumann family was close-knit and pious; the Wormgoor family was too.

In all—it wasn't a competition, mind you—it looked like the Wormgoors were as loving as the Neumanns, and they enjoyed hiking and the great outdoors to boot.

Dale had absolute confidence in his role as leader of the Neumann family and in his interpretations of the Bible. But a mild discord began to arise between the two families when it emerged, over the course of a few months, that Randall, despite his warm, fuzzy appearance, also had confidence in his role as family leader and in his own, sometimes different, interpretations of the Bible.

From the pulpit of their nascent ministry, Dale told the Wormgoors that there was a direct cause-and-effect relationship between sin and sickness. But Randall did not believe that sin caused sickness. Leilani supported Dale, and, of course, Althea supported Randall. Althea, with thick glasses brushed by the bottom of mousy brown bangs, spoke with a husky voice. If she was being 100 percent honest, she also thought the Neumanns focused an awful lot on demons.

Dale and Leilani tried to talk sense into the Wormgoors. They pointed to the ample biblical and contemporary examples of divine healing: at Unleavened Bread Ministries, infertile couples were conceiving and cancer patients were getting well, all through the power of prayer.

The Neumanns had even experienced such miracles themselves. In addition to relieving Dale's chronic back pain, prayers had moved God to alleviate Leilani's allergies. Kara hadn't been to a doctor since she was three years old. "'Whenever I started to get the sniffles,'" Kara told Leilani, "'I would just start praising the Lord, and they would go away.'" Leilani told Althea about the time one of her sons had gotten sick and prayer had helped him to vomit his demons out of his body.

Despite all these powerful testimonies, the Wormgoors simply refused to be persuaded that faith was the One True Cure.

The problem wasn't the praying. The Wormgoors were all for prayer, but they also made ample use of evidence-based medicine. The Wormgoors seemed to feel that treating sick children with prayer rather than medicine was even morally problematic. Althea later characterized the Neumann approach to healing as "basically, you pray and do nothing but pray."

The debate represented a difference of opinion within the broader Pentecostal community. God's ability to heal is almost universally recognized, but the idea that one should therefore renounce science-based medical care is held by only a small minority of Pentecostals.

Finding themselves on the opposite side of this argument from the Wormgoors didn't sit well with the Neumanns. Their relationship cooled, the disagreements over the Bible spilled over into disagreements over the business, and by March 2008 the coffee shop partnership had fallen apart. The two families were still cordial to one another, but the bad feelings threatened to turn into active feuding.

Neither family knew it, but the Wormgoors were about to see exactly how effective prayer could be.

It would take an act of faith and an act of courage.

.:.

As the most popular and influential book ever written, the Bible retains more sway over individuals' decisions than you might realize. An estimated 7.7 billion copies have been printed, and 100 million more are printed each year, which means people are printing Bibles more quickly than God is printing people. That helps explain why 90 percent of Americans have prayed for health—but the majority coexist quite happily with hospitals that they believe are among God's many creations.

In 2021, my search for an inside look at faith healing led me to a steamy June weekend in Miami. This was where, in 1956, a rotund and freewheeling Pentecostal faith healer named Jack Coe told a couple to remove the leg braces of their toddler because Coe had just cured him of polio. When they did, the boy suffered debilitating pain, and the parents sued Coe. A Florida judge found in favor of Coe, but God did not; a year later, the healer died of polio himself at the age of thirty-eight.

On a Friday evening, I drove just north of Miami to Margate and parked where no one would see my rental car. Small lizards leapt for the safety of the brush as I walked through a church parking lot, passing an old prison bus that had been converted into a ministry cafe.

The church had been rented by a group called the Last Reformation for a two-day event that would teach the faithful to heal chronic pain, asymmetry of the legs, mental conditions, drug addictions, cancer—really, anything that might afflict them.

The message of the Last Reformation's charismatic leader, Torben Søndergaard, boiled down to a few simple, emphatic precepts. First, a belief in God demanded that one become an active disciple of Jesus. Second, one became a disciple by learning how to create more disciples; this was done through a combination of baptizing them, healing them, and casting out any demons that had taken up residence in their bodies.

And third, when it came to a postmortem entrance into the kingdom of Heaven, you were better off the more people you had healed and baptized. God keeps score.

Because followers were so incentivized to create more followers, Torben's system functioned like a faith-healing pyramid scheme. As a skeptic, I thought it seemed silly and pointless—not that I, a hopeless addict of both board games and puns, was one to point fingers.

But silliness crosses a line into toxicity if it harms the public health by convincing people to forgo medical care. In 2019, Søndergaard had been dragged publicly in Denmark for this very thing. A Danish television station sent two undercover journalists to one of his events and produced an episode that accused him of telling people with mental illness to throw away their medicine.

The broadcast repeatedly aired a quote from Torben, whose bald head glistened: "God is always stronger than medicine."

In a video response posted on his YouTube channel, Søndergaard told his viewers, "To take a few words out of context, it's just so crazy." The thing that really got under Søndergaard's skin, he said, was that the subject of medicine would never have come up without the meddling of the hidden reporters.

"We never talk about medicine," he said. "The only reason I talked about medicine with that undercover journalist was because she asked a lot of questions about medicine."

.•:ˊ

BEHIND THE LARGE, ORNATE DOUBLE WOODEN DOORS OF THE CHURCH in Margate, Florida, the air was blissfully cool. People filtered down a short passage that contained a decorative alcove and into an auditorium with a stage in front and folding tables selling Last Reformation swag in the back.

I had decided that although I wasn't actively identifying myself as a journalist, it would be unethical to outwardly lie about it. My plan was to simply observe anonymously. The event was open to anyone who bought a ticket, and no one had asked me about myself.

Soon, Torben was addressing the audience through a microphone. It's hard to describe him as anything other than a beamer, with constant smiles that focused happy energy with a laser-like power.

"Okay!" he beamed. "I am going to say welcome and looking forward to spending some time with you!"

His Danish accent was, I had to admit, undeniably adorable.

"If you need to be baptized in water, get baptized tonight," he told us. Baptisms carry their own logistical challenge, because to Pentecostals like Torben, the gentle sprinkling of water from a fountain was just not adequate; only a full-body immersion will get the job done. He'd used lakes and streams, a black plastic tub filled with a garden hose, even the ocean.

"We have water fourteen minutes from here—I don't know," said Torben. "There is water someplace."

I knew that the nearest body of water was the canal across the street, part of a twenty-two-mile system carved from the porous limestone of the Biscayne Aquifer. The canals were also alligator highways. Just a few miles away, a family of alligators living in that same canal system had been removed after repeated incidents with a family of humans living in an adjacent apartment complex. One of the gators was thirteen feet long.

It would be really kind of terrible if an alligator bit someone during the baptismal process, I thought.

I definitely did not want that to happen. Even if it would help me sell books. How many books would it help me sell? I reflected on it a moment and concluded to myself that it was probably a lot. It would probably help me sell a lot of books. It would be really terrible though.

And, I thought with a sort of admiration of my own saintliness, *I would not want that to happen.*

⁘

TORBEN'S FLOCK WAS AS DIVERSE AS A DOVE SOAP COMMERCIAL: OLD AND young and of various apparent ethnicities. Everywhere I turned, there were smiles and hugs. A handful of young men in pressed dress shirts spoke quietly with lilting African accents. A woman with a complicated cloth strapping system held an adorable Kewpie doll of a child to her stomach, face out. White men with an aura of hard living smiled with relief, their clothes less worn than their faces.

They were, in short, nicer dressed than me, more interested in self-development and spiritual growth than me, and more motivated to give of themselves to help the world.

From what I could tell during the early going, this was a very loosey-goosey version of a traditional church service. There was no sign of cultishness, no high-pressure sales tactics. Money was raised through the sale of swag, a gate fee, and the passing of a collection box but no more aggressively than I'd seen at many other churches or at secular events.

What am I doing here?

But then, Søndergaard introduced, with great fanfare, a young man named Jeremy.

"We're gonna teach you how to heal the sick," said Jeremy, the smoothness and confidence of his patter indicating that he was a regular speaker. If you sat next to him on an airplane, you would have to listen to him talk about Jesus for the duration of the flight and need to make sure your wallet was still in your pocket when you landed. Jeremy told the crowd that ten years before, while addicted to street drugs, he had been on seven different medications, including Suboxone and antidepressants. During a church sermon, Jeremy had experienced a sort of epiphany.

"I felt like I was—do you guys not understand? The Bible says that we're healed. Why are we on medications? Why are we living on crutches? We're healed!" he said. "And it seemed like no one else got it. No one else understood it. But I did."

Then, Jeremy told us, he took immediate action.

"And I went home and I just took all my medication and threw it in the trash can," he said. "All seven medications and threw them in the trash can." Next, Jeremy took out his phone and told his doctor he was done taking his antidepressants and other medicines, due to divine saving.

"I said, 'I will never come back to see you again.'" He added with a cocky chuckle, "'Not for diseases at least. Maybe to talk about Jesus.'"

Jeremy said that he hadn't taken any medication of any sort since.

"You guys," he told the crowd, "can do the same thing."

And adorable Torben Søndergaard, who two years before had been so offended at the very idea that he had told mentally ill people to throw away their medicine, beamed.

After about an hour of testimonials, Torben retook the stage with what was starting to seem like the smile of an impenetrably smug Cheshire Cat.

By then, my nervousness about being detected had melted into abject boredom. Book sales were no justification for an alligator attack, but when you added in the mental benefits of relieving monotony, the moral equation seemed much murkier. Søndergaard announced it was time for everyone to heal through prayer. Phew.

Then it struck me.

Had he said—everyone?

I slouched lower in my seat, no longer bored.

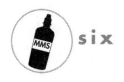 **six**

THE ALIEN'S DRINK

PHYSICIAN, n. One upon whom we set
our hopes when ill and our dogs when well.

—Ambrose Bierce, *The Devil's Dictionary*, 1906

W ITH THE INTERNET IN FULL SWING AND A HOME COMPUTER IN his hands, the alien in Jim Humble's skin devised a plan to circumvent the sinister forces arrayed against him and bring his Miracle Mineral Solution directly to the inhabitants of planet Earth.

Step one: Put the life-saving humanitarian message about MMS on a website, for all the peoples of the world to see.

Step two: Actually, hang on.

The alien was having a hard time with step one. Nothing in his billion-year existence had prepared him to create a website, and so he decided to outsource it. He sold a patent on what he called "a special process for recovery of gold" for $17,000. He spent $14,000 of those earnings on a software company that said it would build a webpage for his One True Cure. But the webpage never happened. The alien in Humble's skin said the software company screwed him over.

This sort of thing seemed to happen to the alien quite a lot. He found a partner, who helped finance further efforts to build a website. They hired a web designer, who quit and sued them. They hired a grant writer, who, the alien noted sourly, "also began working against us."

Somehow, this happened four more times, with four different employees. They "all bombed out and took our money and produced nothing," the alien in Humble's skin complained. It was almost as if they were agents of Planet of the Gods ruler Manzanora, sent to foil his mission.

But the immortal being couldn't give up, not when popularizing his One True Cure was so close he could taste it. And in fact, he did taste it. His partner bought him a hundred-pound drum of sodium chlorite, which he used to keep experimenting with different formulations of MMS, adding hydrochloric acid to activate it and then diluting it in an acidic liquid, like lemon juice. He tested it, using the human body he inhabited.

This went spectacularly wrong at one point, when the intergalactic alien accidentally burned his own eye with MMS. For a time, the alien's human eyeball seemed as if it might actually fall out of its human socket.

"The skin around my eyes dropped and stretched downward about an inch," noted the alien in Humble's skin. "I was worried, but it cleared up in a few days."

Finally, the alien settled on a formulation that looked like pale yellow lemonade and tasted a bit like swimming pool water. In 2003, he sat at his kitchen table and used a lab scale to portion out hundreds of bottles of MMS, each containing 450 doses.

By the alien's calculations, the total batch added up to well over a million doses, but there was no one to take them. This was frustrating. Larry Lytle, Toby McAdam, Robert Young, a thousand others—seemingly everyone was selling their One True Cure on the internet, but somehow he was left out of the equation.

With a webpage nowhere in sight, the alien in Jim Humble's skin began emailing people in other countries, seeking help to administer MMS without having to navigate the US government. Which led him to the continent of Africa, where, far from the prying eyes of the FDA, he began his campaign to help humankind.

．∵∵

IN 2004, THE ALIEN IN HUMBLE'S SKIN TOOK MASS QUANTITIES OF MMS to the hospital of a Christian mission in Kakamega, Kenya, where he had convinced those in charge to let him treat malaria patients. The alien put on a white lab coat with the words "The Malaria Solution Foundation" embroidered in gold on the front.

"I wore my hat, light tan pants, and white shoes," he said. "I looked like a doctor."

Never guessing that the doctor was actually an alien in disguise (and lacking medical credentials), several hundred people showed up to be treated. Helpers lined up twenty or thirty glasses at a time, and the alien went down the row three times, first using a measuring spoon to add MMS to each glass, then pouring in vinegar, and finally topping off each dose with pineapple juice.

After Kakamega, he flew to Nairobi. Then to Kampala, Uganda. The alien eventually visited Sierra Leone and Tanzania, dispensing MMS to anyone who would swallow it.

He wanted to do formal clinical trials, which he sensed could pressure the medical establishment to accept MMS. But the ways in which human scientists conducted ethical clinical trials seemed to be incomprehensible to his otherworldly mindset. For example, most human scientists would not look upon a population of Malawi prisoners as consenting participants in testing an unproven medication that had almost allowed an eyeball to jiggle out of its socket.

"Someone had suggested that doing clinical trials in the local prisons would be the easiest thing to do and the easiest place to get permission," the alien reported. "We decided to give it a try."

He chose the prison in Lilongwe, which had one toilet for every 120 inmates and one water tap for 900. The prison's assistant medical technician gave the alien and his team permission to do their version of clinical trials. "We slipped him a few dollars at several different times and he was quite cooperative," the alien in Humble's skin later wrote.

The alien may have realized that, in Earth culture, this resembled bribing the nearly powerless to do medical experiments on the totally powerless. And so the alien amended his statement, implying he was instead due a pat on the back. "Actually, it is only fair to mention that he was quite cooperative even before we slipped him a few dollars," the alien wrote, "but he was such a nice man that we thought it would be nice to help him out a bit."

The following morning, the alien gave ten prisoners his regimen of MMS, vinegar, and pineapple juice. Soon after, they checked the temperatures of the subjects.

"The first thing we learned was that those ear thermometers simply do not work in Africa. I think it is because ears in Africa, especially in prison, are cleaned differently, or not at all," the alien wrote, somewhat racistly.

After the prison experiments, the alien and his helpers treated people in various small villages, where residents lived in thatched huts. There, the alien in Humble's skin said, many of the people they gave MMS to "vomited worms, and some had dead worms in their stools."

The alien found this to be fascinating. He concluded that vomiting and diarrhea were, in many cases, a part of getting well.

As word of MMS spread, public health advocates pushed back, fueled by reports of people getting sick after taking it. They said the active ingredient in MMS was actually industrial bleach, which the alien found to be downright slanderous.

"Chlorine dioxide is used in more than 1000 public water works to kill the diseases of mankind," the alien in Humble's skin wrote. "Why would anyone refuse to believe that it can be used to kill the diseases in the water of the human body?"

Seeking to spread the word of MMS further, the alien in Humble's skin began penning a book that was part autobiography, part history of MMS, and part a summing up of the alien's views on the American government.

"There are those who want to kill the human race," the alien in Humble's skin wrote. "They have been working at it for a lot longer than you would believe if I told you. It's not an easy job, killing the human race, but they have been at it for a god-awful long time."

The alien also said that, while there were some natural diseases, there were also dozens if not hundreds of new diseases that were "traceable back to laboratories of the Government."

.•:˙

THE ALIEN IN HUMBLE'S SKIN WASN'T THE ONLY ONE WHO SUSPECTED that the United States government was manipulating the public health system on behalf of corporate interests. The details differed, but nearly all the alternative healers I spoke with were convinced that the FDA was simply a Big Pharma puppet.

Where did this idea come from?

I am sad to say that there is a kernel of truth to it.

The FDA is a creation of the nation's laws, and those laws are made by the nation's duly elected lawmakers. And the pharmaceutical industry spends lots of money to influence this process. The number of registered Big Pharma lobbyists—1,270—significantly outnumbers the lawmakers themselves.

The nonpartisan watchdog Center for Responsive Politics reported that between 1998 and 2005, Big Pharma spent $900 million on lobbying. A separate analysis of public data, published in *JAMA Internal Medicine*, showed that between 1999 and 2018, Big Pharma spent $6 billion on campaign contributions and lobbying. That's a lot of money, but it was only 0.1 percent of the $5.5 trillion spent on prescription drugs in the US over the same period.

This is also a problem at the state level. A Center for Public Integrity report demonstrated that Medicaid pays inflated prices for medications that patients do not need, as a result of Big Pharma meddling. It cites examples of drug companies influencing the committees that advise states on Medicaid by buying members lavish dinners, hiring them for consulting gigs, convincing speakers to give favorable testimony without disclosing financial ties, and even "helping" doctors fill out the paperwork needed to get costly drugs approved by state Medicaid programs.

We know all these systemic flaws exist because a robust network of media and patient advocacy groups tracks and reports such things. And yet, this same watchdog network has never found evidence of what would be the biggest story ever reported: a secret plot of government and Big Pharma to sicken or kill the human race.

Which brings us back to a certain ancient alien god.

.·::·'

WHILE THE ALIEN WAS WRITING HIS BOOK, SOMETHING UNEXPECTED happened.

In 2005, the alien was working on the roof of a building at the old Nevadan gold mine when he fell off the roof and broke both his back and his neck. At this point, the alien uncharacteristically put himself in the hands of the (FDA-approved, Big Pharma–controlled, Manzanora-manipulated) medical establishment that he believed was actively trying to kill him.

A government-subsidized helicopter airlifted him to Reno, where a titanium screw was used to immobilize the second cervical bone in Jim Humble's spine. After six months, doctors told him he would need to undergo another operation to put in more screws.

The alien did not want another operation. And even outside MMS, he had tools in his toolkit to help avoid surgery. For example, he had also developed a technique for healing by touch.

"The basic theory is that the brain controls all the healing in your body," he explained. "So if you can increase the communication between the brain and the area that's bad, it will heal faster. In minutes sometimes."

The alien did not heal his neck by touch. Instead, he pursued yet another advanced healing method unknown to science. He bought some of the strongest magnets on the market, powerful enough to cut through any bipedal carbon-based life-form.

"Magnetism must have a completed magnetic circuit through the body in order to get maximum healing power," the alien later wrote. For five days and nights, with spaceships whizzing by overhead on their way to Area 51, the alien sat in an upright position with the magnets in place. He said this is what healed his bones.

When the alien finally completed his book, *The Miracle Mineral Supplement of the 21st Century*, he encouraged people to make their own MMS. First, he said, they should obtain hundred-pound barrels of sodium chlorite, which cannot be legally purchased by individuals.

"You might be able to find a local business that will receive the sodium chlorite for you and let you use their name," the alien wrote. He also had advice for those wary of ingesting a bleach-like solution based on the say-so of a best-in-the-world-but-somehow-cash-strapped gold assayer selling ebooks on the internet.

"If it scares you to take it," he wrote, "try giving it to your dog first."

After a couple more false starts, the alien finally established a web presence. He gave the first half of his book away for free and charged $9.95 for people to download the second half. Soon, he was taking in $350 per day on (half) book sales, and various independent suppliers who had heard his message were selling Americans an estimated eleven thousand bottles of MMS each month.

.•:

ONE OF THE MANY PEOPLE WHO HEARD THE WORD FROM THE ALIEN IN Humble's skin was Mark Grenon. He'd gone to high school in New Hampshire in the 1960s and described himself as "an average little punk kid." He worked at Kmart and grocery stores and then with his dad on construction gigs. When he was seventeen, he and a buddy traveled through California, Washington, and Oregon, picking apples and meeting all kinds of people. He got married and fathered eight boys. He became very religious and in 1993 set up a residential mission in the Dominican Republic.

I spoke with Grenon multiple times. "The same people who own the TV station own the pharmaceuticals," he told me. "So this is what we're dealing with, bro."

Grenon's first major experience with MMS was when he used it to successfully treat himself and his kids for a MRSA infection. This added further proof to Grenon's long-held belief that the medical establishment, and vaccines in particular, were ruining the world.

"You know these movies about zombies?" he asked me. "It literally is gonna happen."

At this point, though Toby McAdam had also independently brought up zombies to me, I did not realize that zombies were a thing. And so I asked Grenon, with a tone of disbelief, how vaccines could turn people into zombies.

"Because it's literally rewriting their DNA," he told me.

Even a rogue researcher like Robert Young, I thought, could not have come up with anything half so bizarre as Grenon's explanation: The vaccines contained nanoparticles that were shed into the body. The nanoparticles "corrupted" the DNA. And those with corrupted DNA would have malfunctions in the brain that induced violence and a taste for human flesh. Grenon implied that he had personally witnessed such things.

"I've seen some really crazy shit," he said.

After his positive experience with MMS, Grenon followed the instructions in the alien's book and began distributing it in the Dominican Republic and Haiti. He eventually established a correspondence with the alien in Humble's skin. In 2010, the alien, flush with online book sales, agreed to go live in Grenon's missionary compound. He sent Grenon $25,000 and asked him to arrange for private living quarters that would allow him to write more books.

Two months later, the alien in Humble's skin arrived in the Dominican Republic. By then, authorities were beginning to crack down on MMS producers, and the movement was in danger of fizzling. The two sentient beings decided to put their heads together and figure out the best way to fulfill the alien's humanitarian mission: to make MMS go mainstream.

And *then* things started to get weird.

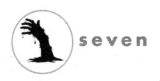seven

AMERICAN HEALTH CARE

An old acquaintance who knew well the character of a celebrated empiric, said to him, while standing at the door, "Prithee, doctor, how is it that you, whose origin I so well know, should have been able to obtain more practice than almost all the regular bred physicians." "Pray," says the quack, "how many persons have passed us while you put the question?" "About twenty." "And pray how many of them do you suppose possess a competent share of common sense?" "Perhaps one out of the twenty." "Just so," says the doctor, "and that one applies to the regular physician, while I and my brethren pick up the other nineteen."

And how often have we seen the contemptible ignoramus raised by the voice of popularity above the level of the learned and accomplished physician, and boasting of nineteen twentieths of the practice.

—James Thacher, *An Essay on Demonology, Ghosts and Apparitions, and Popular Superstitions*, 1831

THE FDA'S 2002 FLURRY OF ENFORCEMENT WAS MEANT TO BE A flex showing that thousands of bureaucratic, unlikable, stick-in-the-mud science addicts, whose very lunch breaks were tightly controlled by the ungainly *Operations Manual*, could make the world safe for the public and dangerous for hawkers of One True Cures.

In the past, between the 1960s and 1990s, similar periods of stepped-up enforcement had portrayed the FDA as a devastatingly effective monster, hunting down scofflaws and chewing them up like Flintstone vitamins. But now, the statistics that ruled their lives painted a very different picture.

The 1994 Dietary Supplement Health and Education Act combined with the internet to stock the country with thousands of One True Cures that, like shoals of herrings, afforded each other protection through their sheer numbers.

The FDA may have been a fearsome and frumious beast, but it was also slow. It soon found itself embroiled in a massive game of whack-a-mole. It would invest the resources to shut down an adulterated brand of dietary supplements only to see those same toxic pills resurface at different URLs, with different brand names, selling to the growing number of Americans who were turning to the internet for health solutions.

Consider illicit online pharmacies, which represented just one tiny slice of the fraudulent-cure landscape. Because they sold actual drugs, they were a top concern for the FDA, which in the early 2000s was targeting roughly four hundred websites annually, resulting in a few dozen arrests per year.

That was pretty good by 1999 standards, when the National Association of Boards of Pharmacy estimated there were a total of four hundred online pharmacies sending drugs to American consumers. But it was like wrestling Gremlins out of an Olympic-sized swimming pool—by 2005, the number of pharmacies had ballooned to 11,000. (Funnily enough, though they nearly all claimed to be selling less costly Canadian versions of American drugs, only 214 of the 11,000 were actually registered in Canada.)

The proliferation was a straightforward example of free-market economics. One study showed that illegally selling sildenafil (a drug that causes erections) through a bogus online pharmacy was two thousand times more profitable than selling cocaine and was also less likely to result in criminal penalties.

In every conceivable corner of cyberspace—dedicated websites, online storefronts of legitimate retailers, internet forums and emails, not to mention brick-and-mortar operations—Americans were also being bombarded with illegally inflated sales pitches for tainted supplements, bogus medical devices, and dangerous health treatments. People like Larry Lytle, Toby McAdam, and Robert Young (and aliens like Jim Humble) were selling their lasers, homemade pills, alkalizing supplements, and water purifiers as One True Cures with impunity. The *Operations Manual* instructed FDA agents on the proper way to walk across a set of train tracks (at right angles, without stepping on rails), but for this it had no answer. With so much illicit activity, the FDA's enforcement wing was like a fierce old tomcat drowning in a sea of mice. The agency tacitly admitted that it simply couldn't bring everyone to justice when it formed a triage team that sifted through the complaints to find the most egregious pills and medical devices and health services that would be investigated for possible formal warnings and criminal convictions.

Bureaucrats at the FDA, the CDC, the Justice Department, and professional medical organizations knew they had to evolve. They began revising their methods, trying to figure out how to best drop the hammer on One True Cures once and for all. If the agency could only get its hooks into a small percentage of the lawbreakers, it was clear that it had to, at a minimum, shut those operations down emphatically and make them an example that would deter other perpetrators.

But the One True Cures were evolving too.

And the battle of wills between the FDA and One True Cureists would have unintended consequences for an entirely different crowd: antivaccine advocates.

.•::

BY THE EARLY 2000S, THE WORST THING ABOUT BEING IN THE ANTIVACCINE movement was that there was no longer an antivaccine movement to speak of.

Sure, every time a new vaccine was rolled out, it sparked fresh public fears, but the problem was the dang things kept working. Over decades, the Numbers Junkies behind the vaccines racked up victory after victory—polio, smallpox, diphtheria, tetanus, pertussis, all wiped out by successful public vaccination campaigns. In the 1950s, roughly a third of Americans were vaccine hesitant. But now? The antivaxxers watched glumly as the most recent childhood vaccination achieved a 97 percent coverage rate, which resulted in zero cases of measles in the US in the year 2000.

It was enough to make an antivaxxer feel very blergh.

Without any financial engine behind the antivaccine message, about the only folks still refusing vaccines were owners of composting toilets, a sprinkling of parents who kinda-sorta heard they caused autism, and fringe members of minority religious groups like the Amish. And Mark Grenon.

Even the Neumanns, well on their way to eschewing all medical care, vaccinated each of their four kids, and if the Neumanns weren't gettable for antivaxxers, then what was the point?

The problem was that the antivax movement relied on tired old arguments. People simply didn't think vaccines were unsafe, or bad for the environment, or sacrilegious. But then something kind of wonderful happened for them.

In 2005, in Los Angeles, there was an alternative-healing expo, one of those events where attendees pay a few dollars to wander rows of booths rented by sellers of organic lip balm, hypnotism services, dietary supplements, and healing crystals. These sorts of events happened all the time, especially in New Age–friendly California, but this particular one was the brainchild of Indiana-based supplements manufacturer Wendell W. Whitman. Whitman was, like Robert Young, a graduate of the Clayton School of Natural Healing, and in an effort to advance the prospects of alternative healers in Washington, DC, he had branded this event as the first-ever "Health Freedom Expo."

The expo, organized by Whitman's lobbying group, the HealthKeepers Alliance, featured a typical lineup of alternative-health speakers, including Hulda Clark (whose One True Cure included a $350 "Zapper" to kill the parasites she believed caused all disease), Charlotte Gerson (whose diet-based One True Cure, Gerson Therapy, cost up to $15,000), and Kurt Donsbach (who, among other dubious enterprises, ran a One True Cure alternative hospital for terminal illnesses in Mexico).

But the lineup also included some atypical names: medical-freedom activists like attorney Diane Miller of the National Health Freedom Coalition, and Joan Vandergriff, leader of the Sunshine Health Freedom Foundation (and former seller of a "pH Balancing plan" on audiocassette).

These activist speakers were there to bring a message to the alternative-healing community: One True Cures could be made much more profitable through the idea of "medical freedom." For years, the healers had been desperately trying to defend the crappy science behind their various One True Cures, but under the banner of medical freedom, it was not about the remedies' efficacy in treating disease. It was about the consumer's right to buy the treatment they wanted.

Medical freedom wasn't an entirely new idea, of course, but the proliferation of One True Cures in the internet age gave rise to a whole class of American entrepreneurs who had a vested financial interest in beating back the regulations that were designed to protect the public. Fueled by their raw energy, the Health Freedom Expo was an enormous success for all involved, spawning dozens of similar events across the country. In evolutionary terms, if the internet caused the species quack to become so immensely prolific that regulatory predators couldn't keep pace, the medical-freedom activists now invited them to herd up and act as one for mutual protection and benefit.

Thanks to these sorts of grassroots actions, diverse sellers of One True Cures began speaking in a single voice. When Robert Young had a chance to meet President Barack Obama at an event, he didn't start talking about the science of acid and alkaline diets. "Freedom is a God-given right," he told the president. "It's about the right to choose between complementary or alternative or conventional treatment." Health freedom was also how the alien in Humble's skin, now joined by human Mark Grenon, began to describe the extraterrestrial mission of distributing MMS. Toby McAdam said he merely wanted to exercise his rights to sell supplements; Larry Lytle argued that the ability to purchase lasers was "a private right"; and Pentecostals like Dale and Leilani Neumann began defending faith healing as an exercise of their constitutional religious rights.

As sellers of One True Cures were converted into medical-freedom advocates, a side effect was the creation of a political space that welcomed the fringe actors remaining in the antivaccine movement. They were, like alternative healers, eager to move on from scientific debates and instead talk about the rights of Americans to choose. And they were happy to point to One True Cures as solutions to the communicable diseases that vaccines were designed to prevent. Within two years the speaker lineup at Health Freedom Expos had incorporated antivax activist leaders, including Dr. Joseph Mercola, who asserted in a 2006

New York Times best seller that the avian influenza pandemic was government fearmongering to control the populace. Mercola was himself marketing a wide variety of health care and wellness products with bogus health claims.

.•: :•'

IF ALTERNATIVE HEALERS AND ANTIVAXXERS WERE HAPPY TO HAVE FOUND A label to rally around, imagine how happy it made the people who had created the label in the first place. This was another fringe group, the ones who had already defined what medical freedom means in America: libertarians.

It's hard to think of two cultures more different than a touchy-feely New Age alternative-healing movement that celebrates mindfulness, and the free-market, small-government libertarian capitalists that celebrate mind-your-own-businessness. But the medical-freedom label formed an unprecedented bridge between these two worldviews.

Libertarians had articulated a clear and comprehensive vision of medical freedom, one that went far beyond weakening federal vaccination programs and allowing unregulated sales of One True Cures.

The 2000 political platform for the national Libertarian Party advocated for "a complete separation of medicine from the state. We oppose any government restriction or funding of medical or scientific research. . . . We support an end to government-provided health insurance and health care." If the United States adopted this pure free-market approach to health care, it would be the first nation in the world to do so.

The Future of Freedom Foundation, a libertarian policy think tank, published an article that staked out the parameters in more detail, blasting the National Organ Transplant Act of 1984, which ensures that donated organs are allocated according to medical need rather than financial resources.

"Why?" asked the article's author, Laurence Vance of the Ludwig von Mises Institute (and the Libertarian Christian Institute, and the International Society of Bible Collectors). "Why do Americans not have the medical freedom to buy and sell organs?"

Vance called for such lovely human rights as "the freedom to dis-criminate," "a free market in medical devices," and "a free market in ambulance services," which means that if you live in an area that can't financially support ambulance coverage, you should pack your sorry, heart-attack-having ass into the car and drive to the hospital yourself. Though, since medical-freedom activists also advocate for the right of an emergency room to refuse service for nonpayment, you'd better not forget your wallet.

The government's responsibility for public health was cemented back in 1901, when the US Supreme Court ruled seven to two to uphold a mandatory vaccine program to combat a deadly smallpox epidemic; in its ruling, the court established the right of the government to use po-lice powers to control epidemic diseases.

But in the libertarian vision of medical freedom, there are no medical-licensing laws, no Medicaid or Medicare, no federal grants for medical research, and no federal programs to combat public health threats like HIV/AIDS. To achieve this, they plan to shutter every federal laboratory in the country and forever abolish the FDA, along with the Department of Health and Human Services and the National Institutes of Health.

The guiding principle of medical freedom is that a person's health and safety are the sole concern of the individual, not the government, which is one of the very best imaginary concepts out there.

That bit of whimsy often collides with the fact that society has a sig-nificant stake in an individual's health, as a 1980 Massachusetts court noted in a case involving mandatory helmet laws for motorcycle riders. "From the moment of the injury, society picks the person up off the highway; delivers him to a municipal hospital and municipal doctors; provides him with unemployment compensation if, after recovery, he cannot replace his lost job; and if the injury causes permanent disability may assume the responsibility for his and his family's continued suste-nance. We do not understand a state of mind that permits a plaintiff to think that only he himself is concerned."

I suspect that targeted surveying would reveal that 100 percent of healthy libertarians proclaim their intentions to do without all these luxuries, while 100 percent of libertarians lying injured on the pavement admit that, yes, such societal services are kind of necessary, now that they think of it.

.•:·'

As the leftist, New Age creators of universal energy, herbal cures, meditation, and pyramid pendants adopted the libertarian medical-freedom label, they paid a price for their newfound clout: large segments of the alternative-health movement drifted away from their cultural and spiritual roots and embraced a more commercial version of healing. What they really wanted was the right to sell their products to the public; in pursuit of that, they were signing on to a much broader idea of medical freedom that wanted to dismantle key parts of the social safety net.

Meanwhile, as libertarians absorbed the political power of the alternative-healing industry, their calls for medical freedom gained sway with mainstream Republicans. Elected leaders who could not have been persuaded to endorse lasers or pH miracles in any circumstance were suddenly rallied to their cause.

Perhaps Republicans got on board because of their long-standing vision of a more limited form of government. Or maybe it was because they had the same exact vested interest that the purveyors of the One True Cures did: product sales.

During the aughts, national politicians—almost exclusively Republicans—began monetizing the email lists of their campaign supporters by partnering with for-profit corporations to sell supplements. An exposé by journalist Ben Adler for the *New Republic* found that a typical transaction involved about a hundred dollars per one thousand names, allowing campaigns to pull down millions of dollars. (Democrats tended to monetize their lists in other ways, such as renting them to explicitly political causes and candidates.)

Because of this, tens of millions of rank-and-file Republicans were deluged with targeted, shady health-marketing claims from the presidential candidates they trusted. Herman Cain urged 330,000 supporters to buy TestoMax 200, a One True Cure for erectile dysfunction. Pat Robertson's crowd was tempted with an age-defying protein shake. Ben Carson's voters heard all about the Mannatech dietary supplement line. Mike Huckabee sold his followers heart disease fixes and a diabetes solution kit, while Newt Gingrich pitched a cancer cure that cost just seventy-four dollars per year, and Alan Keyes began hawking Prevennia, a supplement that could supposedly prevent the cell mutations behind six thousand diseases.

America had, quite by accident, created a real clusterquack.

WHEN THE SELLERS OF ONE TRUE CURES BEGAN TO IDENTIFY AS medical-freedom advocates, the change in messaging and tone didn't raise any immediate alarms at the FDA and the other enforcement agencies tasked with protecting the health of the American public. Enforcement agents didn't care about the political rhetoric and stances of potential fraudsters. They simply went on pounding away at the violators, as they always had. That's what guiding documents like the *Operations Manual* told them to do.

But a small minority of public health officials did see the downsides of their own inherent stodginess and were beginning to realize that being mind-numbingly boring was an impediment to influencing an American public that, in the digital age, wanted its important information to be sugarcoated with entertainment value.

Public officials had to somehow find a space for themselves on the fun side of the cultural landscape. Over on that end of the zeitgeist, far from droning recommendations about handwashing and sunblock, something even sillier than medical freedom was rising from the grave.

Long after the George Romero films (*Night of the Living Dead*, *Dawn of the Dead*, and others that mention *Dead*) defined zombies for moviegoers as slow-moving people eaters, images of them lingered in the corners of the public imagination. The Romero films eventually spawned a whole subgenre of low-budget horror movies from up-and-coming directors. Before David Cronenberg, Sam Raimi, and Peter Jackson directed *A History of Violence*, *Spider-Man*, and *Lord of the Rings*, they cut their teeth helming zombie flicks like *Shivers*, *The Evil Dead*, and *Dead Alive*.

As movie monsters go, zombies make for slightly boring characters, on account of their not having functioning brains. A vampire has pathos, romance, and morally shaded characters; a werewolf is a semitragic victim of its own disease. But a zombie is just a dangerous bag of meat.

And yet, interest in zombies grew. The 1990s saw the release of 46 zombie movies; in the 2000s, it was 172, with offerings ranging from A to Z (that's *Aaah! Zombies!!*, a film told from the perspective of the zombies themselves, to *Zoombies*, about a zombie outbreak among zoo animals). During the 2000s, the number of zombie books quadrupled, scholarly papers on the academic platform JSTOR increased fivefold, and mentions in the *New York Times* increased eightfold. Through 2008, Google had fewer searches for zombies than for vampires or wizards; in 2009 and beyond, it has had more than five times as many zombie searches than vampire and wizard searches combined.

For the first time in history, usage of the word "zombie" in English-language books outstripped usage of the word "apocalypse." Clearly, the idea of a zombie apocalypse was completely overshadowing the original Judeo-Christian meaning of apocalypse—a time of divine revelation when the corrupt world would be blasted apart but with the important upside of the faithful being rewarded with an everlasting kingdom. By wallowing in images of a zombie-laden world, America was instead taking its apocalyptic coffee black, with no revelatory cream or divine sugar.

Why were zombies gaining such appeal? The features that define them give us hints. As threats go, they are a vacuum—they have no evil plans, no power of speech (or thoughts that would necessitate speaking), no lairs to retreat to, no desire for self-protection, no capacity for bargaining or negotiation. They are amoral, decentralized, and driven by a single craving—brains.

The mystery of zombies' enduring charisma drew the attention of various academics, including Daniel Drezner, a Tufts University political science professor who studies the whys and wherefores of zombie culture. Drezner suggested that the uniquely American take on zombies—in which governments have invariably been toppled and rendered impotent—reflects modern fears of massive global threats that are impersonal and indiscriminately deadly, like viral pandemics and climate change.

If zombies are indeed a metaphor for global threats, there is also something undeniably silly about their lurching slowness and stupidity; dressing up serious threats in this way is empowering, like putting a clown nose on a Nazi.

And so, while lots of people were talking about zombies, few were taking them seriously. It would require a keen mind to actually recognize them as a force that could be harnessed to achieve political gain.

And just such a keen mind existed. It lay in the cranium of a worker at the Centers for Disease Control and Prevention.

PART THREE — ACUTE PANGS

In which the system tries to break One True Cureism

When I was ill you came to me,
Doctor, and with great urgency
A hundred students brought with you
A most instructive case to view.
The hundred fingered me with hands
Chilled by the blasts from northern lands;
Fever at outset had I none;
I have it, sir, now you have done!

—Martial (Marcus Valerius Martialis),
"Patient and Doctor," c. AD 40

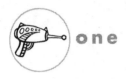 **one**

LARRY LYTLE'S LASER LIGHT LEADS TO LIFE

When a doctor does go wrong he is the first of criminals.
He has nerve and he has knowledge.

—Arthur Conan Doyle, *The Adventures
of Sherlock Holmes*, 1892

NOT REALIZING THAT HE HAD LEFT A SELF-INCRIMINATING VOICE-mail with the feds, Larry Lytle continued trying to hold the government at arm's length while selling exorbitantly priced lasers to old people with health conditions.

The FDA was eager to address Lytle's One True Cure so that it could move on to the next in an unwieldy and growing queue of fraudulent remedies. And so agents got serious. Their seriousness was apparent because they sent Lytle warning letters full of capitalized letters that Meant Business. A warning letter is a sign that the FDA has gathered evidence of serious violations but it doesn't have the appetite to invest more resources in physical seizures or criminal prosecutions. It's basically the sheriff telling a mob member to go home peacefully so that the sheriff won't have to discharge one of the six remaining bullets in his revolver.

But Lytle didn't want to walk away. By then, he had sold at least twenty thousand devices, reinforcing his self-image as a legitimate businessman with a deep-rooted financial stake. So he decided to show the government that he, too, Meant Business.

He wrote the FDA an earnest letter. The good news was that he agreed to stop selling lasers to the public. The bad news was that, according to Lytle's very Lytle-centric interpretation of the relationship between medical freedom and the law, Americans could spend ten dollars to join private membership associations, or PMAs, in which membership came with the benefit of being able to purchase a laser directly from Lytle. Either consciously or unconsciously using the language of the medical-freedom movement, he wrote that conducting such transactions was the right of American citizens. Because he was selling lasers to PMA members and not the public at large, he said that the FDA had no jurisdiction.

In 2012, when a pair of FDA investigators who very much believed that they did have jurisdiction showed up on Lytle's doorstep, he turned them away, explaining that because of his legal dodge his business was no concern of theirs.

The FDA decided that it could not waste any more time, which means that it spent three more years pursuing the case against Lytle, during which time he continued to sell his One True Cure.

Finally, at the behest of the agency, a federal court in January 2015 issued a preliminary injunction freezing Lytle's entire operation. The Tri-Tech manufacturing facility cut off his supply of lasers. He wasn't allowed to sell a single Q1000. It was a painful time for him, and not just because of the lasers. About a month earlier, Lytle's son and business partner, Kip, whom he had saved from the rushing waters of the 1972 flood, had died of brain cancer.

It seemed like a good time to retire. It seemed like a good time for the FDA to move on.

But he didn't. So it couldn't.

⸪

AT THE TIME OF THE COURT INJUNCTION, LARRY WAS SITTING ON AN inventory of somewhere between six hundred and one thousand lasers, each worth thousands of dollars. That was a lot of money for Larry to walk away from, and why would he? Because a bunch of shortsighted, manxome investigators couldn't see the healing light?

The ruling came down on a Wednesday. The following Tuesday, Lytle talked it over with Ronnie Jr., who by this point had founded Laser Wellness Inc., a Q1000 distributor.

Technically, Ronnie's corporation owed Lytle hundreds of thousands of dollars for lasers he had previously taken on credit. They agreed that he would keep selling, to pay off the debt.

Lytle also brought in Irina Kossovskaia, who had once worked as an eye surgeon in a bleak monolithic hospital in Nizhny Novgorod, a large, frigid city on the banks of Russia's mighty Volga River. At some point, Kossovskaia faced a choice: she could keep cutting into eyeballs in the frozen tundra or shoot for something larger. In Russia, they have a saying: take yourself into your hands.

And so, Kossovskaia left Russia to become a "holistic MD"; she specialized in energy healing devices, regeneration, and age reversal, and was associated with various wellness businesses, including a laser company selling Q1000s.

For Lytle, bringing in Kossovskaia, who had a deep list of contacts within the industry, was critical. Would she take him up on his offer? In Russia, they have a saying: without effort, you won't even pull a fish out of a pond. Kossovskaia was in.

It's hard to imagine someone doing less to comply with a court order than Lytle and his coconspirators did. The court ordered Lytle to stop selling; instead, he gave a list of his distributors to Kossovskaia, who began offering them lasers from Lytle's enormous stockpile.

The court ordered Lytle to refund the money of every customer he'd ever had; instead, he had a contractor call the customers and try to squeeze them for more money, which amounted to a fraudulent debt-collection scheme.

The court ordered Lytle to surrender his remaining lasers; instead, he sent a letter to the FDA, telling them that, two weeks before the court issued its injunction, he had made a personal decision to proactively shut down operations and quickly sold off all the firm's assets.

"There is no inventory of QLaser products," he wrote.

The FDA suspected that Lytle still had some lasers, but—critically—they did not know where the lasers were. Though Lytle told distributors that they were being held in a warehouse in Rapid City, the FDA could find no evidence that such a warehouse existed.

Keeping one step ahead of the FDA, in March Lytle called his investment advisor in Rapid City and asked him how to manipulate his assets in order to evade their seizure. He bought a pair of $50,000 Ram pickups. He worked to open new bank accounts—a local one under the name Old Cap Trust and another offshore account with a bank in Belize.

Lytle bought thousands of $20, half-ounce silver bullion coins commemorating the Battle of the Coral Sea. He also bought sixty-one $200, one ounce gold bullion coins commemorating the same battle. (As an interesting side note, these bullion purchases were likely an example of Lytle falling prey to the same sort of hucksterism that he himself was accused of. In the same way that the internet and conservative media channels were creating a profitable synergy around selling alternative health care, various Fox News personalities were personally profiting by pushing bullion as an investment against the supposedly impending doomsday that would be caused by the collapse of the economy and the government. In some cases, gold was being sold at 300 percent of its true value, often to conservative seniors who trusted those talking heads more than they trusted their bankers.)

Lytle, Ronnie Jr., and Kossovskaia began to secretly move lasers out, and money began to flow in. Though the government could not find the laser stockpile, individual units were turning up in the homes of buyers in Chapel Hill, North Carolina, in Billings, Montana (where Toby McAdam was in his own increasingly tough battle against the FDA)—seemingly everywhere.

Ronnie was also continuing to hold laser-selling "seminars" for small audiences of elderly people. His first check to Lytle, a payment against his debt, was for $32,945. Kossovskaia pressured distributors to buy their Q1000s before the FDA made such sales illegal.

In April, more FDA investigators showed up at Lytle's door, asking a lot of questions about the location of the lasers that Lytle said no longer existed. They found nothing, but once they left, Lytle decided that his mountain of remaining lasers was no longer safe in Rapid City. He convinced a former employee to obtain 537 lasers, with an estimated street value of $4 million, from the secret location where they were stored (which appears to have been the Rapid City home of a Lytle family member). The worker took the lasers on a twenty-two-hour road trip to Buffalo, New York, near Kossovskaia's Canadian base of operations. Several days later, Kossovskaia sent an email to the various distributors, telling them that she had more lasers available for purchase. The FDA was making it difficult for the trio to do business—but not impossible. Since the crackdown, Ronnie Jr. had sold 258 QLasers for $810,244.

Late that summer the FDA showed up to perform yet another inspection of Lytle's facilities. When the agents brought up the missing stockpile of lasers, Lytle gave them an invoice that supposedly documented their liquidation into cash. It was dated January 2, twelve days before the court had issued its injunction. According to the invoice, a final inventory of six hundred QLasers had been sold and shipped to Universal International, a company based in Allahabad, India. Court documents do not name the owner of the company, but Lytle had contacts there who had once conducted human trials of QLasers on people with diabetes.

Lytle also produced a letter, signed by the Allahabad distributor, saying that the distributor had traveled to Rapid City to pick up the lasers and had promptly removed them from the country (and, conveniently, from the reach of the FDA). Also conveniently, there was no shipping record because unknown representatives of Universal International had collected the lasers from the office when no one had been there.

The inspectors left empty-handed. The trio continued to sell Q1000s. Kossovskaia wired $25,380 and then another $28,888 from her company, Mediscen Niagara Inc., to Lytle's Old Cap Trust bank account.

In October a federal judge made the injunction permanent, sparking a fresh round of media interest. Lytle told *BuzzFeed News* that it wasn't about his ability to make money. It was a matter of the American public's right to freedom. "Church members can claim ways to treat diseases within their church," he said. "I don't know why I am the target."

Lytle went to his alma mater, Chadron State College, for the homecoming festivities, where he was honored with the Family Tree Award.

In the 1950s, he'd led the Chadron Eagles basketball team in scoring for two years running, posting 1,093 career points, third best in the college's history. Now he posed for a group picture with his family, his posture erect, white hair flowing like qi into his close-cropped beard to form a continuous snowy mane. He was eighty-one years old. Even then, he could have retired. He had everything.

And still, he pushed for more.

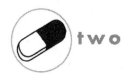 two

TOBY MCADAM'S SUPPLEMENTS SANCTIONED

By medicine life may be prolonged, yet death
Will seize the doctor too.

—William Shakespeare, *Cymbeline*, c. 1611

ONE DAY, TOBY SURPRISED ME BY MENTIONING THAT HE OWED A great debt of gratitude to Elon Musk, hero to libertarian capitalists everywhere.

"I would have to say Elon Musk is probably the one who inspired me," he told me. "If I ever see him again, I will thank him. . . . He's responsible for what I did."

Toby saw himself as a sort of colleague of Musk—a businessman driven by a higher ethic who influenced policies and laws along the way. But Toby was realistic. He didn't have Musk's star power, and he knew that Musk would never give him a meeting. So when the FDA was closing in, he did the next best thing. In the summer of 2013 he found Musk (whose mother, nutritionist Maye Musk, is a spokeswoman for an "antiaging" nutritional supplement that "revitalizes mitochondria") at an economic summit, and he made sure he was among the first in line to address Musk from a microphone set up in the auditorium aisle.

Toby related the conversation to me multiple times, recalling it with what seemed like crystal clarity. Toby explained to Musk about the roadblocks being thrown up by the FDA. "I said, 'How would you do it?'"

Musk's answer gave him hope.

"Elon said, 'Fight it.'"

Toby said that the FDA was making it hard. They were threatening him with consequences for noncompliance and not answering Toby's questions.

"'If they're not going to respond, just keep doing it,'" he remembered Elon telling him.

"I listened to what he said. I respected the guy. I fought it."

Sharing the stage with Musk was Montana senator Max Baucus, a Democrat who had been unhelpful in brokering an agreement between Toby and the FDA. Toby said Baucus tried to interject in the conversation between Toby and Musk, but Toby shut him down.

"I said, 'Oh no. You were part of the problem.'" It was clearly a memory Toby cherished, the public smackdown he had given Senator Baucus.

"In front of the whole crowd. I said, 'You lied.' I got asked to leave the summit."

Toby was happy to leave the summit. He'd gotten what he wanted: validation and inspiration from one of the greatest capitalists in the world.

I wished I had been there to see it myself. So I found video of the exchange on YouTube. It was not what I expected.

•:•

IN THE DARKENED AUDITORIUM, AS A WOMAN FANNED HERSELF WITH A pamphlet, Musk finished a standard keynote address and then fielded a handful of questions. Most questioners were up and down quickly. Musk joked about how he became an entrepreneur: "I guess I'll have to start a company, because I can't get a job anywhere."

As the witticism drew a laugh, Toby approached the microphone, wearing glasses, a shapeless brown hat, and a white V-necked blouse-type shirt that displayed a healthy amount of snowy chest hair. He carried a yellow folder and poked at his nose as he talked.

TOBY: My name's Toby McAdam, I have a company called RisingSun Health. I deal with, uh, government regulations. What do you think of them?

(The audience chuckled.)

TOBY: I've actually been dealing with the FDA, and after talking to Senator Baucus, I've had fifteen attorneys, they spent three and a half million dollars, we're in the middle of a consent decree. . . .

(Toby's voice kept coming in and out of hearing, so someone asked him to get closer to the microphone.)

TOBY: Oh, they have fifteen attorneys, after I talked to Senator Baucus and Senator Tester, they ended up with fifteen attorneys on the FDA. They've signed a consent decree. But government regulation? What do you think of those? Are they too strict? 'Cause, with the FDA, they haven't had a [unintelligible] since 1995, but they keep changing the rules, and right now, in the last three years, more fatalities have been than the previous fifty.

MUSK: Yeah, I think we probably are getting a bit too regulated. You know, um . . .

(Audience chuckled and clapped.)

TOBY: How would you recommend going about it? Because I've tried with Senator Baucus and Senator Tester. And I just keep getting attorneys. I'm suing—I've actually had to file papers against the FDA myself.

MUSK: Right. Well, I dunno. I think generally, with laws and regulations, I think they all ought to come with some sort of a sunset clause . . .

TOBY (interrupting): Do you think they should set standards?

MUSK: . . . because otherwise they just have an independent life.

TOBY: Right. Do you think they should set standards for all companies to follow?

MUSK: I do think there ought to be standards for bodies. I'm not completely libertarian in the sense that "I don't think there should be regulations at all." I just think that the natural bias of regulations is to last forever. [Argues for default sunset clauses.] So, in fact, I think it would generally be a good idea to have it such that it's hard to establish a rule and easy to remove one.

TOBY: What you're saying is that rules should be consistently used to all companies.

MUSK: Well, sure, of course, absolutely, that's fair. Like—

TOBY: Senator Baucus?

MUSK (uncomfortable laughter): Yeah.

TOBY: That's my point. Thank you.

Musk moved on to the next questioner, who wanted to know how Musk was working to solve the health impacts of zero gravity on the human body for the Mars colony.

That was it. Musk had not urged Toby to fight in any sense of the word. Maybe Toby's version of events is correct, and maybe the video of a completely different version of events is correct. There's really no way to tell.

However it went down, Toby exited the economic summit with a firm belief that Musk had told him not to kowtow to the bureaucrats that were closing in on him.

And so, he fought the law. (Spoiler alert: the law won.)

Because he was under a court-ordered consent decree designed to freeze his business operations, his primary method of fighting the law consisted of secretly selling his products to anyone who would buy them. He wasn't just passing a couple of bottles of bloodwort tincture in shady street deals. He sold an estimated sixteen thousand units for $140,000 over the course of a year or two, mostly through online retailers.

Toby's strategy had a couple of glaring weaknesses, the primary one being that some of his secret sales were actually super-secret purchases by agents of the FDA—two bottles of Lugol's Iodine to an undercover FDA employee, followed by a bottle of Bloodroot Immune Support Capsules to a different undercover FDA employee, and, on the same day, another bottle of Lugol's Iodine to yet another agent, all through RisingSun's Amazon storefront.

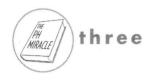 **three**

ROBERT O. YOUNG'S
PH MIRACLE HELPS

> The statements made regarding these products have not been evaluated by the Food and Drug Administration. The efficacy of these products has not been confirmed by FDA-approved research. These products are not intended to diagnose, treat, cure or prevent any disease. All information presented here is not meant as a substitute for or alternative to information from healthcare practitioners. Please consult your healthcare professional about potential interactions or other possible complications before using any product. The Federal Food, Drug, and Cosmetic Act requires this notice.
>
> —Robert Young, on his website

"WHEN I FIRST GOT DIAGNOSED, I DIDN'T WANT TO DO THE conventional route."

Dawn Kali appeared vibrant and healthy against the lush green backdrop of the gorgeous pH Miracle Ranch. She was shooting a promotional video for Robert Young about her breast cancer journey. Her long neck, flowing white blouse, and honey-blonde hair spoke to her all-natural, bohemian aesthetic.

"I started researching alternative treatments," she said, "and out of all the alternative treatments I found, Dr. Young's made the most sense to me."

Kali grew up a "powerful, hard-to-manage teenager" in a San Francisco Bay Area community that was down on doctors and heavily into homeopathy. By 2007 she was a single mother juggling three kids (all unvaccinated, per Kali's upbringing), two waitressing jobs (one at a raw-foods restaurant), and a drinking problem. Her doctor, Nima Grissom, told Kali she had an aggressive strain of breast cancer and recommended she seek additional treatment through an oncologist.

This was problematic advice for Kali, whose understanding was that oncologists were the devil. She had never actually met an oncologist before. But she knew their work from stories told by her favorite aunt, who had also been diagnosed with cancer. The aunt had, against her better judgment, submitted to a single round of radiation, and she told Kali that the radiation caused a mass of necrotic tissue to form on her neck. The aunt had been working with alternative practitioners ever since.

It was a potent cautionary tale, and so instead of an oncologist, Kali explored alternative cancer remedies, which led her to pick up a pH Miracle book by Robert Young, who was steadily building his national brand.

Kali began living the pH Miracle lifestyle, starting with an all-liquid diet of vegetable smoothies supplemented by Young's pHour Salts, purified water drops, and some green powders. She got to the point where she was drinking a gallon of juice each day and taking alkaline water and supplements.

In November of 2009 Kali made an effort to sort out her life. She was in her early thirties. She knew that waitressing wasn't going to pay the bills forever. She got a real estate license and rented out half her condo to help make ends meet.

That's when she saw an ad for a weeklong microscopy course, taught by Young at the fabled pH Miracle Ranch. Like Lytle and McAdam, Young had spent years building his One True Cure brand without significant FDA interference, and he was using that freedom to explore all sorts of entry points into his pleomorphism-based beliefs. Teaching microscopy courses—at a cost of $10,000 per student—was proving to be a lucrative facet of the pH Miracle Ranch. Kali thought that with the course under her belt, she could professionally analyze other people's blood and help them through their own battles with cancer.

"I just felt like it was my calling," she said. She borrowed $10,000 to cover the course, left her three kids with their father, and made travel arrangements.

"Sun shining on my face as I meditate," she posted on social media. "Going to meet Dr. Young (who has saved my life) for the first time."

She entered the ranch's wrought-iron gates and sat in a classroom with a handful of other students, nervously awaiting Young's entrance. And suddenly there he was—with the fitness of a former tennis pro, the nonchalant confidence of a person who has performed for the queen of England, and the brilliant vocabulary of one of the world's foremost research scientists.

I kid, but to Kali it was a frabjous moment.

"I teared up," she said. "I thought he was like my dead father and Jesus Christ in one. Like my savior."

During the class, Young taught her Antoine Béchamp's terrain theory—that all sicknesses were the result of overacidification of the blood and tissue. One of his favorite metaphors involved a hypothetical ailing goldfish: If you had a sick fish, would you treat it directly, or would you change the water? It was the same for people. Change the body's environment by reducing its acid, and diseases would disappear. Young also told the students that they could buy a darkfield microscope from him, with special components, for $7,000.

Kali returned home with $17,000 in debt, a microscope, and plans to start her own business. But a month later, she felt a small lump in her left breast, which sent her into a downward spiral.

One night, "I'd thrown up," she said. She had bulimia. "And was getting ready to do it again. I was in this horrible place." She sat down and emailed Young "a sad letter."

She reminded him of her participation in the microscopy class and explained her situation. She was four months pregnant with her fourth child, in dire financial straits, and desperately, desperately afraid. When she woke early the next morning, at six a.m., Young's response was in her inbox.

"She was down and out," Young later recalled. "I love helping people. So I made her an offer to come to the ranch, and she could stay there."

Since she couldn't afford to pay Young in cash, he proposed a six-week residential work trade.

For Kali, this was a life preserver. Dr. Robert Young, teacher of classes, grower of hair, triple PhD, and, according to his growing resume, member of the California Farm Bureau (membership number C118341), was welcoming her into his orbit and offering personal treatment.

She couldn't get to Valley Center soon enough.

Young reviewed her lab results and told her she should avoid prenatal vitamins and stick to the low-acid diet more strictly. Although he disputes what exactly he said to Kali, his theory was that if cells were too acidified, the body responded by binding them up and walling them off to protect the rest of the body. Removing a tumor was like picking at a scab. It could disturb the area, allowing the cancer to spread even further. The same logic applied to biopsies—they could just make things worse.

The arrangement worked out very well. After shadowing a patient care worker to learn the ropes, Kali worked hard to please Young, and her sunny disposition and all-natural, Californian lifestyle were a good face for the ranch. She got to know the staff—Dr. Ben Johnson, whose medical license allowed him to administer IVs legally, and general manager June Asisi, who was also being treated by Young for her type 2 diabetes.

Asisi was privy to all the inner workings of the ranch because she sat on the executive committee of Young's corporation, pH Miracle Living, which also included Young, his wife, and attorney John Baird.

Kali, who made a point of making friends, quickly became a familiar face. She soaked up everything Young taught—for example, because negative, uffish thoughts could actually inhibit success, some patients did poorly after falling into the trap of "stinking thinking."

That was just a little phrase Young had come up with. He was always borrowing or coining such terms and working them into his educational materials—stinking thinking, "The New Biology," alkalarianism—to see what might catch on.

Kali's pregnancy made it difficult to stick to the all-liquid diet, but she took her mind off her hunger by reminding herself of the wonderful journey she was on.

"I would sit in the sauna at the ranch, reading alternative cancer treatment books, and come away thinking, 'Yes, I'm going to be the poster child and show them.'"

She also got to see different sides of Young's personality. In some ways, he seemed to love the trappings of status—he enjoyed having matching watches and matching shoes and driving his Mercedes. But he could also be relaxed, showing up in a T-shirt, shorts, and sneakers to lead an exercise class or playing tennis on the courts with his kids. He was charming and funny in a goofy way that she found to be utterly disarming.

During the morning exercise classes, which included a round of "Younga Yoga" (another Youngism) for anywhere between three and ten participants, he would sometimes be playful, making faces and dancing to the background music with exaggerated motions.

"I have these fond memories. There was this one night, I forget where it was, but we went to a bar and he did a karaoke. He couldn't wait to get up there." Kali said he chose David Guetta's "Sexy Bitch" and hammed it up to great applause. "He's a performer. He got up there and he did a great job."

His conversations with Kali were, according to her, often laced with jokes, amounting to what she saw as a sort of ineffective, low-grade flirting. He had a thing for pregnant women and she was sexy, ho ho. She was his girlfriend, pregnant with his child, ha ha.

She kept it friendly without letting it go there. She joked back. His wife would kill her, har dee har har.

But really, it didn't make her fearful.

"He was a Mormon, with this wholesome feel about him, even at his worst," she later said. Youthful hair notwithstanding, he was significantly out of her ideal dating age range. "He had this kind of church-boy wholesome purity about him. He wasn't a ladies' man. He didn't have a smooth way about him."

But the awkwardness of it left her disappointed.

"I was sad, in fact. Because I wanted him to be more like a daddy to me," she later said, scoffing at her own naivete. "My dad died when I was thirty. Not too long before this happened."

And if she was being honest, the attention from her idol made her feel special. And led to perks.

"I felt like I could get away with more from him," she said. If there was a pH Miracle event that piqued her interest, she would say, "I think I should go," and he almost always said yes. He took her to group cleanses and even on a wellness retreat to Thailand.

One day, Young fired the guy who handled the ranch's incoming emails.

"I could do that," Kali told Young. And "within an hour I was in the office, getting hired. That's when my career took off there. I was getting a commission on sales. I was doing well, selling something I believed in."

She made $80,000 that year, more than she'd ever made in her life. And the ongoing treatment advice from Young was an equally valuable benefit. He paid for Kali to undergo lab work, including ultrasounds, thermography, and blood counts. Each time, she had the lab send the results to Young, and he would review them with her.

When Kali saw Dr. Grissom, the surgeon expressed concern for her health, but Young and Kali's aunt had prepared her for this. Of course the doctors were going to try to scare her. Doctors knew nothing about disease—the entire medical system was ignorant of the alkaline diet, and the alkaline diet was everything.

When she went to Grissom's office, she would take her aunt along. Together, they peppered Grissom with questions. Doesn't chemo cause cancer? Doesn't radiation cause cancer? Doesn't doing any sort of imaging cause cancer?

The surgeon didn't know what to say.

Young eventually invited Kali to give glowing testimonials on camera.

"Cancer cannot survive in an oxygenated environment with a high pH," she told his audience. "I left my cancerous tumor in my body, which was supposedly classified as aggressive, and left it alone."

She echoed Young's teachings.

"As Dr. Young says, when the fish gets sick, do you treat the fish, or do you change the water? I changed the water and maintained a healthy pH, and my body remained in balance."

There were other patients at the ranch, many faithfully battling their own cancers with the alkaline diet.

There was the unforgettably named Genia Vanderhaeghen of West Perth, Australia, a woman in her sixties who arrived in December 2012 with a whole clan of Vanderhaeghens—her husband, Maurice (an engineering consultant for the oil and gas industries), her two daughters, her sister, and her son-in-law, all on the program and paying for their stay. Genia had metastatic pancreatic cancer and an expected life span of two weeks. In addition to the standard IVs, juice, and pureed food designed to bring her acid levels down, she was receiving colon hydrotherapy and lymphatic massages to flush and work the existing acid out of her body.

One day, Kali saw Dan Barkin, a Las Vegas man in his late sixties, through a window. She knew he'd been there for months, spending every dollar he possessed on everything the ranch had to offer—specially prepared food, colon hydrotherapy, light therapy, nutritional therapy, colonic therapy, lymphatic massages, and lymphatic drainage. The exercise classes for the day had ended, but Kali saw Barkin out there alone, jumping on a trampoline, over and over, clearly gassed but not giving up. He did it all the time. Something about it just seemed so brave.

It made Kali realize that those who were coming to the ranch were betting something much more precious than their money on the pH Miracle. They were betting their time, which in many cases was a scarce commodity. For most, days spent at the ranch were days lost with family. The ranch, Kali saw, could be lonely.

She was reminded of this again during a chance encounter with another patient, Naima Houder-Mohammed, a captain in the British military with advanced breast cancer.

"I met Naima briefly. It was sad," Kali said. "She was alone on the property just wandering around. She looked very sad to me."

Genia Vanderhaeghen outlived her two-week prognosis, but the aggressive treatments failed to fully restore her health. She lingered for three weeks, four, five. Then she asked Young to join the Vanderhaeghens at a family meeting on the ranch. She had chosen to discontinue the program and stop eating. She and Maurice asked Young if it would be okay for her to die at the ranch.

"And I had a hard struggle with that," Young later said. "But, you know, Maurice became a friend. His wife became friends. And how could I refuse her request that she wanted to pass quietly and peacefully at the ranch. . . . So, you know, they made a choice. And I agreed to allow her to continue and pass there on the ranch."

In January 2013, nearly two months after her arrival, his friend Genia Vanderhaeghen died, never to be forgotten.

⁘

THOUGH KALI WAS EARNING A LOT OF MONEY AND THE YOUNGS WERE taking in millions a year, she began to worry about the financial viability of the Miracle Ranch.

The property itself—the avocado farm and the palm trees and the bougainvillea and the grapefruit trees—was "absolutely stunning." But Kali grew increasingly puzzled at the little signs of budgetary constraints and decay. The car dedicated to picking up patients from the airport—patients paying up to $5,000 a day—was kind of beaten up. They gathered to eat breakfast in a garage with few frills.

Kali said the ranch was split between managers who wanted to do everything by the book and those who would indulge Young's more free-wheeling way of doing things. Baird, the lawyer, repeatedly stressed that only Dr. Johnson should administer IVs. Asisi, who managed day-to-day finances, asked people not to give Young cash. But to others on staff, Young could do no wrong.

"He considered himself, and he still does, the biggest research scientist in the world," Kali said. "He would say it all the time. 'I'm a research scientist.' His science was going to be groundbreaking. You were a pioneer in this new biology. You felt lucky to be next to him."

The money issue came home to Kali in 2012.

Young and his wife took Kali and another worker to set up a pH Miracle booth at the Health Freedom Expo, which took place in a suburb of Chicago at the Renaissance Schaumburg Hotel. There were booths from two hundred alternative practitioners, each representing one or more people eager to sign on to the idea of medical freedom.

"It's about how our health freedoms are being taken away, and it's about exposing the truth," said Kevin Trudeau, one of the expo's featured speakers and an "honored recipient of the Health Freedom Expo Hall of Fame award." Trudeau was billed as a consumer advocate, but in fact he was a consumer predator. He had thirty-two thousand infomercials under his belt and was en route to declaring bankruptcy because of a $37 million judgment against him for misinformation contained in his book, *Natural Cures "They" Don't Want You to Know About.*

Young and his wife were both also featured speakers. In the promotional information, his bio billed him as "widely recognized as one of the top research scientists in the world," while her credentials ended with "and, yes, she is the sister of actor, director and founder of Sundance, Robert Redford."

Kali and her coworker did the heavy work—lugging boxes of supplements and promotional materials to the booth and then staffing it for the three-day event. It was rough on Kali's back, which was spasming painfully.

She had done other expos for Young before and had an idea of what to expect. They sold supplements and signed up coaches and received a percentage commission. She estimated that she and her coworker would earn about $800 each.

But, conspicuously, there had been no mention of payment. At the end of the event, they asked Young to stop by their hotel room to discuss the finances. Kali's coworker asked when she would be paid. That was when Kali saw yet another side of Young.

"He tore her apart," Kali said.

He told them that no one was being paid for the Chicago event and that they were lucky to be there. He called them ungrateful and said they were being greedy. Kali's coworker, he said, was too overweight to represent the lifestyle.

"'You're not a good look for this place,'" he said, according to Kali. "He was just seething. He was just yelling at her."

Kali was worried. She was worried about her relationship with Young. She was worried about the financial viability of the Miracle Ranch. She was worried about how that could impact her own finances.

But what she should have been worried about were the painful spasms in her back.

.∴.

ONE JANUARY MORNING IN 2014, YOUNG WAS RUNNING AN EXERCISE CLASS, IVs were being prepared, and the kitchen was churning out a steady stream of alkalizing smoothies.

Suddenly, four men wearing bulletproof vests and bearing AK-47s barged into the gym. Outside, two helicopters hovered over the compound, providing air support to a group of roughly forty law enforcement officers led by the US Marshals' San Diego Fugitive Task Force. Every entrance was blocked.

It didn't feel like real life. "Am I in a movie? This was surreal," said Young. "Let's see. What are we doing? Teaching people how to eat, how to live, how to exercise."

It was ridiculous. Young was a teacher. A research scientist. A recognized avocado grower certified by the California Avocado Commission. And here were a bunch of government thugs, acting like they were storming a drug kingpin's compound. They ransacked the ranch. They took his computers, his printers, his files.

The argument against the alkaline diet is essentially that it does not work—the body's mechanism for regulating alkaline and acidic substances, namely absorbing them into the bladder and pissing them out, prevents your diet from having much of an impact at all.

But still, there was little sense that Young's theories posed any urgent threat to society. The bulk of Young's advice—eating a healthy vegetable-based diet and getting plenty of exercise—is universally acknowledged as beneficial. Even the one time he'd been arrested in Utah, back in 1995, his case wasn't treated seriously. He'd pled to a misdemeanor, paid a thirty-dollar fine, and walked free.

Not this time.

"My poor son was handcuffed, as if he had done something wrong," Young later recounted angrily. "He was totally naked when they arrested him."

After the arrest, Investigator James Clark of the San Diego District Attorney's office reached out to Kali and asked if she had any knowledge of Young crossing the legal line. Had Young offered her not lifestyle advice but medical advice? Had he personally given her any IVs?

She told Clark that she wished she could help, but she hadn't seen anything like that. The only medical care she had received or witnessed had been legally performed by Dr. Johnson, the member of the ranch staff who had a medical license.

She was lying.

.•:

YOUNG WAS CHARGED WITH SEVEN COUNTS OF PRACTICING MEDICINE without a license and two counts of grand theft. He initially pled not guilty but eventually struck a deal in which he agreed to go to jail for several months for unlawfully diagnosing and treating four people, including Dan Barkin and Genia Vanderhaeghen.

As part of the deal, the prosecutor insisted on a specific condition: Young had to make a public declaration, which he read aloud in court.

"I, Robert O. Young, declare freely and voluntarily, under penalty of perjury that: I do not have any post high school educational degrees from any accredited schools. I am not a microbiologist. I am not a hematologist. I am not a medical doctor. I am not a naturopathic doctor. I am not a trained scientist."

That hurt.

He was incarcerated for five months at the East Mesa Reentry Facility. He was served with divorce papers from Shelley Redford Young, perhaps a delayed reaction to the fact that Young had fathered a child by another woman in 2010. He was relegated to the bottom bunk of his cell, which didn't even have a window. It was a low time.

"The first three months, I never even saw the sun," said Young.

But he was determined not to let it break him. He believed in himself. Somewhere out there was a truckful of bottlefuls of great, and he knew he could find his way back behind the steering wheel.

"Life can either make you bitter or it can make you better," he said.

And there was one thing that made prison a bit more bearable. Something about the other inmates that he would remember, years after his release, with something approaching fondness.

"They called me Doc," he said.

The ranch's medical professional, Ben Johnson, was stripped of his license by the California state medical board and ordered to pay $20,000, some of which went to reimburse the office of Attorney General (and future vice president) Kamala Harris for the cost of prosecution.

Young suspected he was being targeted in an expression of Big Pharma's efforts to stifle the pH Miracle. And so, as soon as he got out of prison, after a three-week trip to Spain to clear his head, he took some steps to protect himself.

He put the ranch into the name of a trust, headed by his son Adam, with himself named as one of the beneficiaries. He shuttered pH Miracle Life and started a new company, pHorever Young, that continued to sell supplements out of the ranch warehouse. Another new corporation, PHM Life, was run and owned by his daughter's husband, Matthew Lisonvee. Young got 10 percent of the gross sales.

These measures were implemented none too soon. Because very quickly, in December of 2015, he was sued in a San Diego court for an obscene amount of money by someone who accused him of perpetrating an obscene amount of harm. The person alleged fraud and negligence and said Young should pay compensatory and punitive damages.

It was Dawn Kali.

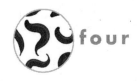four

ALICJA KOLYSZKO'S LEECHES SUCK

"Wounded? A fiddle-stick's end!" said the doctor. "No more wounded than you or I. The man has had a stroke, as I warned him. Now, Mrs. Hawkins, just you run upstairs to your husband and tell him, if possible, nothing about it. For my part, I must do my best to save this fellow's trebly worthless life; Jim, you get me a basin. . . . And now, Master Billy Bones, if that be your name, we'll have a look at the colour of your blood. Jim," he said, "are you afraid of blood?"

"No, sir," said I.

"Well, then," said he, "you hold the basin"; and with that he took his lancet and opened a vein.

A great deal of blood was taken before the captain opened his eyes and looked mistily about him.

—Robert Louis Stevenson, *Treasure Island*, 1883

THE LEECH QUEENPIN SAT OVER AN EMPTY PLATE IN THE BALEEN restaurant, holding court as servers slid in and out of her orbit with the perfect balance of deference and quiet dignity. They perhaps sensed her greatness, without understanding that said greatness sprung from bloodsucking parasites.

Maybe that was for the better.

There are people, Alicja told me pityingly, who know nothing about leeches.

Alicja herself can talk leech trivia all day. She will give you precise details about their anatomy, from teeth to testes. A group of leeches is called, collectively, a slither. Their behavior in the wild is strangely tender—as hermaphrodites, any two leeches can breed; in some species, the parents make little nests out of leech moss, lay eggs, and help their tiny baby leeches feed for the first time by opening a wound in a prey animal.

She also has an encyclopedic knowledge of all the players in the leech market, not just in the United States but globally. Alicja tracks the scientific literature, taking note whenever a new study weighs in on hirudin—the anticoagulant present in leeches' salivary glands—or identifies yet another chemical compound in those extraordinarily complex organs. Though more research isn't needed to do what she does, she sees the information as helpful to her ultimate goal of gaining widespread public acknowledgment.

"The benefits for the human body are immense. However, you know nothing can be implemented without research—whether false or true but accepted," she said.

Alicja doesn't doubt that the government, working on behalf of Big Pharma, has persecuted alternative healers of various disciplines. But she isn't talking about the other modalities I am writing about.

"I'm not talking about the other modalities you are writing about," she told me. "I am speaking of hirudotherapy."

She believes that, as the One True Cure, hirudotherapy is in a class of its own.

"For Big Pharma, we are the biggest enemy," she said. "Think about it."

Alicja herself is so far inside the leech bubble that a lack of even basic knowledge on leeching is kind of unfathomable. But leech ignoramuses are at least harmless. Much more dangerous are those who try to capitalize on the amazing power of the leech to heal, without really understanding what the hell they are doing.

In this category, Alicja includes the United States government. It turns out that, even as other fly-by-night One True Cures were being shunted en masse into the FDA's enforcement wing, advocates of the original One True Cure were knocking on the door of the FDA's regulatory division, crowing like the crowd and asking to be included as part of the evidence-based regimen of medical practices.

To understand why, we have to dip once more into the bloody history of the Victorian medicinal leech craze brought about by people like French military hospital administrator François-Joseph-Victor Broussais.

.•∴

WHEN HUMANS BEGAN TO RAPIDLY DEPLETE WILD STOCKS OF LEECHES, A new industry was born: leech farming.

As with the similarly questionable art of cat skinning, there was more than one way to grow a leech. Some people raised them in large holding tanks, rather like the $400 million salmon farm built in the 2010s on an old tomato field in Homestead, Florida. Others walled off portions of existing leech-laden marshes and tried to harvest them sustainably. Still others stocked ponds with thousands of leeches, hoping they wouldn't misbehave.

Sometimes the leeches misbehaved.

In one notable case in the late 1800s, a local newspaper reported that a group of people woke up in the middle of the night in their low-rent Californian tenement building, only to find that a disquietingly large slither of leeches had escaped from a neighboring leech farm and into their beds.

Nowhere in the world was the leech-growing business more vibrant than in France, and nowhere in France was it more vibrant than in the Bay of Arcachon, on the edge of the Celtic Sea, where huge populations of leeches were kept in meres, or lakes.

To feed the leeches, livestock were driven into the shallows and then allowed to leave when the leech farmer judged that the animals could stand to be drained of no more blood.

For a time, there was a significant debate over what sort of livestock was best used to feed the leeches: horse, ass, or cow? Each was a viable option; horses had the upside of bearing the cheapest sticker price, but the others also had virtues that could be talked out. Of one's ass, the upside was unmatched endurance, but as was noted in a contemporary journal, "when at length it falls into the water under the storm of its numerous enemies, it becomes mad with terror." And of the docile cows it could be said they had an end-use value: beef for human consumption.

Ultimately it was a matter of taste. Like asses, or dislike them in general, it was clear that when it came to leeching, they were too volatile, often kicking. Asses, many leech farmers concluded, were just not working. Asses off the menu, these leech farmers were left to choose between horses and cows. When it became clear that horses "wear out too soon—the veins opened by the leeches did not heal; and so the life's blood could not be renewed," most settled on cows.

As the journal noted:

Now, the cow has to do duty as nurse to the young annelides. Frightened, haggard, but resigned, the animal submits, with a stupid kind of astonishment, to the attacks of clusters of leeches hanging on her legs; and when the moment of utter exhaustion comes she is sent off to her pastures to renew life, and furnish a fresh repast. Two weeks suffice for each process, alternately carried on, until death puts an end to being eaten in detail. The owner of about eight acres of marsh supplies yearly two hundred cows for the nourishment of eight hundred thousand leeches: he buys the animal for about two pounds and sells the carcass for 16 shillings.

While that was the dominant viewpoint, I am compelled to note that cow use was not universal, and some farmers stuck with the ass. It was simply a matter of corralling it tightly, covering the ass with leeches, and afterward being sure to take the animal to pasture and watch the ass munch contentedly on grass until it was, once again, a fat ass.

The Arcachon Bay region, which exported 1.5 million leeches annually to Bordeaux alone, had an economy that was very leech dependent. But when global trade collapsed, doctors turned elsewhere, and farms began to go bust.

Some leech farmers persevered, but after more than a hundred years of decline, by the 1980s anyone who wanted a fabled Arcachon Bay leech had just one place to turn—Jacques Desbarax, the last leech farmer, who had survived in part by shifting to low-cost man-made breeding tanks. But business wasn't very good, and Desbarax was getting older, with no heir apparent to carry on the mantle.

To solve that problem, one day he bought a stuffed animal. He took that stuffed animal (I'm not sure what it was, but almost certainly not a leech) to a dinner he had arranged at the home of an old friend, a biologist. Desbarax knew that the biologist's daughter, Brigitte Latrille, would be there.

To many in France, Latrille was a hero. She was a four-time Olympian fencing champion, a smooth terror with the foil who, under the bloodless swordfighting allowed by the International Olympic Committee, left her foes in theoretical tatters.

Desbarax presented the stuffed animal to Latrille, whose best swordfighting days were by then behind her. She was a thirty-three-year-old single mother who was burned out at her job at Air France. Desbarax told her the toy was a present for her son, three-year-old Hector. Then he smoothly asked her if she wanted to come see his leeches.

This was not a come-on. It was a business proposition, and when Latrille did go to see his leeches, she saw promise in the broken-down relic of a farm that relied on a trickle of orders from around the world. In 1992, she bought it and renamed it Ricarimpex, which signaled her intention to brand her leeches as a modern medical product, on par with the pills and injections promoted by Big Pharma.

One of the long-term customers that Latrille inherited from Desbarax was a medical supply shop in New York City run by a scrappy Holocaust survivor and serial entrepreneur named Rudy Rosenberg. Rosenberg moved about a thousand leeches a month, mostly to small-scale traditional healers from Eastern Europe. In the late 1990s, Rosenberg enlisted Latrille in his biggest (and possibly dumbest-sounding) entrepreneurial scheme yet: if they could convince the FDA that leeches were a valid medical treatment, their inventory of leeches would skyrocket in value. It was, essentially, an exercise in capitalism. As the once-mighty leech industry crumbled, it left behind vestiges, people whose financial interests were still tied to a supply of a little-used product and who needed to stimulate demand or face economic extinction.

Rosenberg and Latrille submitted a formal request asking the FDA to sanction the use of leeches in medicine. The idea was absurd. No one had ever suggested that an animal should play this sort of role in health care.

Surely at least one FDA administrator upon whose desk the leech proposal landed wanted very much to laugh it off. But this was the FDA.

Though the *Operations Manual* doesn't explicitly forbid laughing, there is a sense it is very much frowned upon.

And so, agents at the FDA gritted their teeth and gave the formal request formal consideration.

But which department should field the matter? Were leeches a biological product, like vaccines and donor blood? Or were they medical devices, like stents and stethoscopes?

This question of jurisdiction occupied them for weeks. Committees were formed. Phrases were parsed. Papers were written. Precedents were searched for, and definitions were analyzed. Finally, a decision came down from Mark Melkerson, acting director of the Division of General, Restorative and Neurological Devices.

"The eating of blood" is how Melkerson characterized what a leech does. "Those are mechanical processes."

Therefore, the agency began to process the application as though leeches were, like lasers, medical devices. They essentially viewed them as little machines that ran on blood instead of electricity.

The FDA initiated an extensive review of the usage of leeches in medicine. They found the expected standard body of academic research that exists around any perennial quirky treatment: documentations of the historical use of leeches, mostly in other countries (as when Andrea Bocelli, the famous Italian opera singer, underwent a leech treatment on his eyeballs that he hoped would restore his sight, which it didn't).

However, quite unexpectedly, they also found something else: a case study by Dr. Joseph Upton, a well-respected doctor from Boston Children's Hospital who became familiar with the use of leeches while serving as a surgeon overseas in the Vietnam War. Back in the states, Upton used leeches to treat a child whose ear had been bitten off by a dog. Upton reported that he was able to reattach the ear thanks to the leeches, which he said promoted healthy blood flow by secreting an anticoagulant—hirudin—and sucking blood.

Upton was not alone. Leech use was exceedingly rare, and yet there were a handful of well-respected practitioners who for one reason or another reported success using leeches in a modern medical setting. These weren't quacky fringe healers. They were establishment practitioners. The university trained. The Numbers Junkies.

In Asheville, North Carolina, a doctor used a leech to assist in reattaching a thumb that had been blown off the hand of a seventeen-year-old boy by a firecracker. Leeches helped in a case where a Virginia man lost his ring finger in a freak accident involving a homemade pull-up bar. They also helped in the case of an Ohio cancer patient who was having her nose reattached. Leeches had even played an oft-overlooked role in one of the most scandalous surgeries of the day. Following the infamous involuntary penectomy of John Wayne Bobbitt at the hands of his abused wife, surgeons reportedly had leeches on standby in the procedure to reattach Bobbitt's penis.

The more the FDA bureaucrats looked at the evidence, the more difficult it became to ignore the facts: when it came to promoting blood flow into areas that needed oxygenation, leeches were uniquely delicate, and therefore, as Alicja asserted, a totally superior modality to anything on the market.

And so, in 2004, the FDA made a stunning announcement. A species of leech—*Hirudo medicinalis*—was the first biological organism to be approved as a medical device.

"Sheesh," commented one wag on a panel of FDA observers. "The FDA's reputation for incompetence remains intact."

As a result, a little-known feature of many modern hospitals is a leech tank squirreled away in the basement; for reasons of squeamishness, the tanks are often spoken of only on a need-to-know basis. And with no leech farms in the US, many of those leeches come from Latrille, who, as one of the only authorized providers of medical-device leeches, was soon selling eighty thousand leeches a year to the United States, many of them through Rosenberg.

.•∴

THE FDA RULING UPENDED THE WORLD OF MEDICINAL LEECHING, AND IN some ways that benefited Alicja. The leech was gaining legitimacy, and Alicja got work as a consultant for various hospitals that wanted to know how to manage a medical device that could have a bowel movement.

But the FDA ruling was also a frustration.

It had approved a single, extremely narrow use for the leech, but Alicja believed that leeches were the One True Cure, good for treating inflammation of all sorts, disorders of the blood and heart, and even terminal illnesses like cancer and diabetes. And it could be done gently, without resorting to an invasive surgical procedure of the sort that hospitals sometimes use leeches for.

She and a colleague took another leech-based proposal to the FDA: they sought to prove that medicinal leeches could treat diabetic neuropathy. There were conversations and presentations, but when the logistics and costs of the required medical trials emerged, it was clear the strategy would never work.

Even when she served as a consultant, she said, the culture gap led to frustration.

"They won't follow my direction because they have no idea about noninvasive hirudotherapy," she said. "They don't know anything about it. They only know about invasive hirudotherapy. They don't understand the concept."

How to explain to the FDA that the unique combination of all the hundreds of chemical compounds in leech spit, including some that are likely undiscovered, will produce good health?

"And for that you have to present to the FDA. How many diseases do we have? Do you have to prove every single one?" she asked, scornful. "It's like trying to build artificial leeches. It's millions of dollars for this nonsense. You cannot copy nature."

This underscores a fundamental disconnect between evidence-based science as administered by the FDA and One True Cures. The scientific establishment has, through thousands of studies conducted over hundreds of years, moved inexorably away from the idea of systemic ills and their corresponding silver-bullet systemic cures. As evidence has mounted, the idea of using a single treatment method to restore the balance of bodily humors, or qi, or acid levels, or spiritual absolution to achieve a state of perfect health yielded to the recognition of the human organism as prone to a collection of discrete, diverse symptoms that require discrete and diverse methods of treatment. Data has broken people down into assemblages of flawed objects—strained tendons, inflamed corneas, septic blood—that can be repaired or replaced to alleviate problems.

The FDA's approval of leeches was not an abandonment of its allegiance to evidence-based medicine; it was, rather, an unprecedented effort to pound a squishy round peg into a rigid square hole. So it's not surprising that ever since authorizing leeches the FDA has struggled to coexist with the chaos inherent in a biological organism, which is not sterile and cannot be precision engineered. Introducing wild animals into surgical settings led to all sorts of problems. It was like Jurassic Park, but there was no Jeff Goldblum, and also the people who got eaten were, at the end of the day, fine.

Leeches squirmed uninvited into body cavities to feed in peace. They sometimes developed resistance to antibiotics and conferred it back to the patient. And some became vectors for things like harmful bacteria.

In one case, a five-year-old boy whose left middle finger was hanging on by a stretchy bit of tendon (due to a sliding-door injury) was aided by a single leech, which fed near the nail bed for twenty minutes. Afterward, the little boy's finger bled unabated for fifteen hours, and he needed an infusion to stay alive. (The boy eventually lost the finger.) Doctors warned that the rare case of "profound, ongoing, life-threatening bleeding after a single leech application" was a reason to carefully monitor leech patients, particularly children.

After the FDA approved *H. medicinalis* as a medical device, researchers uncovered a massive taxonomic error. It turned out that the leeches everyone in America was using in surgery were not *H. medicinalis* at all. They were of a closely related species, *H. verbana*. This meant that the leeches in hospitals weren't legal, and the leeches that were legal weren't in hospitals.

The FDA has stood by its decision, troubleshooting as quickly as trouble can be shot. But all these problems underscored the fundamental cultural breach between the medical establishment and practitioners of alternative treatment. As a result Alicja sees the FDA primarily as leech meddlers, using their little bit of narrow knowledge to muddy the waters of a One True Cure. She is confident that over time her truth will out.

"It is spreading, mouth to mouth," she told me. "We are totally on the verge right now."

But the FDA is only one example of leech bobbling.

The resurgence in leech use generated by the FDA helped Alicja build her business, but it also buoyed those whose leech-based businesses are less scrupulously run. Alicja said that in addition to scoffing at the FDA, she's battling the seedy underbelly of leechdom: the leech underground.

five

THE NEUMANNS' PRAYERS RAISED

DOCTOR: Foul whisp'rings are abroad. Unnatural deeds
Do breed unnatural troubles: infected minds
To their deaf pillows will discharge their secrets.
More needs she the divine than the physician.
God, God, forgive us all!

—William Shakespeare, *Macbeth*, 1623

LEILANI.

Dale.

She mothered. He fathered.

She prayed fervently. He preached passionately. Faith cured her anxiety. God healed his back. She worried about her youngest. He, too, noted Kara's listlessness.

Leilani said Kara was eating less; Dale saw her drinking more water. Leilani thought it might be puberty's onset; he remembered Ariel had exhibited similar symptoms. As a Pentecostal, Leilani believed demons caused sickness; Dale agreed prayer could drive the demons out. On Good Friday, Leilani closed the cafe at six; Dale headed home with a McDonald's dinner for Kara. Leilani found Kara wearily doing homework at the kitchen table, where Dale fed her a McChicken sandwich and half a milkshake.

Together, they decided they would pray for their eleven-year-old daughter, who had the March flu, or a demon.

Many parents would have seen Kara's tiredness as a nagging late-winter flu, brought on by that year's (it was 2008) persistently cold and dry February and March; there had only been a few days above freezing since the previous fall. Dale and Leilani had a lot else going on to occupy their minds. The dissolution of the partnership with the Wormgoors disquieted Leilani and set back their plans for a ministry. Happier news came from California: Leilani's younger brother had just gotten married to a woman named Ariel Neff. It was fun that their kids would have an Aunt Ariel who was, at eighteen, just a few years older than their Ariel.

On Saturday morning, the day before Easter, Kara woke up, thirsty and ready to go to Monkey Mo. But she still didn't look quite right. Kara admitted she still felt tired, so Leilani told her to stay home with Dale, who was working on the family's taxes.

When Dale took a break from the paperwork, he thought Kara looked off.

"Are you okay?" he asked.

"'Just tired,'" she said.

He told her that she could rest in her parents' bed. She went to lie down.

When Leilani came home from Monkey Mo around four p.m., as soon as she touched the doorknob of the family home, a foreboding jolted her. "The spirit of death," she felt, was inside the house.

Frightened, she ran upstairs to where Kara's form lay, motionless, in the master bedroom. Leilani touched Kara's arm apprehensively and was relieved to feel the warmth of her daughter's skin. But Kara was shockingly worse off. She was extremely weak and pale; her breathing was labored; her legs were skinny, blue, and cold.

Leilani swung into action—it was now clear that, for some unknown reason, her daughter was under some sort of spiritual attack. She and Dale began to pray fervently, with Leilani massaging warmth into Kara's legs. Kara said she wasn't hungry, so Leilani brought her a glass of water and made her a smoothie, which Kara consumed.

Because the Neumanns' personal prayers to God had not healed Kara, they decided to bring in the big guns: agreement in prayer.

Agreement in prayer is a shorthand nod to a biblical verse in which the faithful are told that if two or more people ask for something, it will happen. The common understanding among Pentecostals is that the more people who come together, the more powerful the prayer.

Leilani began to work the phones, calling relatives and Bible study members—but not the Wormgoors, not after their falling out. She phoned Carolyn Neuen, Lynn Wilde, and Dan and Jennifer Peaslee.

Dale's mother, Elvera, said it sounded like the flu; Leilani's father, Leo Gomez, and her new sister-in-law, Ariel, promised to lend their prayers. So did Evalani, Leilani's mother.

Dale sent a mass email out to ubmadmin@americaslastdays.com, a LISTSERV run by the Pentecostal group Unleavened Bread Ministries. "We need agreement in prayer over our youngest daughter, who is very weak and pale at the moment with hardly any strength," he wrote.

One UBM member replied by thanking God for giving "Dale and Leilani the faith to hold fast." The member commanded "that spirit of infir-mity to loose Kara now, leave her body, leave her home, and go back from where it came and stay there."

Dale and Leilani asked that the message be forwarded to UBM preacher David Eells. He was known for mixing his fringe religious ideas with his hyperconservative politics. Just a year before, he'd promoted a dream by one of his followers that Hillary Clinton was pregnant with "a long, green gangly alien/demon-looking creature growing inside." Eells also subscribed to various conspiracy theories, including the idea that Big Pharma and the medical establishment were in cahoots with the government to hurt the American public. He saw evidence of this in deeply aberrant behavior by disturbed individuals, like a 1991 case, reported by the *Los Angeles Times*, of a sixty-one-year-old woman who attacked her eighty-seven-year-old mother by biting her at least twenty times on the face and arms, in some cases chewing down to the bone, until the daughter's nightgown was soaked with blood. On his website, Eells blamed Big Pharma, though he did not yet have a complete theory of the case.

Despite his eccentricities, Eells was unquestionably true to his faith. He, his wife, and his five children had also eschewed doctors for God, who had cured their every ill, including bone fractures.

Family members called more family members. Word spread. Prayers joined prayers, a huge invisible network that wrapped young Kara in warm intentions. The Neumanns hoped that powerful prayers from Eells could put them over the top.

.•.:

WHAT WAS ACTUALLY HAPPENING INSIDE KARA'S BODY WAS SOMETHING much worse than a cold and much more physical than a demon.

The human body produces the hormone insulin, which is needed so the body can effectively absorb sugar into muscles and other tissues. This is the process that fuels us with energy. Kara's body was not producing enough insulin because she had diabetes. That meant she wasn't able to tap into the sugar in her system as an energy source, which explained some of her tiredness.

The body has a backup strategy for periods when it can't access those energy-providing sugars. It releases other hormones that break down the body's fat and uses it as fuel instead. This produces a series of by-products that are collectively known as ketone bodies, or ketones.

A whole raft of fad weight-loss plans, such as the Atkins Diet, chase this fat-burning process, a state that is referred to as being "in ketosis." Because of the lack of sufficient insulin being produced by Kara's body, she was in a form of ketosis called diabetic ketoacidosis. She had been for weeks, possibly even months.

Robert Young, with his pH Miracle Diet, suggests that acid in the body is the cause of all ills. That's not true. But in Kara's case, her blood was so saturated with acidic ketones that the buildup of acid was a real danger. Left untreated, ketoacidosis can cause someone to slip into a coma or even die.

The Neumanns were praying. Science suggests that prayer, like meditation, does indeed afford various beneficial health effects: boosting the immune system and self-esteem, lowering blood pressure and heart rate, and decreasing stress levels.

Though the beneficial effects of prayer and meditation are real, they are often overstated in the literature because of a series of common experiment flaws that can be particularly difficult to iron out of studies of health and prayer. These confounding factors include the unrelated but invariably contiguous benefits of receiving emotional support (which can include an enhanced awareness of symptoms); the random fluctuations in severity of illness that can coincide with prayer; the Hawthorne effect (that people change behavior and self-descriptions because they are being observed, which means that someone might just say they are feeling better); the Rosenthal effect (in which investigators elicit the responses they are looking for); and, of course, the placebo effect, which demonstrates that if a patient believes they are taking medicine, their health can improve, even if they're swallowing only a sugar pill.

But even discounting these problems, the scientific evidence suggests that Kara's diabetic ketoacidosis was exactly the sort of condition that cannot be cured by the positive mental effects of prayer. It would seem impossible for someone's mental state to have significant sway over the high levels of ketones running rampant throughout her body. Absent medical care, only actual divine intervention could cleanse the body of the ketones.

And divine intervention was exactly what the Neumanns were counting on. Their phone rang. It was Eells, responding to their email plea for help. He agreed to pitch in.

"They did not seem overly concerned because they had had healings before. This is not an unusual kind of request to us," Eells would later say. Given his beliefs about Hillary Clinton, he must have had a pretty high bar for what counted as unusual.

Around seven p.m., Dale and Leilani called for a break in the praying. It was getting late, and their other three children—Luke, Hamilton, and Ariel—needed to eat. They left Kara lying in the master bedroom and sat down for dinner.

At some point Ariel got up to use the bathroom and found Kara lying on the bathroom floor, pants around ankles. She had tried to go to the bathroom but had fallen off the toilet.

Dale rushed upstairs, scooping Kara into his arms, and carried her to a couch in the living room, where they could keep an eye on her. She breathed raggedly, as if running an endless race.

"Do you love Jesus?" Leilani asked her.

Kara moved her eyes back and forth and moaned a response.

"She might have said yes. I know for sure she was acknowledging it. What sounds came out, I don't remember," said Leilani. "She was making noises. . . . My focus definitely was to pray."

After midnight, Dale and Leilani finally decided they needed sleep to keep functioning. They would later say they "were exhausted . . . [from the] non-stop praying and just continually trusting in the Lord."

The kids stayed with Kara, who lay limp and unresponsive on the couch, and continued a vigil that consisted of ongoing prayer. Two of them—I'm not sure which two—slept beside her all night, praying until the darkness took them.

.•::

IT WAS FIVE A.M. ON EASTER SUNDAY AND PITCH BLACK OUTSIDE WHEN the kids came in to wake Dale up; he'd gotten only a few hours of sleep. The kids were excited on this day of miracles. They told him that Kara kept kicking the covers off the couch, exhibiting more life than she had shown in the night.

Dale went to check on Kara, who still lay on the sofa. He tried to sit her up, but she couldn't hold herself in a sitting position. When he called her name, she only moaned faintly. But her breathing *did* seem less labored than it had the previous night. Her hands were also much warmer.

"Whatever this is, Lord, it's going to burn out of her," Dale said.

As Dale, and then Leilani, assessed Kara, outside, the first glimmering of sunrise began. Up above the Earth, in the heavens, the night's celestial bodies began to dim.

Someone realized that Kara had peed on herself; Dale carried her upstairs and laid her on the bathroom floor so he and Leilani could give her a quick sponge bath. Her eased breathing gave them some measure of confidence, but they sensed that more work was needed.

Leilani called the Peaslees and Lynn Wilde and asked them to come pray over Kara in person.

On the phone, Leilani's father suggested that she should give Kara Pedialyte; Leilani responded that to do so would take away from the glory of God. However, perhaps as a sort of compromise, Leilani tried to feed her daughter soup and water through a syringe. The liquid just dribbled out of Kara's mouth.

Reinforcements began to show up.

At nine a.m., Lynn Wilde arrived and began praying over Kara. But still, something was missing. Dale and Leilani began to discuss an unpleasant thought.

What if Kara's sickness was the result of their falling out with the Wormgoors? Perhaps God was punishing the sin of pride, or perhaps this crisis was meant to revive the idea of a partnership that would grow into an important ministry.

Leilani didn't want to call Althea and Randall Wormgoor—it was a bitter pill to swallow. But she would do anything for her daughter. And she would do anything for God.

Althea answered the phone, reticent, reserved. Leilani told her that Kara wasn't eating, drinking, or talking and was lying on the floor. Leilani told them her suspicions, that this was God's effort to mend a fence between them. She thought it might be the lack of forgiveness between the two families.

"Will you come over and pray?" asked Leilani.

Althea said they would.

Around eleven thirty, Lynn Wilde and Leilani carried Kara upstairs to the bathroom for another sponge bath. Dale put a futon in a room just off the kitchen for Kara to lie on. When the Peaslees arrived, Jennifer went upstairs and was shocked to see Kara pale, her breathing once again audible and labored.

Downstairs, Dan Peaslee was shaken by Dale's appearance. Passionate orating aside, the aspiring minister was usually in total control of himself. But now he was visibly upset, with red nose and eyes. Dan suspected he had been crying.

Kara was carried back downstairs—light and limp, an ashen bag of wheezes—and laid on the futon. They gathered around her and shared communion, breaking bread together.

Those in the Neumann home didn't realize it, but two thousand miles away, Kara's illness was causing ripples in the extended family.

Dale's sister, Susan Neumann, had spoken on the phone to Ariel Neff, who had become Leilani's sister-in-law just two days before. When Ariel heard that Leilani was trying to give Kara fluids via syringe, she worried that Leilani could inadvertently drown Kara. But unlike the rest of the family, the eighteen-year-old didn't feel bound to defer to Leilani and Dale. She decided to do something about it.

AROUND ONE THIRTY, SHORTLY AFTER THE PEASLEES LEFT, THE WHOLE Wormgoor family pulled up to the Neumanns' gray house in the woods. Althea, for one, had not believed for a second that Kara was as sick as Leilani claimed. Neither had Randall. Their wariness was understandable; part of the falling out had been about the efficacy of faith healing, and now, here they were being asked to participate in a dramatic, high-stakes round of faith healing. But how could one refuse?

Once inside, the Wormgoors realized that Leilani had not been exaggerating. Kara was on the futon, eyes partially open but unaware.

When they gathered around Kara, Leilani said it was a chance for God to show his power. If human frailties had torn the Neumanns and Wormgoors apart, they were ready for God to restore Kara's health and reunite them in a common, sainted purpose.

Meanwhile, at about two p.m., Ariel Neff began to call authorities in Wisconsin, trying to get someone to do a wellness check on Kara. Her first call, to a nonemergency department, led nowhere, not on Easter Sunday. Ariel hung up.

Next, Ariel called 911 and got through to a dispatcher named Stacey at the Marathon County Sheriff's Department in Wausau, about ten miles from the Neumann home. The center handled some thirty-two thousand emergency calls each year for seventy-eight police, ambulance, and fire departments spread throughout a sixteen-hundred-square-mile area.

Stacey didn't know the Neumanns, and because Ariel didn't have a proper street address for the family, she couldn't help. Ariel hung up again.

Back in the Neumann home, Leilani put her hands in the air.

"Oh Lord," she said. "You can heal diabetes. You can heal cancer."

And—perhaps miraculously—Kara's breathing grew stronger. When God showed his power, Leilani said, her little girl would come back ten times better than ever.

Time continued to race by. A few minutes past two thirty, Randall pulled Dale aside and broached a delicate subject. If it were one of his three daughters in this condition, Randall said, he would take her to the doctor. Whether from the stress of the situation or the difficulty of taking advice from Randall, Dale snapped at him.

"Don't you think that crossed my mind?" he asked.

Dale later said that he understood where Randall was coming from. But at the same time it was an expression of doubt, and doubt—the enemy of faith—was the last thing Kara needed.

"We just weren't doubting the Lord," Dale later said. "The Word says that we shall be healed."

At almost this precise moment—the sort of momentous coincidence that inspires belief in the divine—Ariel Neff placed the third in a holy trinity of calls to the authorities. A dispatcher named John answered. It was 2:33 p.m. Ariel gave him a brief summary of the situation.

"So I was hoping maybe somebody could go over there or something?" Ariel said.

Time was ticking away.

"Can you go over it again, since I don't know what you talked about with Stacey," said John. "You're going to have to tell me everything."

"Okay," said Ariel. She apologized. Then, once again, she began to explain.

"My sister-in-law," said Ariel, "she's very religious. She doesn't—she believes in faith instead of doctors. And she called my mother-in-law today and we're all in California. And she explained to us that she believes her daughter is in a coma now. And she's relying on faith."

"So this person that's in a coma is not in a hospital," said John. "She's at home?"

Tick, tick.

"She's at home," repeated Ariel. "And she's eleven."

Ariel gave John the Neumanns' address, which he read back to her.

"So you want me to send an ambulance over there, right?" he asked.

"Please," said Ariel. She warned that Leilani would be resistant to medical personnel showing up on her doorstep.

"I'll get somebody going," said John.

Ariel was relieved. "Okay," she said. "Wonderful. Thank you so much." They hung up. It was 2:35 p.m. on Easter Sunday. The entire exchange had taken only two minutes. Two precious minutes.

Tick.

.•:·

DISPATCHER JOHN MOBILIZED POLICE AND AMBULANCE VEHICLES. THE Neumanns were fortunately situated, just six miles from Ascension St. Clare's Hospital on Ministry Parkway. The ambulance left St. Clare's campus and hooked an immediate left onto Weston Avenue, a four-mile straight shot along low, flat land where marshes pooled dark waters beneath shrubs and immature trees. Birch bark showed gray against white snow.

It was unclear whether the responders represented salvation for Kara or damnation for Dale and Leilani, who could be accused of mistreating their daughter. Just as Randall and Dale were sidebarring about the possibility of taking Kara to the hospital, Althea Wormgoor gazed down at the thin little girl. She saw Kara's lip twitch. It was hard to describe, but the movement frightened Althea.

Agonal breathing is a reflex reaction, a gasp triggered directly by the brain when a person's body is not getting enough oxygen to survive. One of the Wormgoor girls said what no one wanted to believe—Kara had stopped breathing.

Panic descended. Althea, not knowing that emergency personnel were already on their way, decided to call 911, but she couldn't remember the Neumanns' address. She began looking for an envelope or anything with the house number on it. Randall punched 911 into his phone instead.

"Jesus!" Dale fell to his knees and held Kara to himself. He cried out, "Jesus, Jesus!" He cuddled her. "Jesus," he moaned.

It was around 2:40. Ariel had hung up with the dispatcher five minutes earlier.

"Hello?"

Without any preamble, Randall spit out the address to the 911 dispatcher.

"Maplewood?" asked the dispatcher. The Neumanns' living room was now a pandemonious din.

"I can't hear you," said Randall.

The dispatcher said that emergency services were en route; an ambulance, fire vehicle, and an officer.

"Do you need something?" the dispatcher asked.

"A girl is not breathing," Randall said.

After verifying the address again, the dispatcher tried to direct Randall.

"Do you know how to do CPR, sir?" he asked.

"Okay," said Randall, obviously distracted. "Hello?"

"Yes, can you hear me?"

"Yes."

"Okay," said the dispatcher. "Do you know how to do CPR?"

"I don't know," said Randall. "Nobody here is doing it. Nobody's doing it." He addressed the room. "Anybody?"

At a stop sign, the EMTs turned left onto County Road J, a shaggy median on the left, an Arby's in a field on the right. The ambulance had insulin on board, more than enough to treat even advanced ketoacidosis.

The dispatcher, now talking to Leilani, confirmed that Kara was not breathing.

"No, I don't think," said Leilani.

"Now, what I want you to do is tilt her head back," the dispatcher said. He told her to feel by Kara's nose, for breath.

"Tilt her head back," Leilani said to Dale, who was cradling Kara's body. "Tilt her head back, okay. Tilt her head back. Put your head by her mouth. Tilt her head back."

"Just feel by her nose," said the dispatcher, "and see if she's breathing."

"Okay," said Leilani. She spoke to Dale, frantic. "Is she breathing?"

Then, as he checked, "Is she breathing? Is she breathing?"

"No," Dale said.

"No, she's not," Leilani reported back to the dispatcher. Then, more hysterically, "She's not breathing. Okay, she's not breathing!"

Tick, tick, tick. The ambulance slipped neatly under the overpass of State Highway 29, then past undeveloped fields, on the left a car dealership, on the right the Highland Community Church, whose members called doctors to treat their sick children. It crossed the Eau Claire River on a little bridge with rusty gray guardrails and then picked up speed on a straight, worn strip of blacktop guiding them out of the marshes and onto dry land, where the trees grew taller and more dominant.

Leilani relayed instructions from the dispatcher to Dale. Two breaths into Kara's mouth at a time.

"Keep breathing into her mouth. Keep breathing into her mouth. Breathe into her mouth," said Leilani.

"Try to calm down, okay?" the dispatcher asked Leilani.

"Okay," she said.

Tick, tick. Outside, the temperature hovered at thirty-two, the line between thaw and melt. The ambulance took a sharp right onto the winding and curving Roble Lane, and finally, after a couple of blocks, onto Maplewood Drive.

"Did she—did she respond to the breaths at all?" asked the dispatcher.

"No," said Leilani. "No. No. I don't think so."

She turned to Dale again.

"Did she respond to the breaths? Did she respond?" Then back to the dispatcher. "No, I don't think so."

"Okay," said the dispatcher. "What I want you to do—is she lying flat on her back?"

"Yes," said Leilani. But then she suddenly lost interest in the voice on the phone. She had seen the vehicles arriving in the driveway, the emergency personnel exiting their vehicles and hurrying up the steps.

"Here he comes!" she said. "Here he comes! They're here!"

As the dispatcher tried to clarify, Leilani shouted to the people coming in the front door.

"Over here," she called. "Over here! Over here!"

It was 2:44 p.m.

As the door swung open, Officer Scott Marten hurried in, trim and middle-aged with sandy brown hair and a friendly face. He absorbed the chaotic scene—Dale pushing ineffectually on an extremely skinny, prone form, attempting CPR. Two EMTs, Jason Russ and Hyden Prausa, hustled in behind Marten and quickly confirmed that Kara had no breath of life. No pulse. Bluish-gray skin. Warm to the touch.

At 2:45, the wind began to rise outside and shifted to the north, gusting and cold. As Kara was rushed to the hospital, Russ noticed a sweet fruity odor around Kara's mouth, which caused them to check her blood sugar; it was eventually determined to be five times the normal level.

The Neumanns followed behind the ambulance, making an emergency call of their own. When David Eells picked up, they asked him to pray for God to spare Kara.

"I did," said Eells. "I called on our prayer ministers and elders to pray for her too."

They got to the hospital at three p.m. Kara's body was taken into a trauma room, and staff worked to revive her. At three thirty, Choon P'Ng, the emergency room doctor, declared her dead.

The Easter Sunday miracle had not been brought about by fierce faith expressed in relentless and fervent group prayer.

It had not been brought about by reconciliation with the Wormgoors.

It had not been brought about at all.

Madeline Kara Neumann was dead.

In that instant it became clear that, with internet-based communities egging each other on to ever more radical expressions of religious freedom, the consequences were real, and tragic, and of concern to the broader public.

The doctor and an autopsy agreed that her death, logged at three thirty p.m., was the result of diabetic ketoacidosis resulting from untreated juvenile-onset diabetes mellitus, the most advanced case the autopsy team had ever seen. High blood sugar, high blood acid, and high hemoglobin levels indicated weeks of poor control of the levels of sugar in her system.

Dr. Ivan Zador, a pediatric endocrinologist at Marshfield Clinic who specializes in diabetes, reviewed Kara's records and concluded that she could have been saved "very late into the day of her death." Even if she had been breathing, as she had been five minutes before the EMTs arrived, her prognosis for survival would have been very good.

The surviving members of the Neumann family walked in circles around her bed, praying over Kara's lifeless body. John Larson, the county medical examiner, summoned from his home, said the body would have to be taken to Madison for an autopsy.

"You won't need to do that," Dale and Leilani said. "She will be alive by then."

Dale was hopeful: "Well, Jesus raised Lazarus from the dead. So I'm hoping. Yeah. I'm trusting. I'm believing that there would be a resurrection."

Customers who arrived at the coffee shop the next day, while Kara's autopsy was being performed, found a sign that said it was closed "due to a family emergency."

Not until Tuesday's autopsy did Dale and Leilani seem to fully understand that Kara was gone. Dale described himself as "very sad. Very, very sad."

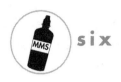 **six**

THE ALIEN'S DRINK BLEACHES

Disclaimer: These statements have not been evaluated by the Food and Drug Administration. MMS (Master Mineral Solution) has not been FDA approved to diagnose, cure, mitigate, treat, or prevent any disease.

—Jim Humble, www.jimhumble.co

Jim cannot take responsibility for any adverse detoxification effects or consequences resulting from the use of any suggestions he may give.

—Jim Humble, www.jimhumble.co

In a Colombian compound around 2010, a human and an extraterrestrial sat down to agree on a legal definition of MMS.

Though MMS could cure cancer, Alzheimer's, autism, Parkinson's, multiple sclerosis, and HIV, Mark Grenon and the alien in Jim Humble's skin knew they couldn't call it a drug.

If they did, the FDA would be too limiting to their freedom.

MMS could boost one's immune system like a vitamin regimen, but they wanted real freedom, not the halfhearted compromises the FDA allowed the supplement industry.

Instead, they wanted the freedom of constitutionally protected speech or, even better, religion. Should they distribute MMS under the legal shield of a sympathetic church? No, an organized church breathing down their neck would also be limiting. It was okay to be accountable to God, of course, but here on Earth, they wanted to hold themselves accountable, at their discretion. Answering to religious leaders—that wasn't freedom. They wanted to *be* religious leaders.

Yes! Grenon and the alien in Humble's skin could be religious leaders!

But not the sort of religious leaders who were tied to Sunday worship, and hearing confession, and some of the other services and baggage and paperwork that came with running a traditional church. That wasn't real freedom either, was it?

The alien, having originated on the Planet of the Gods, didn't have the traditional view of God as described in the Bible, but he did have relevant experience, back when he was in one of his earlier bodies and saw a spaceship crash to the Earth. The immortal alien and some friends found a single survivor, a young woman. They laid her on the ground and used their advanced technology to straighten out and heal her broken bones and other injuries.

The aliens were about to leave when they realized they had never caught her name. And when they asked her, it turned out to be Eve. As in Adam and Eve. True story! (Says the alien in Humble's skin.)

Needless to say, this sort of thing had given the alien a somewhat broader worldview than was allowed for in the Bible, and he did not consider himself a traditionally religious person. Grenon, on the other hand, was an ardent Bible student and had been preaching the word of God for years.

It was a pretty big difference.

"But we worked together," said Grenon later, "because we had a common goal."

And so they agreed on a common (though very uncommon) strategy to freely distribute MMS through a church of their own invention.

At its heart, the idea of the separation of church and state is meant to allow one to engage in the spiritual practice of one's choice without being persecuted by the government. But at the outer edges of this sphere of protection are bad actors who refuse to stay in their lane. The idea of an MMS-centric church was a different brand of fringe medical freedom than the one that had killed Kara Neumann, but it was an equally audacious perversion of the concept, one that sought to fuse religious extremism with the emerging juggernaut of the One True Cure industry.

THE GENESIS II CHURCH OF HEALTH AND HEALING, FOUNDED IN 2011, was unlike any other church on the planet. There were no in-person services, no physical edifices, no communions or baptisms or confessions or last rites. Grenon was the cofounding bishop. Not to be outdone, the alien in Humble's skin was the cofounding archbishop.

They wrote the church's doctrines, which blended scientific speech reminiscent of that uttered by Robert Young, the potent fervency displayed by the Neumanns, and a hyperinflated emphasis on the idea that cleanliness is next to godliness (a maxim which, incidentally, does not appear in the Bible).

A core belief of the church was that "our individual spirits live within our temple or our PHYSICAL body and therefore need to maintain said temple in a clean manner as God, our Creator demands." To achieve this purity of the soul, church members had to scour their bodies with MMS.

The church did not sell MMS, according to the church. However, it did accept twenty-dollar donations. The government says that in exchange, donors were given four-ounce bottles of the church's signature miraculous sacramental cleansing water. But the church claims it didn't sell it. That would be illegal.

The donation program was an instant success. Bottles of MMS began flying out the door, and thousands began to tune in to the church's online events.

The key to the growing number of converts was Grenon, whose image as a gruff, tenacious bandersnatch proved to be a magnetic draw. "I'm just a fighter," Grenon would say. "That's not saying I'm a hero or anything. But I hate evil. I love facts. And I love God. I'm not afraid." On popular social media platforms branded to the Genesis II Church, Grenon talked scripture for hours and could seamlessly transition between the Bible and the news of the day, all with a sense of humor and authenticity.

One of Grenon's sons, Joseph, helped with promotions. Another son, Jonathan, was responsible for manufacturing and bottling MMS out of a backyard shed in a family home in Bradenton, Florida. A third son,

Jordan, was the distributor, filling orders and handling conversations with customers—or receiving donations and sending sacraments to church members.

Church officials strategically built a network of people who had a vested interest in MMS by hosting seminars around the world; attendees paid as much as $450 to become Genesis II health ministers, who were authorized to make and disseminate MMS themselves. Grenon also set up an MMS "Restoration Center" in his residential compound in Santa Marta, Colombia, where MMS-focused retreats cost $5,000 per month.

Grenon and the alien in Humble's skin had words of disagreement in 2015, and the alien left the church to live in Mexico. But Genesis II's operations no longer relied on the extraterrestrial.

Grenon and his sons continued giving seminars and correspondence courses; in all, they trained two thousand Genesis health ministers from 145 different countries. Soon, they were reading MMS testimonials on a weekly Genesis II radio broadcast, G2Voice, which racked up 250,000 downloads and three million views. ABC News ran a story in which Lindsay Wagner, an actress who had played the Bionic Woman in the eponymous 1970s television series, credited MMS with clearing up her debilitating case of hives.

With so many health ministers and church members supporting MMS that it would be virtually impossible for the government to shut them all down, it was time for MMS to go to the next level.

.·: :

ONE THEORY THAT PROVED TO BE COMPATIBLE WITH MMS WAS PLEO-morphism, which at the time was spreading through One True Cure communities like a virus, demonstrating that the ideas of the cat-jarring Antoine Béchamp had, like his victims, nine lives.

The alien in Humble's skin, who had several friends in common with Robert Young, wrote that pleomorphism explained not just MMS's ability to cure systemically but the workings behind all sorts of One True Cures, each one being stymied by the FDA, the FTC, and the AMA (American Medical Association).

The alien continued to explore the limits of MMS. He knew that drinking it was good. But there were other methods of ingestion and other patient populations to consider. He experimented with MMS colonic cleanses and inhaling MMS-laden vapor. There was MMS to brush your teeth. MMS for pregnant moms and unborn babies. MMS for animals.

Finally, the alien came up with an idea for the ultimate MMS treatment: injection.

To test it, he added a single drop of MMS to 150 milliliters of saline solution and administered it to himself via an IV.

An hour passed. There was no effect. Had he done something wrong?

No, not unless you counted injecting a cleaning fluid into his body.

About ninety minutes after the injection, it hit him. He began to feel cold and to shiver uncontrollably. He also had an urge to vomit. These symptoms are exactly what one might expect the human body to do in response to a toxic chemical. But the alien saw the shivers and nausea as signs of efficacy.

"I was sick, but quite elated," he said. "Something different was happening, and this had never happened before."

After further experimentation, the alien decided that his reaction was a result of the MMS destroying foreign agents in the body, releasing poisons in the process. Some poisons, he concluded, were so deeply embedded in the body that simply swilling MMS couldn't get to them.

"That could only be because the chlorine dioxide is going deeper into the body tissues," he wrote.

These deeply embedded poisons, he said, were "laboratory-generated diseases," invented by the US government.

The alien's breakthrough was not universally rejected. One woman charged $2,000 per session to treat cancer patients by injecting them with MMS in her garage, causing a nasty blood clot for at least one breast cancer patient. But gaining broad public acceptance would be an almost impossible lift, even with help from a masterful MMS advocate like Mark Grenon.

About the only path forward would be for Grenon to convincingly present MMS to someone who was very, very powerful but also very, very silly. The right person had to be really big, bigger even than the Bionic Woman. Ideally—and this was just pie-in-the-sky spitballing—someone like the president of the United States would go on live television and tell the world that infusing the body with bleach could be helpful.

That would really change the whole ball game, if something that crazy were ever to happen.

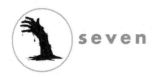seven

AMERICAN HEALTH CARE A REFUGE

We can find most of the old beliefs alive amongst us to-day, only having changed their dresses and the social spheres in which they thrive. . . . Names are only air, and blow away with a change of wind; but beliefs are rooted in human wants and weakness, and die hard. . . . What shall we say of the plausible and well-dressed charlatans of our own time, who trade in false pretences . . . without any fear of being fined or whipped; or of the many follies and inanities, imposing on the credulous part of the community, each of them gaping with eager, open mouth for a gratuitous advertisement by the mention of its foolish name in any respectable connection?

> —Oliver Wendell Holmes, "The Medical Profession in Massachusetts," 1869

FOR A CENTURY, DOCTORS HAD RESTED ON THE BEDROCK OF SCIEN-tific surety fueled by the Numbers Junkies; what they had to offer the American public was an evidence-based constellation of procedures and recommendations, including vaccines, that demonstrably led to a dramatic increase in the life span of the human organism.

Standing on that bedrock, the medical profession took the public's trust for granted—medical doctors routinely expected patients to accept extreme cures like mind-altering pills, anesthetization to allow strangers to rummage around in their insides, and the stabbing of their children with needles filled with tamed versions of deadly diseases.

A century of fringe One True Cures had failed to destroy this trust, but the culture of health care was changing. Patients with cancer and other serious illnesses were flocking to Larry Lytle's laser seminars, to Toby McAdam's virtual storefronts, to Robert Young's Miracle Ranch, to

Pentecostal faith-healing events, and to the new alien-founded church, which became known to critics as the Church of Bleach.

But of course they were just a few small actors in an endless swamp of profit-driven medical misinformation. By 2011, it seemed clear that the medical establishment was getting its ass kicked by a shadow health empire that it barely knew existed. That year, for the first time in American history, more adults were taking supplements than not. The use of probiotics had quadrupled over the past decade. Roughly one in two hundred Americans who boarded an international flight did so to receive health care in places like Costa Rica, often getting treatments that would be illegal in the US. That translated to nearly a million people, a ninefold increase over 2003. More people were choosing not to go to their doctor, and a national survey showed that 60 percent of these off-grid patients never told their doctor about the alternative treatments they underwent, whether leeches, lasers, or low-acid liquid diet.

The most heavily trafficked alternative-medicine website in the world in 2011 was mercola.com, run by antivaccine activist (and Health Freedom Expo speaker) Dr. Joseph Mercola, who in 2009 stopped practicing medicine and in 2010 sold $7 million worth of supplements (such as "Dr. Mercola Vitamin K2," which he did not adequately test for adulterants) and medical devices (including "telethermographic cameras," about which he made unfounded medical claims). The website's stance against Big Pharma was articulated alongside articles pimping things like so-called horny goat weed for erectile dysfunction. That year, Mercola's website drew 1.9 million visitors a month (as many as the website of the National Institutes of Health), many of whom came back multiple times a week.

The proliferation of One True Cures had serious consequences. If an individual winds up in the emergency room because they took a dietary supplement laced with a dangerous drug or toxin, we can all make fun of that person for not being more careful about what they swallow. But it's not just one person. In 2015 alone, twenty-three thousand Americans went to the emergency department after taking bunk dietary supplements to lose weight or improve their sex lives or boost their athletic skills.

Meanwhile, it was clear that the FDA, formidable as it might be, was doing little to deplete the vast flocks of quacks running amok. By 2014, nearly one in four Americans had purchased items from online pharmacies, and thirty-six million of them did it to get drugs for which they had no prescription.

Worse, academics and watchdog groups began to point out just how ineffective the FDA was, even when it had a violator in its grasp. Between 2007 and 2016, the FDA identified 746 brands of supplements that were laced with prescription drugs—but only 360 of them were recalled. The rest were still available for sale within the framework of the unstoppable juggernaut of America's retail system.

In one study that was particularly embarrassing for the FDA, researchers took a closer look at hundreds of products that had been recalled between 2009 and 2012 and found that dozens of them were still available for sale a year after they had been recalled. The researchers bought and analyzed those products and discovered that two-thirds of them were still adulterated with the same ingredients that had prompted the recall. In 2014, one US congressman ruefully noted that penalties were steeper for counterfeiting a designer purse than a designer drug.

And even when the FDA pursued a case through the criminal court system, operators like McAdam, Lytle, and Young were able to continue making money for years.

∴

WHEN EVENTS LIKE THE HEALTH FREEDOM EXPO SUCCESSFULLY MERGED New Age healers with cutthroat medical-freedom values, it was as if they'd successfully brokered a wedding between Oprah Winfrey and the Grinch. Their quacky offspring raked in massive amounts of loot, some of which was inevitably diverted into efforts to undermine America's regulatory system in the name of medical freedom.

That meant showering antivaxxers with cash. People like Mercola joined conservative political donors to fund grassroots organizations like Texans for Vaccine Choice or Oklahomans for Vaccine and Health Choice. Mercola, whose net worth ballooned to more than $100 million, funneled $4 million into the National Vaccine Information Center, which fought against vaccine mandates by arguing in part that they violated a Christian tradition of freedom or liberty. (Though some said liberty and some said freedom, science had never settled the difference between the two, mostly because no one has ever found a true example of either.)

The FDA and the medical establishment had been doing all they could to drop the hammer on One True Cures. It occurred to them belatedly that One True Cures might figure out how to drop the hammer on *them*.

Taking the fight to the medical establishment—this was the next evolution of the health-freedom movement. As these groups promoted all sorts of One True Cures (the primary qualification for which seemed to be that they were not vaccines), they successfully lobbied twelve states to pass laws weakening vaccine requirements. Between 2000 and 2015 measles coverage dropped from 97 percent to 92 percent of kids nationally; it became as low as 86 percent in some areas.

Several years later a group of researchers from the University of Idaho would set out to learn why, during this time period, large numbers of literate Americans began rejecting vaccines that had been proven effective. Conventional wisdom was that people were individually losing faith in institutions and then banding together under the banner of medical freedom, which had been adopted by the Republican Party.

But in fact, their research proved the opposite: political identity dictates vaccine opinions, not the other way around.

This meant liberals didn't support vaccines because they loved science; it was because political influencers told them that vaccine support made them good liberals. And rank-and-file conservatives didn't begin to rail against vaccines because they had an inherent distrust of doctors. They opposed them because a dense network of influential alternative healers, political leaders, and entertainment personalities told them that doing so made them good conservatives. It made little difference to them that those same healers, political leaders, and entertainment personalities were earning money from products—bogus supplements, fraudulent medical devices, and quack-informed wellness services—that sold better when distrust in mainstream medicine was rampant.

It's enough to make the medical establishment huff in indignation. But before they allow that indignant air to puff over their petulant, deliciously self-righteous lips, it would behoove them to remember something: it's their fault.

.·:

OR AT LEAST, PARTLY THEIR FAULT.

In his 2019 book *Ruined by Design*, the outspoken, visionary designer Mike Monteiro argues that most of the problems that run rife through Big Tech and society at large—everything from toxic speech and harmful misinformation on social media platforms to disenfranchisement of poor and minority voters—should not be thought of as mistakes or free-floating problems. Instead, he says, they are the inevitable outcomes of systems that are designed to produce those effects, whether the system in question is Twitter or the Electoral College. If we took an ethical, thoughtful, and inclusive approach to designing (or redesigning) those systems, he writes, most of the problems would simply evaporate.

The proliferation of One True Cures is kind of like that: an inevitable product of poorly and inequitably designed systems. In this case, the systemic failures of the misinformation-friendly internet, soft-on-supplements legislation, and the ineffectual FDA were compounded by another flawed system, one that was not so much a failure as doctors' on-purpose prioritization of all the wrong values.

Low vaccination rates and high use of alternative medicine are both associated with rural areas, where Americans tend to make less money, have fewer educational opportunities, and have less health insurance coverage than their urban counterparts.

These are the areas that need doctors most, and yet they are the very places that suffer from chronic doctor shortages. As one 2000 study noted, about 20 percent of Americans live in rural areas, but only 9 percent of physicians practice in those communities. Roughly 25 percent of rural residents told pollsters that they had recently had trouble accessing medical services, either because of cost or because the services they needed were too far away. The problem has gotten worse since the turn of the century. Between 2005 and 2022, more than ten rural hospitals closed each year, and only 1 percent of medical students say they want to practice in rural communities.

When medical professionals leave a territory, One True Cures and antivaccine messaging move into the vacuum that is left behind. And the absence of medical professionals in rural areas is not a fluke; it is an integral part of the field, as designed by the American Medical Association.

In the mid-1800s, soon after the AMA was formed, it ran doctors for state legislative positions across the country. Once elected, they worked to address what they saw as the most pressing problem of the profession: too many doctors and not enough patients. By imposing stricter licensing requirements and preventing the chartering of new medical schools, they successfully slowed the number of doctor graduates, almost entirely based on the argument that reducing supply would increase demand, which would increase their own wages. This was, perhaps, a defensible position when doctors carrying black bags on horseback to house calls could barely make ends meet, but the appetite for money considerably outlasted that era. No matter how high wages got over the next one hundred years, the AMA continued to lobby to further narrow the pipeline of doctors.

It has been strikingly effective. In 2020, the average self-employed physician earned more than $350,000. And the doctor supply is so small and poorly distributed that Mississippi had just 191 licensed doctors per 100,000 people, roughly half as many as work in New York, Vermont, Rhode Island, or Maryland. And even those states compare unfavorably to the 400 doctors per 100,000 enjoyed by the residents of the Russian Federation, or Italy, or, of all places, Kazakhstan. (Greece had 550 doctors per 100,000 people, and Cuba had 840, the most in the world.)

By making American doctors so precious, the AMA inflated the social and financial status of its members, which introduced another, unintentional obstacle to access. Degreed doctors now comprise an intimidating elite culture, one that breeds mistrust and misunderstandings as hallmarks of medical care for rural patients nearer the low end of the socioeconomic ladder.

Had the health care model that the AMA so aggressively designed and sold to the public included an ample flow of doctors whose pay didn't create a massive class gulf with so many of their rural patients, quackery would have lacked a friendly medium for its growth.

.∵

So, BY 2011, THE DESIGN OF AMERICA'S HEALTH CARE SYSTEM WAS, FOR many people, great.

It was great for doctors, who earned ridiculously high wages.

It was great for the healers who were making money off One True Cures.

It was great for the antivaccine movement, which was gaining converts every month.

It was great for libertarians, who in medical freedom had struck upon a resonant rallying call that mainstream Republicans found difficult to ignore.

And it was great for Republican political leaders and conservative media outlets, who welcomed alternative healers into their ranks and in many cases made money from alternative-health products themselves.

All these groups coalesced around a narrative: Big Pharma runs the government, so cutting government regulations and enforcement capabilities hurts Big Pharma.

That basic premise gained lots of fans—including Big Pharma.

After all, the massive corporate pharmaceutical companies had been butting up against government mandates ever since Pharma first got Big. The industry has spent decades fighting Democratic-sponsored reform measures that would lower drug prices by importing cheaper drugs from Canada, imposing price caps, and negotiating Medicaid/Medicare prices.

And so, the ability of libertarians to co-opt alternative healers meant that America's health care system was also great for Big Pharma.

It was not so great for patients.

When vaccination rates dipped, a bevy of infectious diseases that were waiting in the wings rushed back onto the American stage. In 2000 measles was eradicated; in 2014 there were twenty-three outbreaks in low-vax areas, and in 2015 a woman died of measles. Vaccine refusal was also associated with outbreaks of chicken pox, pneumococcal disease, and whooping cough.

Even worse, the lack of trust in doctors hurt cancer patients. A group of Yale researchers examined 840 cases in the National Cancer Database and compared those who chose conventional cancer treatments like chemo, surgery, and radiation against those who chose One True Cures and other alternative therapies. The difference was stark—in fewer than six years, twice as many lung cancer patients who'd chosen alternative treatments were dead. Those with colon cancer died at four times the rate. Those with breast cancer died five times as often.

David Gorski, an oncologist with the Barbara Ann Karmanos Cancer Institute who has tracked such trends, told journalists the study showed that "alternative medicine kills cancer patients. It is basically no different than refusing treatment altogether and much more expensive and troublesome."

He traced the blame to the medical-freedom movement.

"Appeals to freedom," he said in one published account, "are like the gateway drug to pseudoscience."

.: :

THE YEAR 2011, A TIPPING POINT FOR ALTERNATIVE HEALING, WAS IMPORTANT for another reason.

Deep beneath the Pacific Ocean, the edge of one tectonic plate was being jammed beneath the tectonic plate that held Japan. This wasn't news. It had been happening at a rate of three inches a year since long before humans had invented the concept of news. But that March, it became news in the biggest possible way, when a chunk of the underlying plate suddenly gave way, causing the seafloor to pop up by about fifteen feet and the plate holding parts of Japan to suddenly drop by about three feet. The magnitude 9 Tohoku earthquake was so big it shunted Japan eight feet to the east. It was so big it shifted the Earth six inches on its axis. It was so big it sped up the rotation of the planet (only by 1.8 microseconds a day, but still—your days are now just a tiny bit shorter. Thanks Obama!). The earthquake and resultant tsunami also wreaked havoc on human systems—transportation systems, energy systems, water systems, telecommunication systems, and that most important of all human systems, the biological system that allows us to slobber, reproduce, and contemplate the irrationality of high baby-formula prices (usually in that order).

The tsunami killed more than twenty thousand people and caused multiple nuclear meltdowns, a disastrous toll for everyone except sellers of supplements, who pivoted to prey on the baseless fears of Americans living thousands of miles away from the radiation. Toby McAdam, still selling his RisingSun products, told the local newspaper that he doubted the radiation would drift to Montana—"but it could." He recommended that his "Lugol's Iodine solution" be applied to the skin daily as "an ounce of prevention." Though public health officials said people self-treating with iodide supplements were more likely to harm than help themselves, orders spiked so sharply that Toby's website crashed.

The multifaceted nature of the tsunami-caused chaos makes it perhaps appropriate that the event also marked the beginning of the United States' descent into a full-blown zombie apocalypse.

The June following the earthquake, the CDC began a conversation about emergency preparedness on Twitter that led to a handful of people jokingly tweeting that they would like the CDC to weigh in on a catastrophic zombie attack.

This led to the predictable wave of lols, rofls, and laughy-face emoticons, but it also sparked an idea for Dave Daigle (a CDC communications administrator) and Dr. Ali S. Khan (a CDC expert in disaster preparedness).

With Daigle's input, Khan wrote a piece for the CDC website explaining how to prepare for a zombie apocalypse. This neatly demonstrated the humanity of the person on the other side of the icy-cold stethoscope even as it leveraged the innate appeal of zombies to teach real-life strategies to cope with actual disasters.

It turned out people were hungry for messaging about people hungry for brains. The CDC zombie apocalypse preparedness plan was an instant hit, racking up so many views that the CDC server froze up, overwhelmed by all the traffic.

This bit of fun was so successful that a team of researchers from the University of California, Irvine, published a congratulatory paper in the journal *Emerging Infectious Diseases* urging other public health officials to follow suit. It argued that zombies were an opportunity "to capitalize on the benefits of spreading public health awareness through the use of relatable popular culture tools and scientific explanations for fictional phenomena." They proposed that the medical establishment build on those efforts to stimulate the conversation and do better public education on a variety of health topics.

Suddenly, zombies were everywhere in public health and safety. The CDC, the Department of Homeland Security, and the Federal Emergency Management Agency all published in-depth zombie-related literature. Finally, public officials were seizing the initiative and taking back the cultural space they had inadvertently ceded to promoters of One True Cures.

Also in 2011, a Harvard Medical School physician and aspiring novelist named Steven Schlozman appeared on the radio show *Coast to Coast AM*, which spun tales of conspiracy and paranormal phenomena to a large and credulous national audience from two a.m. to four a.m., seven days a week. Because *Coast to Coast AM* was the most popular late-night radio show in the country, with ten million listeners, it was a great opportunity for Schlozman, who was there to promote his latest work, *The Zombie Autopsies: Secret Notebooks from the Apocalypse*. In the book, Schlozman drew on his medical knowledge to describe "Ataxic Neurodegenerative Satiety Deficiency syndrome" as the medical cause of zombies (it was of course a fictional work of fictitious fiction). The format of the show required that Schlozman spend the opening stretch talking about the events of his novel as if they were real, before shifting to an acknowledgment that it was all pure fantasy.

Daigle, Khan, and Schlozman were helping people learn a bit of science in a fun way.

But their efforts quickly ran up against a problem: there is more than one way to view a zombie apocalypse.

.·.:·

ONE FACT THAT THE CDC AND ITS FELLOW AGENCIES FAILED TO FULLY appreciate was that, in zombie properties like 2009's feature film *Zombieland* and 2010's hit television series *The Walking Dead*, very little screen time is given to public health concepts like water sanitation. The action takes place after most health authorities have had their faces eaten, leaving individual survivors to run around attacking infected people with baseball bats, crossbows, and shotguns as a means of self-preservation.

That's why other groups were quickly lining up to enlist the hot new cultural craze into their own, very different agendas. Zombies became the centerpiece in gun advertisements and were a major part of the NRA's annual conventions, where shooting at the undead carried none of the moral baggage that came with shooting at human targets.

"Because the zombie canon focuses so squarely on the apocalypse, its spread into popular culture can erode faith in the resiliency of civilization," wrote Daniel Drezner, the Tufts University professor and zombie expert. "The zombie narrative, as it is traditionally presented, socially constructs the very narrative that agencies like the CDC and FEMA are trying to prevent."

Drezner documented the way that zombie references became a sort of dog whistle for gun rights—those on the outside glossed over a quirky head-scratcher while targeted audiences became fired up, even though they would clearly never need to shoot a zombie in real life.

Until some Americans began to ask, *Will I need to shoot a zombie in real life?*

.•:˙

TOBY MCADAM HAD TOLD ME ABOUT THE 2012 MIAMI INCIDENT IN WHICH a man bit the face off a homeless man and then was himself described by authorities as slow to die after being shot. But Toby was not the only person fascinated by that attack. It let the undead cat out of the bag.

Soon after the news broke, a self-described Bitcoin evangelist and promoter of alternative-health supplements doctored a *Huffington Post* article about the incident so that it attributed the cause of the face eating to "LQP-79," a virus that destroys internal organs and makes the host hungry for human flesh.

The fake article went viral, blitzing digital media feeds so thoroughly that LQP-79 was soon the third-most-searched term on the CDC website, forcing the agency to officially deny the existence of a zombie virus.

Around then, communities of zombie-themed survivalists and militias sprang up all across America. One was an offshoot of the well-established Michigan Militia, while others had names like the Kansas Anti Zombie Militia, the Anti Zombie Unified Resistance Effort (AZURE), Zombie-Fighting Rednecks, the Zombie Eradication and Survival Team, Postmortem Assault Squadron, and the US Department of Zombie Defense.

One, a loosely affiliated national group called the US Zombie Outbreak Response Team (ZORT), popularized a strange mishmash of survivalism and cosplay. Its website features pictures of preppers in tactical gear and tinted sunglasses using stickers and goofy accessories to trick out their trucks as zombie-fighting vehicles that would be equally at home in *Ghostbusters* or *Mad Max* universes. It was in some ways good fun. But they also carried real firearms. And engaged in real postapocalyptic survival exercises.

"A Zombie could be anything from a person infected by a pandemic outbreak to a crazy nut job, criminal or gangster who wants to hurt your family and steal your food and preps," reads ZORT's promotional material.

Though ZORT purports to be simply providing tongue-in-cheek cover for legit training that would be helpful in a natural disaster, of course the real difference between zombies and hurricane survivors is that one must be shot in the head and the other should be given a hot toddy and a shower.

Did any of these folks actually believe in zombies?

Probably not. But there was potential.

Drezner cited research showing that when considering paranormal ideas, people look less to the logical evidence and more to whether other people believe in the ideas. This means that even if no one believes in zombies, if some people believe that other people believe in zombies, then some people will believe in zombies. The gaslighting became so effective that the gaslit then gaslighted others, until fear of actual zombies took on an undead life of its own—call it masslighting.

And really, the online picture was becoming quite blurry. At the CDC, Daigle and Khan began getting inquiries about their Zombie Preparedness Plan from concerned citizens who wanted to know what sort of firearm was recommended to repel undead invaders. Meanwhile, after his *Coast to Coast AM* appearance, Schlozman got emails from listeners who wanted to know what medicines could stave off a zombie infection, and whether he had recommendations for how to protect one's home. China's state media had to formally debunk a robust rumor that Ebola victims were rising from the dead as zombies. And in 2014 in the Florida statehouse, a representative formally proposed "An Act Relating to the Zombie Apocalypse" as the name of a bill that would allow citizens to carry firearms without a permit in an emergency.

Shockingly, a 2015 survey showed that 2 percent of American adults thought the most likely apocalyptic scenario would be one caused by zombies.

And zombie references kept popping up in unexpected places. People downloaded audio fitness tracks in which joggers were kept motivated by imaginary zombie antagonists that pursued them as they ran. A man named Vermin Supreme, who sought the 2016 Libertarian Party nomination for president, added a platform plank on "zombie apocalypse awareness." He also advocated using zombies for renewable energy. Even Big Tech was in on it. Buried in Amazon's user agreement for a game-development engine, clause 57.10—a gag, probably?—read that the software should not be used in life-and-death situations, such as in medical equipment, nuclear facilities, spacecraft, or military combat operations. "However, this restriction will not apply in the event of the occurrence (certified by the United States Centers for Disease Control or successor body) of a widespread viral infection transmitted via bites or contact with bodily fluids that causes human corpses to reanimate and seek to consume living human flesh, blood, brain or nerve tissue and is likely to result in the fall of organized civilization."

With zombie stories saturating popular culture, the lore in TV and film began to expand beyond the simple trope of shambling brain eaters. There were zombie rom-coms and zombie mockumentaries. On the CW Television Network, a show called *iZombie* tells the story of a Seattle morgue worker infected by a zombie virus. In this world, zombies retain their personality and capacity for reason, as long as they are well fed (on brains). During the third season, which aired in 2017, a militant group of zombies releases a deadly flu virus in Seattle; local public health officials announce a mandatory flu vaccination, only to find that the zombies have tainted the vaccines with a substance that will turn the vaccinated into zombies.

Vaccines that zombified ordinary citizens?

Luckily for public health, no one would believe that in real life.

PART FOUR CONVALESCENCE (OR DEATH)

In which One True Cureism breaks the system

'Twas in the middle of the night,
To sleep Young William tried;
When Mary's Ghost came stealing in,
And stood at his bed-side.

O William dear! O William dear!
My rest eternal ceases;
Alas! my everlasting peace,
Is broken into pieces.

. . . .

The body-snatchers they have come,
And made a snatch at me;
It's very hard them kind of men,
Won't let a body be.

. . . .

My tender body was pack'd-up,
And in a sack did go;
To be a *little* body at,
Sir Dalley's great depôt.

I was cut up as *Stratford* was,
And *Y-ll-ly* from Carrow;
Came stealing in—and stole away,
My brains and spinal-marrow.

I vow'd that you should have my hand,
But fate gives us denial;
You'll find it there at Doctor *Wr-ght's*,
In spirits and a phial.

. . . .

As for my eyes,—the lovely eyes,
That once beam'd from their sockets;
You'll find them both at Mr. *H-ll's*,
In his *large* breeches-pockets.

My very skull was lent to *St-rk*,
Without any apology;
And all my lumps and bumps he found,
That are in Craniology.

. . . .

As for my feet,—the little feet,
You used to call so pretty;
There's one I know at the *Town-close*,
The t'other's in the *city*.

The *Pupils* dear, them sweet young men,
I vow they wrote on vellum;
A letter to the Doctors *big*,
And got my cerebellum.

. . . .

Don't go to weep upon my grave,
And think that there I be;
They hav'n't left an atom there,
Of my *anatomie*.

—Excerpts from "A Parody on 'Mary's Ghost';
or, The Doctors and Body-Snatchers," 1829

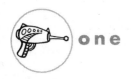**one**

LARRY LYTLE'S LASER LIGHT LEADS TO LIFE SENTENCE

This book has been written and published strictly for informational purposes and should not be substituted for consultation with your own health care professional. . . . The information imparted here is not the practice of medicine.

—Larry Lytle, "Disclaimer and Disavowal of Responsibility," *Innate Wisdom*, 2008

DESPITE THE FEDERAL INJUNCTION AGAINST LARRY LYTLE'S LASER operation, 2016 went on in much the same way that 2015 had, with Ronnie Weir and Irina Kossovskaia selling more lasers from their secret stockpile to distributors and members of the public, and sending more cash to Lytle's Old Cap Trust account.

A new year, 2017, dawned, bright with the promise of healing light. Lytle's hidden stockpile of lasers was shrinking, but surely it would be possible for the trio of conspirators to identify a new manufacturing partner.

Near the end of January, there was a knock on Lytle's door. It wasn't an FDA inspector. It wasn't an FDA investigator. It wasn't someone bearing a certified mail envelope with a capital-letter-laden warning letter inside.

It was a group of enforcement officers from the United States Postal Service. And the Postal Service does not play. They had guns, handcuffs, and a criminal indictment from a federal grand jury against one Robert Larry Lytle for eighteen criminal counts, including conspiracy, obstruction of the FDA, criminal contempt, providing false documents, mail fraud, wire fraud, and obstruction of agency proceedings.

Kossovskaia was arrested in New York and transported to Rapid City over the weekend. Lytle's longtime live-in partner, Fredretta Eason, who had been listed as the registered agent of Old Cap Inc., was charged with criminal contempt.

And where had the federal prosecutors gotten their key piece of evidence? From one Ronald "Ronnie" Weir Jr. In exchange for a reduced charge, Ronnie had told prosecutors that, on Lytle's behalf, he and his employees fielded phone calls from interested consumers and fed them misinformation. Sick people would ask whether the Q1000 could cure leukemia, gout, or some other disease. Ronnie affirmed that they all received the same answer: "The QLaser could safely and effectively treat it."

It didn't take Kossovskaia long to follow Ronnie's lead in cutting a deal. She was sentenced to fifteen months and Ronnie Jr. to two years, mostly in Pennington County Jail. When he got out, he was able to rejoin his wife and land a job in Rapid City's real estate market.

Lytle had far less leeway to make a deal. During his trial he was combative and erratic. He fired his lawyer for misrepresenting him. He tried to withdraw his guilty plea at one point, and he filed a suit in state court against his prosecutor.

When it finally came time for Lytle's testimony, he lied. He equivocated. He shifted blame. Nearly all the devices, he said, were sold by thirty-three other companies (his distributors), not by him. He said the lasers' efficacy had been proven in a diabetes study, though he couldn't produce it. Sure, he said, the Q1000 might not have worked all the time, but it was completely harmless in any case.

"I make no apologies for the QLaser," he said. "I believe in it."

But the case against Lytle was formidable.

Prosecutors said Lytle and his coconspirators had intentionally targeted elderly people with chronic, serious medical conditions. They presented thousands of pages of victim-impact information. A fifteen-year-old girl testified that her mother had forgone cancer treatment in favor of a QLaser system. Her mother's death, the teen said, "shattered my world." In all, the prosecution documented sales of twenty thousand lasers to thousands of elderly consumers for sales totaling $16.62 million between 2010 and 2015 alone.

Finally, in late January 2018, about a year after his arrest, Lytle pled guilty in a deal that won him little concession other than an assurance that the criminal contempt charge against his septuagenarian girlfriend, Fredretta, would be dropped. As part of the deal, he surrendered his trucks and his commemorative gold bullion. Prosecutors had already taken $239,711, spread over six different bank accounts, and Lytle forfeited another $637,000.

The only question was what society should do with Coach Larry Lytle, once a young boy in a sod house on the prairie, once a heroic civic leader building his community back from the ravages of a flood, once a well-respected dentist, but also someone who was so singularly minded that he seemed unable to operate within the bounds of the law.

Lytle and his daughter told the court that his freedom was vital to his continued health. He needed access to his QLaser, and he controlled his illnesses with diet and exercise.

The court clearly wrestled with the morals of the situation—it felt wrong to lock up an old man with murderers, but Lytle had displayed such a determination to flout the law that setting him free seemed likely to result in further mischief. The court considered his contribution to society as a dentist and as a member of the Rapid City Council. Ultimately, the eighty-three-year-old Lytle was sentenced to twelve years in prison.

The laser show was over.

Lytle immediately surrendered himself to US marshals and was transported to join the seventeen hundred inmates buried within the smothering heap of rock known as the Federal Correctional Institution, Gilmer, in West Virginia. For months he sat in a bleak cell. His millions of dollars were gone. His gold bullion was gone. He spent his eighty-fourth birthday behind bars. Then his eighty-fifth. A variety of age-related health problems began to steal over his body.

Records from the Bureau of Prisons showed that Lytle found it increasingly difficult to hear people speaking to him. He had diverticulitis, a condition in which little bits of food get caught in the intestinal walls, causing infections and inflammation that can be extremely painful. He had a disorder of the prostate and hypertensive heart disease. When he slept in his prison bed, he suffered from apnea, a medical condition that sometimes causes a person to stop breathing until a great, explosive gasp reestablishes the flow of oxygen. At some point, the pain of osteoarthritis in his hip caused him to begin using a wheelchair.

Lytle said he wanted to treat himself with a laser, but instead prison authorities addressed his various medical conditions in the way institutions do. They gave him a breathing apparatus to help his apnea, which Lytle said he couldn't plug in. They offered him eye exams and medication for his blood pressure, which he refused.

Lytle submitted an application for compassionate release, which allows for the discharge of prisoners who have not yet served out their sentence but are suffering health concerns that are inconsistent with incarceration. In order to qualify for compassionate release, an applicant must suffer from age-related chronic or serious medical conditions, or must be deteriorating to the point where they can no longer function within the institution.

Prison bureaucrats weighed what to do with Larry Lytle, who was wasting away while in their care. Would keeping the eighty-five-year-old behind bars make America safer? His case showed that even when the justice system invests the resources to finally put a purveyor of a One True Cure behind bars, there is no easy answer.

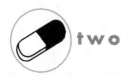 **two**

TOBY MCADAM'S SUPPLEMENTS SANCTIONED BY FDA

"Is there no hope?" the sick man said.
The silent doctor shook his head
And took his leave with signs of sorrow,
Despairing of his fee to-morrow.

—John Gay, "The Sick Man and the Angel," 1727

AFTER A LENGTHY LEGAL PROCESS, IN DECEMBER OF 2015 TOBY McAdam finally cut a deal and pled guilty to contempt of court. He was fifty-seven. Nine years had passed since the FDA first told him to stop selling products under false pretenses. Toby agreed to pay an $80,000 fine he had previously been assessed, plus $5,000 in attorney fees. He was sentenced to four months' incarceration.

Following court orders, Toby booked a plane ticket in early 2016 and boarded a flight to Englewood, Colorado, where he presented himself to the Federal Corrections Institution, a low-security prison for men.

"I never thought I would wind up in prison," he said. Even when he was sentenced, Toby had assumed he would ride out his four months in a local county lockup. "That's like putting somebody that jaywalked into state prison with felons."

During the check-in process, prison staff confiscated some painkillers he had made for himself for his bothersome sciatic nerves. Like the other inmates, he wore jeans and a blue shirt with prison-issued boots.

The prison contained an odd and eclectic mix of high-profile inmates who were either trying to live down, or up to, their reputations.

Less-well-known inmates whispered about Jeff Skilling, the former CEO of Enron, serving twenty-four years. Walter Lee Williams, a gender studies professor and human rights activist, was serving five years on charges related to sex acts with two underage boys. Scott Lee Kimball, who looked like an extra on *Sons of Anarchy*, had spent his time as a free man selling organic beef and committing murders. Armed robber Steve Nigg, a Wisconsin tough, enjoyed the twin distinctions of having been shot with a jury-rigged zip gun in an Arizona prison and playing Santa Claus at a hometown event between periods of incarceration.

Then there was Blago, the nickname for the former Democratic governor of Illinois Rod Blagojevich, imprisoned for various forms of corruption, including attempting to sell a US Senate seat. After Blago was forced to resign from office but before he was jailed, he appeared on the TV series *Celebrity Apprentice*, in which famous contestants were eliminated or retained based on their competence at executing business-related tasks. Before Blago was cut by the game show's host (for overseeing a Harry Potter–themed project that incorrectly called its famous fantasy castle "Hogwards"), a member of the public recognized him and said, "You're a disgrace. Enjoy prison!"

The thing was, in some ways Blago *was* enjoying prison. For three years he had been working with other inmates to help them obtain their GEDs. Another inmate had taught him to play guitar, and he was the lead singer for an Elvis-themed band he'd formed called the Jailhouse Rockers, which performed at inmates' GED graduation ceremonies.

Toby, Blago, and the rest of the inmates also had another pastime that eased the boredom of incarceration: keeping track of the 2016 United States presidential primaries.

Blago actually knew one of the Republican candidates: the former host of *Celebrity Apprentice* was mounting a longshot bid for president. It seemed almost impossible, given the blend of self-promotion and stream-of-consciousness that the host had broadcast on Twitter in the months and years leading up to his candidacy. One tweet: "The Mar-a-Lago Club has the best meatloaf in America. Tasty." Another: "I like Russell Brand, but Katy Perry made a big mistake when she married him. Let's see if I'm right—I hope not."

But of all the topics the game show host liked to comment on, none seemed more dear to his heart than television programming ratings. It was widely speculated that the goal of his candidacy was actually to stimulate viewership for *Celebrity Apprentice* and for a beauty pageant that he had purchased.

The game show host's tweets about ratings were almost obsessive. Oscar ratings were down, he noted. Monday-night *Apprentice* ratings were higher than Sunday-night *Apprentice* ratings. Journalist Lawrence O'Donnell's MSNBC program was an "unwatchable show dying in the ratings." The game show host's *Saturday Night Live* appearance led to the "best ratings in 4 years!"

As Toby got to know the ropes at Englewood, he learned that his fellow inmates were among those contributing to the game show host's ratings. The prison had three recreational rooms, each racially segregated from the other. All three rec rooms had televisions, and the television in each room was frequently tuned to news shows that featured coverage of the Republican primary.

One of Blago's fellow inmates, in a letter praising Blago's behavior, wrote that Blago had once made a math error during a GED lesson. "Well, you guys should take note of this and be encouraged," Blago said, to chuckles. "If I could be Governor, some of you guys could be President."

.·. :

OUTSIDE THE WALLS OF THE PRISON, ANOTHER GROUP WAS ALSO WATCHing the 2016 Republican presidential primaries with avid interest: the alternative healers and antivaccine activists who had joined forces in the medical-freedom movement. After just a decade or so of collaboration between the two groups, signs abounded of their influence on the major candidates. The supplement industry alone spent a record $9.7 million on the election cycle, giving medical-freedom activists a wide choice among candidates with ties to One True Cure–type products and services.

In early 2016, around the time Toby traded his shoes for prison boots, individuals were beginning to drop from the large field of eleven

Republican candidates. On February 1, it was former Arkansas governor Mike Huckabee, who in addition to selling his followers' emails to purveyors of ineffective heart disease cures took thousands in donations from supplement manufacturers. Huckabee's exit was quickly followed by that of Kentucky senator Rand Paul, author of the Health Freedom Act and longtime member of a right-wing medical-freedom group whose members did not believe that HIV causes AIDS but did believe that abortions cause breast cancer.

As the race narrowed, no one knew which of the candidates who owed a debt of gratitude to One True Cures would win. Would it be Florida senator Marco Rubio, who had taken more supplement money than anyone else in the field? Texas senator Ted Cruz, whose family's financial fortunes had once been saved by Mannatech, a religiously inspired supplement company? Mannatech also had ties to another primary candidate: Dr. Ben Carson, a neurosurgeon who took money from and promoted Mannatech, in part by crediting its products with helping treat his prostate cancer (Carson's political supporters received Mannatech-promoting emails).

Then there was the game show host, whose campaign strategy seemed to rely heavily on tweets about television ratings. If TV journalist Megyn Kelly stopped covering his candidacy, he opined, "her ratings would drop like a rock!" He noted that his interview with another journalist, Anderson Cooper, "beat her by millions!"

Other tweets by the game show host had more obvious appeal to the medical-freedom movement, including some that gave credence to the idea of "doctor-inflicted autism." He tweeted that "healthy young child goes to doctor, gets pumped with massive shot of many vaccines, doesn't feel good and changes—AUTISM! Many such cases!" During the campaign, the game show host also met with Andrew Wakefield, the disgraced doctor (and holder of a nutritional supplement patent) whose inaccurate study played a central role in spawning the vaccine-autism myth. The game show host had even himself sold a branded "health kit," which consisted of a pricey and scientifically dodgy package of vitamins and a urine test.

For the health-freedom activists, weirdly, the game show host was a pretty good horse to back. The guy seemed to believe anything.

•˙:˙

INSIDE THE PRISON, IT DIDN'T TAKE LONG FOR TOBY TO SUSS OUT THAT the game show host's campaign had most of his fourteen hundred fellow inmates not just intrigued but burbling with excitement. It was unclear whether Blago's influence played a role, but Toby estimated that 70 percent of Englewood's prison population would vote for the game show host, if convicted felons could legally vote, which was something the "tough-on-crime" game show host was vehemently opposed to.

There were signs that outside the Englewood facility, even the non-Blago-inhabited prisons across the country were full of fans of the game show host. In Maine, one of the few states that allows the incarcerated to cast ballots, a burgling, thieving drug trafficker serving ten years told reporters that he liked the game show host's vision for the economy. And in a couple of years, a first-of-its-kind 2018 poll of eight thousand prison inmates by the Marshall Project would find that the game show host had more support from inmates than any other candidate, a scathing indictment of the idea that humans act in their own interests.

As Toby's fellow Englewood residents became engrossed in the Republican primaries in which they could not participate, Toby drew a light-work detail in the prison's food service system because his sciatic nerves prevented him from lifting more than twenty pounds. In the sweltering-hot kitchen, he mopped floors and stacked boxes of food that had been donated for tax-write-off purposes. One day, it was hundreds of gallons of milk, a week past its expiration. Another day, a pallet of discarded chili from Wendy's that was nine months old.

Toby met a forty-year-old white guy from Indiana who also worked in the kitchen. He was well shaven and soft looking, even a bit flabby. The Indiana man was there because federal investigators had shown up on his doorstep one day with a warrant to search the premises. The Indiana man let them in, knowing that the incriminating pictures they were looking for—child pornography—were stored on a flash drive hidden in a secure location. However, the agents were accompanied by a Labrador retriever named Bear, one of three dogs in the United States that were trained to sniff out electronic media storage devices. The soft-looking Indiana man was sentenced to prison. Of all the inmates who had some sort of notoriety, none drew as much attention as Toby's new workmate. Every time he entered a room, a little ripple of energy flowed through the crowd. Even the guards were a bit starstruck, trying to draw him into friendly conversations.

The man was Jared Fogle, famous for years as the pitchman for the Subway sandwich chain. In the commercials, Jared held up an enormous pair of pants and explained how he had gone from 425 pounds to 180 pounds through walking and eating a Subway sandwich for lunch each day (an ad campaign that was in its way just as disingenuous as One True Cures).

In Englewood prison's kitchen, Toby found Jared kind of likable.

"He's not an arrogant person. He doesn't have that ego," said Toby. "He was actually a pretty nice, easy-to-get-along-with guy. A lot of inmates were."

Soon, Toby and Fogle took to sitting in the hot kitchen together, goofing off for as long as they could get away with. Fogle still had access to money, so he bought whatever he wanted from the prison canteen. Toby offered to go through Fogle's case files and act as his jailhouse lawyer to look for possible legal loopholes. Toby intended to, upon his release, give information about Fogle to TMZ, the news organization that specializes in celebrity dirt. He told me he took pictures of Fogle, hoping to sell those too.

Despite his fame, Fogle was actually in a tough spot. Others saw arrogance in Fogle that Toby did not. And the nature of his charges branded him as a social pariah. In the kitchen one day, Fogle told Toby that other inmates were threatening him.

"Don't worry," responded Toby, who saw himself as a bit of a heavy. "If you have issues, let me know."

Fogle's solution was to pay two large inmates to act as his bodyguards. Soon after, Toby was watching Fogle in the yard as he walked around the track, his two muscled companions flanking him. Also on the track was Steve Nigg, the former Santa Claus and armed robber, strolling in the opposite direction. Nigg walked past Fogle and said hello to him. When Fogle turned to respond, Nigg punched him in the face. Toby watched as Fogle fell down. Nigg kept punching. Fogle's bodyguards did nothing.

By the time the prison guards broke up the conflict, the two men had injured each other. Fogle's nose was bloody, his neck scratched and bleeding, his face swollen and bruised.

Nigg was also in pretty bad shape—he had a small cut on his left hand, inflicted by Jared's face.

Nigg was sent to solitary confinement and became an instant legend among the prison population—and certain segments of the American public. Fogle won continued humiliation and attention for his crimes.

Toby shed no tears for Fogle. But when Toby was released on May 3, 2016, the guards confiscated the photos of Fogle that he'd hoped to sell to TMZ.

.·:·

As a free man, Toby didn't get to see the celebrations of Blago and the other prisoners when the game show host won the final Republican primaries. Before accepting the nomination for president at the party's convention in July, the game show host commented on the momentousness of the occasion. "One of the best produced, including the incredible stage & set, in the history of conventions. Great unity! Big T.V. ratings!"

After accepting the nomination he offered more insight. "The ratings for the Republican National Convention were very good," he wrote, "but for the final night, my speech, great. Thank you!"

The game show host then unexpectedly won the presidency. At his inaugural ball, disgraced antivax doctor Andrew Wakefield showed up with his new girlfriend—Australian supermodel Elle Macpherson—on his arm and threw down the gauntlet to the medical establishment.

"What we need now is a huge shakeup at the Centers for Disease Control and Prevention—a huge shakeup," Wakefield told reporters. "We need that to change dramatically."

It was a sign that the medical-freedom movement was about to be focused, marshaled, and organized through the highest levels of government in an effort to tear down, rather than reform, regulatory agencies and the medical establishment.

In a three-day stretch in early March 2017, the game show host, by then the president, appointed Mannatech shillman Ben Carson to head the federal Department of Housing and Urban Development, saw a massive gas pipeline leak threaten the Alaskan wilderness, and received military briefings on two Taliban bombings in Farah Province and Kabul in Afghanistan, which left twenty-four dead and more than sixty injured.

They were sad times, and so the president tweeted a message expressing sorrow to the American public. "Arnold Schwarzenegger isn't voluntarily leaving the Apprentice," he wrote from the White House, "he was fired by his bad (pathetic) ratings, not by me. Sad end to great show."

•˙:˙•

THE ONLY THING THAT HAD GIVEN TOBY'S LIFE REAL MEANING WAS TO sell supplements. His knowledge constituted a One True Cure that could extend the human life span by decades. His continuing to sell them was his mother's dying wish. It was Elon Musk's directive. It was his most successful career. But now he couldn't do that without going back to prison.

He returned to Billings, Montana, and opened a storefront called Spices of Life Soups for You, also known as RisingSun Soups for You. The soup and organic salad shop, he pointed out, was not using municipal water, which meant his offerings were free of toxins and chlorine. It felt good to say that, but even he had to admit that the healthiest of his soup offerings couldn't cure cancer. As he dished out bowl after bowl, a part of his mind was elsewhere. He'd been incarcerated for what he saw as a minor offense over a principled stance. The FDA had won that battle. But did that mean they would win the war? Toby considered different long-term tactics. Like an organic watermelon gazpacho, his revenge was a dish best served cold.

In the meantime, perhaps inspired by the game show host's improbable victory in the presidential race, Toby decided to reenter the political sphere. As an established system disruptor who spoke truth to power, he expected to send shockwaves throughout the relatively small world of Montana politics.

In July 2017 Toby signed up for a Twitter account to put out the word. "I get involved in politics when the politicians don't get things done and lie," his profile read. "My profession is a master herbalist. I became involved when my mother became ill."

His first tweet read, ominously, "Just getting started. Seem the politicians aren't going to do anything on tax reform. I guess its time to come out of retirement."

Over time he gained two Twitter followers. One was a local newspaper editor. The other was a digital marketing firm. On Twitter and other social media platforms, his tough-talking, derisive posts directed at public officials went unanswered, unretweeted, unrequited, unliked.

The supplements, it turned out, had also been the driving force behind his online audience. Before prison, his latest YouTube video, about bloodroot capsules, had racked up ten thousand views; his first post-incarceration video, about "Eclipse sun tea," had five (not five thousand. Just . . . five).

After about a year, his soup shop closed.

Soup. Politics. They just weren't his calling. He drifted.

Though he considered himself an optimist, it was impossible for him to ignore the dark things happening in the world. Like the control that a shadowy and menacing Deep State was exerting on government. Or the possibility of biological warfare creating real-life zombies, like that guy in Miami.

The Deep State had pushed the Democratic Party away from the Roosevelt roots that had won the support of his departed mother. Though Toby thought the Deep State also had pretty strong hooks in the Republican Party, he voted for Republicans as a lesser evil.

He predicted that the day would come, perhaps soon, for Americans to take up arms against one another en masse. In Montana, every truck had a gun rack, and every rack had one or more guns.

"All hell's going to break loose," he told me one day. "A guy I know says the Democrats are stupid. Who has the guns?"

He told me he had successfully created a turbine that generated power for an electric car. It looked like a little water fountain and held a battery. But vandals destroyed the prototype. Now that he had more time on his hands, he was thinking about rebuilding. He toyed with the idea of a GoFundMe campaign, but it never happened.

One July, he announced that he had invented the first portable personal air cooler, which looked like a beer cooler full of ice that blasted air out through a PVC pipe.

A woman bought one for $600, but after paying him she decided she didn't want it. She didn't take the cooler, but Toby refused to refund the money. When she took him to court, Toby defended himself. He tried to subpoena city officials as expert witnesses but was convicted of theft. He appealed. The amount of restitution he was ordered to pay was reduced from $600 to $540, meaning he was still out 90 percent of the money. But to him, the glass was 10 percent full.

Toby was also absorbing other ideas from the community of medical-freedom advocates and alternative healers. Larry Lytle described universal healing light, Robert Young called it cosmic energy, but to Toby it was life force. The life force persists, he believed, even when a person's physical form expires—a sentiment shared by the alien in Jim Humble's skin. More and more, Toby sensed an emotional register from the otherworld. Unseen forces, he said, were worried and were pushing him to act.

And so, Toby roamed around his Montana home, keeping himself occupied. He tinkered. He puttered. When his phone rang he answered it. He cleaned out a storage locker and sold some of the contents. He played with his dog, Cosmo. Until Cosmo died.

Then Toby's sister, Jeanie, died. She had once sold a pair of sunglasses to Robert Young's (maybe) ex-brother-in-law Robert Redford when he had been in the area to film *A River Runs Through It*. Jeanie liked to tell people she had "touched Robert Redford's ears!" It was a stroke.

Though Toby's relationship with Jeanie had been strained at times, he mourned her, as he had his parents. And his brothers. He was a survivor.

Sometimes he visited his mother's grave and talked to her. As always, Frances was there for him. "I see my mom. I can feel it."

Other times, when he sat on his porch or in a chair, he might feel Cosmo's glossy fur rubbing against the palm of his hand, as though the dog were seeking attention the way he had in life. Or it would be his brother's ghost, grabbing him by the hair of his neck—aggressive but good-natured. These experiences sometimes inspired Toby to come up with an herbal formula. The FDA said he couldn't sell such things anymore, but he jotted them down anyway.

In fact, all the while he had been toiling over pots of soup and portable air coolers and political tweets and ghosts and electric cars and all the rest of it, he had never let go of supplements. He would get back in the game, and the FDA, he felt sure, could not stop him. This would be his revenge.

"Whenever I'm told something can't be done," he told me, "I will do it."

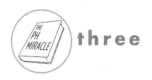 **three**

ROBERT O. YOUNG'S PH MIRACLE HELPS CANCER

> "You really are better, dear, whether you can see it or not. I am a doctor, dear, and I know. You are gaining flesh and color, your appetite is better. I feel really much easier about you."
>
> "I don't weigh a bit more," said I, "nor as much; and my appetite may be better in the evening, when you are here, but it is worse in the morning when you are away."
>
> "Bless her little heart!" said he with a big hug; "she shall be as sick as she pleases!"
>
> —Charlotte Perkins Gilman, "The Yellow Wallpaper," 1892

D AWN KALI'S BODY WAS A METAPHOR FOR THE MIRACLE RANCH itself; she shimmered with positivity and promise, while beneath her skin, cancer.

Her back pain never really went away anymore. Then, in 2013, a few lumps surfaced in her lymph nodes. Kali was determined to stick to the pH Miracle lifestyle, and that was making it difficult to have conversations with certain people outside the ranch, people who just didn't understand that the alkaline diet was on the brink of revolutionizing health care. Her therapist, she felt, judged her for refusing conventional treatment. And then there was Dr. Grissom, the surgeon.

"I'm really afraid that it's finally getting away from you," Grissom said when Kali visited her to approve some blood work. "I just don't want it to get to the point that it's too late."

Kali knew that doubts would just impede her work with Young, so she blocked them out, insulating herself from those sorts of judgments as much as possible.

That's not going to be me, Kali told herself.

Back at the ranch, sunshine poured and smoothies flowed. Kali had a PICC (peripherally inserted central catheter) installed so that Young could infuse her blood with baking soda solutions more easily. When she told Young during an exercise class that the previous night's IV had given her flu-like aches all over her body, he told her that was a positive sign—she was detoxing.

"Any time you got diarrhea, or got sick, that was all detox," she said. "Everything that was wrong was good."

Young, incidentally, has denied under oath ever touching, diagnosing, or giving medical treatment to Kali. He said she was not a patient but a friend that he was helping with lifestyle advice.

Over time, a thread of anxiety began to wind itself around Kali's heart, and she couldn't dispel it. Her back hurt. She craved solid food. She worried that her "stinking thinking" was interfering with Young's program.

Later in 2013, feeling poorly, Kali decided to go see Dr. Garrett Smith, an integrative oncologist who employed both alternative and conventional cancer treatments. Kali arrived with her favorite aunt, the one who had taught Kali that oncologists were the devil.

"I looked around. It didn't feel like Hell," Kali said. In fact, it looked like a spa. "It was this beautiful, artistic—panoramic views, leather chairs, and art everywhere."

Kali's aunt grilled Smith about his credentials and about conventional treatments. Smith took it all in stride. After reviewing Kali's case, Smith told her that conventional treatments were like rungs on a ladder.

"He suggested we try the lowest rung. I said, 'I'm lower than that.' He said okay. He baby-stepped me."

After seeing Kali's lab results, Smith recommended a PET scan, an imaging test that floods portions of the body with a dye for better visibility of the cancer. Over the objections of her aunt, Kali went ahead with it.

The results were horrific. The cancer had spread to various parts of her body—it was in her chest, in her lymph nodes, up and down her spine, which explained the pain and spasms in her back. Her bones were losing mass: 50 percent of her femur was gone, her hip was in danger of fracturing, and Smith said that so much as a sneeze could break her back.

Some small part of Kali had expected this news, but most of her had clung to the hope that Young's opinion about her condition was correct. And so, while sitting in Smith's office, she took out her phone.

"The first person I called was Young."

When he didn't answer, she called the office and told someone to track him down, that it was an emergency. She explained to Young what she was hearing. He told her to follow Dr. Smith's advice.

Even then, Kali didn't believe that Young's theories were wrong—she blamed her own failure to follow Young's protocols.

During a course of heavy-duty chemotherapy, the cancer inside her wilted. Her bones began to heal themselves. She sent Young images from a fresh PET scan, asking him for input into her progress.

A few months later, Kali noticed that Young had published a blog post with images labeled "before" and "after." They were reproductions of her PET scans. He credited the pH Miracle Diet with putting her cancer into remission. It was a small thing. And yet.

For Kali, seeing that post caused a crack in the thick hull of her perceptions of alkalarianism. It was hard for her to view her improvement as a victory for the alkaline diet. She was now working with a nondevil oncologist. His conventional treatments were undeniably the more plausible explanation.

It got her thinking. Which side of the looking glass was she on?

In 2014, as Young's criminal trial for practicing medicine without a license unfolded, she watched Moe Felix testify. Felix had met his wife, Vicki, when they were in their twenties and she was working in Colorado as a ski instructor. They'd been married for twenty-five years. Vicki had received IV treatments at the ranch before dying of breast cancer.

"We desperately were looking for a way to prolong her life," Felix said to Young from the stand. "You, with an air of arrogance and without the blink of an eye, told us you could cure Vicki. You seemed to be the light in the darkness, but you were the darkness."

Kali, by then in treatment for her alcoholism, had a new appreciation for the importance of honesty, to others and to oneself. She cast a fresh eye on all the trappings of authority with which Young had surrounded himself—trappings formed from the densest of smoke, the most deflective of mirrors. As the criminal trial progressed, she realized there were no doctorates. There was no compelling body of research supporting his theories. There weren't even any testimonials, not really. She could only think of a single patient who had claimed to be cancer free posttreatment, and that woman had no documentation.

Far too late, the truth hit her.

"I realized," she said, "that he had almost killed me."

.•:•

To Young, the monthslong sentence in prison had been a ridiculously heavy-handed punishment. But to Kali, it felt like not nearly enough. And so, in 2018, she filed her own lawsuit against Young.

She sought $52 million. Given that, even in extreme cases involving a wrongful death, the median verdict is $2.2 million, it was an insane ask. And Kali was still alive.

As the civil trial got underway, Young had support from both inside and outside the courthouse. One of Young's patients established a Go-FundMe account and raised $32,000 for his legal defense. His son, Adam, and daughter-in-law, Samoni, sat in the courtroom every day. Maurice Vanderhaeghen, widower of Young's deceased friend and patient Genia, told the court that the Vanderhaeghens understood that the ranch provided a "lifestyle treatment" rather than a medical treatment. He said Young was consistently "very kind and caring."

Kali was represented by Bibianne "Bibi" Fell, who taught trial advocacy at the University of San Diego School of Law. Fell, who wore blue suits and had chestnut hair that fell to her shoulders, was known for being dogged in her preparations and quick-thinking enough to turn unexpected moments to her advantage.

Young was represented by Conrad Joyner, who had white whiskers on the scalp of his round head and whose prominent ears gave him the look of an honest, earnest farmer. Joyner (whose father was a beloved local politician and a skilled trial lawyer) had spent the last twenty-six years in courtrooms, mastering the art of delivering folksy authenticity in a pleasing tenor voice.

During the trial, Dr. Smith testified to Kali's medical condition: stage IV cancer had eaten away 50 percent of the bone mass in some areas of her spine. Had she followed conventional treatments when it was at stage I, she would have had a 90 percent chance of becoming cancer free. Now she was incurable.

Kali's health wasn't in question. The real legal question was whether her cancer had spread because of her own poor decisions, or whether it was Young's fault.

Fell's overall strategy was a difficult balancing act. She wanted to show that Young's take on cancer was ludicrous—but she also needed to establish that he was plausible enough for Kali to reasonably believe him. Fell also worried about how Kali would be perceived.

"The jury could hate her because she wound up marketing for Young and bringing more victims to him," Fell later said. "We were walking several different tightropes all over the place."

Joyner's strategy, meanwhile, was simply to show that Young believed in himself. If Young had good intentions and promoted an alkaline diet earnestly, rather than as a fraud, it would dramatically limit his legal liability. Proving that Young believed in himself? Piece of alkaline cake.

The trial had many highlights, but one that went unremarked on by observers came when Young said he couldn't remember exactly what he had told Kali about her blood.

"I would have commented not quantitatively, but qualitatively," he said. "I would show her a picture of what a healthy red blood cell looks like—which is round and symmetrical, even in color, even in shape, even in size—and I would show her a picture of what unhealthy blood looks like, which is uneven in shape, uneven in its color, and its form. And, here again, it's not objective science; it's subjective science."

In just seven words—"it's not objective science; it's subjective science"—Young had inadvertently shown why his theories were not science at all. Long before Louis Pasteur came up with a test for germ theory that could be replicated around the world, even before the Numbers Junkies began to put their stamp on the practice of medicine, from the moment the scientific revolution and the age of reason began, the entire point of science has been to acquire knowledge that is objectively true. Gravity, distance, the speed of light—all these concepts are universally embraced because they can be tested by anyone, at any time.

Objective science has a term for a subjective scientific observation. It's called a hypothesis, which can be proven only with objective tests.

But at the time, Young's comment went unchallenged, and Fell found herself scanning the faces of the jury, trying unsuccessfully to figure out whether they were buying into Young's scientific jargon and authoritative tone. The prospect terrified her.

"He looked good on the stand. He sounded good on the stand. He used all those big words," Fell said. She recognized the image he was projecting.

"All the professorial things we do for our experts, to stand up and use visuals, he did all that. He was a textbook expert. It was scary."

Fell redoubled her efforts to make Young seem unlikable and uncaring. She let the jury see him struggle to remember the names of his deceased patients. She brought up Vicki Felix, whose husband had lambasted Young as "the darkness" during his recent criminal trial.

"Vicki Felix was a client and she passed away?" asked Fell.

"I don't recall Vicki Felix," said Young.

"Moe Felix was her husband," said Fell. "He testified at your criminal trial."

"Oh, yes. Vicki. Yes. Okay," said Young.

"She was a client and she passed away?"

"Yes. After she left the ranch, yes," said Young.

It was up to Joyner to counteract that impression by highlighting Young's very real emotional connection to his other clients.

"What about Vanderhaeghen?" Joyner asked a little later. Surely, the unforgettably named Genia Vanderhaeghen, who had so moved Young with her request to die at the ranch and whose husband had supported Young in his legal trials, would generate an emotion out of Young that would spark some rapport with the jury. "What was the name?"

There was a moment of awful, awful silence.

"What *was* her name?" Young repeated back. He didn't remember.

"Right," asked Joyner.

"I think it's in the record," said Young. "I'm trying to—I think her name was—not Fabienne. That was her daughter." (Fabienne, incidentally, the woman whose name he *could* remember, was a fashion model in her twenties.)

"It's okay," said Joyner, forging ahead gamely. "Vanderhaeghen."

June Asisi, who had stopped working at the Miracle Ranch in March 2013, had testified at Young's criminal trial that she, Young, and other members of the staff routinely hid the fact that Young was administering IVs without a license. Asisi also testified about Dan Barkin, the patient from Las Vegas that Kali had seen at the ranch forcing himself through grueling exercises. According to Asisi, when Barkin ran out of money, he offered to give Young some gold Krugerrands, South African coins worth nearly $2,000 apiece. Young agreed to take them as payment.

A week after Barkin left the ranch, Young told Asisi to drive to Las Vegas to pick up the coins. She made the three-hundred-mile drive, but when she got there she learned that after leaving the Miracle Ranch, Barkin had seen a medical doctor. His cancer had gotten much worse, and he was not parting with his Krugerrands. Kali said Young complained about the nonpayment.

"I give and I give," she remembered him saying. "I can't not help people."

Less than a month later, Barkin was dead.

At the criminal trial more details surfaced about Naima Houder-Mohammed, the determined twenty-seven-year-old British army officer who wrote to Young soon after receiving a diagnosis of breast cancer. He told her that treatments sometimes cost $3,000 per day, and that her "healing program" would take at least eight to twelve weeks of a daily regime plus "hyper-perfusing the blood with alkalinity."

Houder-Mohammed went into a frenzy of fundraising, convinced this was her best chance at life. Her family raided their savings accounts and worked with charities to run fundraising events in the community. Their family business folded.

"One last thing," Young wrote to Houder-Mohammed before she flew to America, "my office needs funds wired to them before you arrive. Have you done this? I hope to see you soon. Regards, Dr. Young."

In all, she paid Young $77,000—everything she had—over three months. When her cancer worsened she left the ranch and checked into a hospital, which soon discharged her to the UK to die among family.

Back at the civil trial, Young seemed to be doing his best to convince the jury that the pH Miracle worked. He expounded on so many medical topics that the judge reminded the jury that Young was not recognized by the court as an expert on medicine, science, or anything else.

In an effort to gain insight into the minds behind the impassive faces of the jury, Fell brought in a focus group to view the courtroom proceedings so that she could consider tailoring her approach in the trial's final phases. "We learned what we already knew, which was that Dawn Kali's involvement was a real problem," Fell said.

Fell, relentless, brought up Young's infidelity, his divorce, and his $200,000 in child support arrears. She documented fifteen of Young's cancer clients who had died, in some cases presenting their death certificates. Fell pulled out copies of Young's books and read excerpts to the jury. She opened his 2013 book, *Reverse Cancer Now*, the cover of which trumpets that it is "scientifically proven to prevent and reverse cancer," and began to quote from it.

"'In fact, to this day, most doctors and many patients still believe that cancer is a physical thing, a tumor. In reality, a tumor is the solution of cancer, not its cause. A tumor is simply a physical manifestation of bound up acidic cells so they do not spoil other healthy cells,'" she read. Then, to Young: "Do you agree?"

"Yes."

Young's words during the trial were the same as they had been at the ranch. But how different they now seemed!

"'Most heart attacks or cancer are brought on by our thoughts,'" read Fell.

"Agree," said Young.

Fell was successfully tagging Young with all sorts of negative attributes—he cared for people too little and for money too much, and he was operating in service of a bizarre theory that was wildly out of sync with established medicine.

Despite all of this, Joyner was accomplishing his main trial objective: Young's testimony showed that he had staked his entire life on his "scientific" beliefs. Whatever character flaws he might have, it seemed obvious that Young believed in the pH Miracle lifestyle himself and therefore was simply offering his purported knowledge to his clients in good faith.

As Fell worked her way through a stack of books written by Young, she quoted some of the more outlandish claims in each, and then set it on the table beside her. When she happened to glance down, she noticed something that had escaped her attention during her extensive pretrial preparations. Spontaneously, she used the court's projector to display an image of the back cover of one of the books, which included a photograph of Young, much younger and—strangely unlike the man sitting in the witness box—bald.

Fell later described Young's reaction as electric. "You could feel his anger. His face got beet red, and I thought he was just going to jump out of that chair and come at me."

Nevertheless, she persisted.

"Is that a picture of you on the back?" she asked.

"Yes, without hair," said Young. Every eye in the jury box went to the full head of hair he sported in the courtroom.

"Have you ever made the claim that you were able to regrow your hair with your diet, nutritional supplements and your program?" asked Fell.

"Well, I have made the claim that hair regrowth can happen if all things are present," said Young. "A proper environment, maybe some seed in order for new hair growth to take place and the right kinds of shampoos and conditioners."

This was actually a point on which under-oath Young and not-under-oath Young differed. When promoting Young pHorever Head pHirst Shampoo as a cure for baldness, not-under-oath Young made no mention that "maybe some seed" was a factor. Not-under-oath Young's message seemed to be that he had relied wholly on his own science during his "personal journey" of "reversing baldness." Fell then posed the key question to under-oath Young.

"And so did you regrow your hair with your pH Miracle system?"

Young was forced to say what Fell already knew. People don't grow hair by drinking vegetable smoothies.

"My hair regrowth and my program in this particular case," he admitted, "started with some transplantations of about 1,000 grafts."

In other words, when it came to treating his own male-pattern baldness, Young believed, as most people do, in paying a licensed medical doctor to use evidence-based science to perform hair transplant surgery. When Fell extracted that simple statement, she showed the jury that Young did not believe in himself, or in the pH Miracle Diet he had sold to Kali for years.

Young was pHucked.

.·:·'

BEFORE ATTEMPTING TO JUSTIFY THE SIZE OF THE $52 MILLION LAWSUIT, Fell asked Young whether he had any remorse for his actions related to Dawn Kali. For what he did.

"What I did," Young repeated. "I pray for Dawn, I love Dawn. It brings tears to my eyes when I think about what's happened to her. I mean, I'm a human being. I care about people. I still care about her."

Young had, either intentionally or unintentionally, responded as if Fell had asked whether he felt empathy for Kali's pain.

"Do you have any remorse for what you did to Dawn?" asked Fell.

He continued to misinterpret.

"Dawn Kali, I have remorse that she's suffering," Young said. "Dawn Kali makes her own decisions. Her situation was her own personal choice. You know, from her aunt and her mother to all of it. I tried to help her every way that I can, financially, emotionally."

"Objection," said Fell. "Nonresponsive."

"It is nonresponsive," agreed the judge. He addressed Young: "Do you understand the question?"

"Ask it again, please?" said Young.

Fell did, emphasizing the relevant parts.

"Do you have any remorse for what *you did* with respect to Dawn Kali?"

Young seemed to lack understanding of the premise.

"I'm not sure," he said, "what I did that would have harmed her in any way."

.∴.

KALI'S $52 MILLION ASK INCLUDED A FEW DIFFERENT CATEGORIES OF DAM-ages. She had already incurred $576,000 in medical bills, the cost of 124 visits with Dr. Smith, who estimated that she would incur about another $280,000. And then she would incur no more.

Kali was also seeking $2.5 million for pain and suffering and $10 million in punitive damages, to deter Young from continuing to treat people.

But the big-ticket item was "future noneconomic damages," the pain and suffering yet to come. The average woman of Kali's age would live for another 38.8 years. Dr. Smith said Kali would live no more than five or six. In an ideal world, said Fell, she would give Kali those years back. But that was impossible.

"All we can do is give her money. That's our system of justice. That is all we have to compensate her for these incredible losses."

Fell suggested that the jury award Kali $1 million for each year of lost life.

"Would she pay a million dollars for another single year with her family?" Fell asked rhetorically. "Absolutely she would do it. Would she pay a million dollars to see her eight-year-old get married? Absolutely she would do it. So for the thirty-three years, $33.8 million."

As the five-day trial wound down and Fell and Joyner made their closing arguments, it was clear that Kali had suffered a terrible tragedy—but was it really Young's fault? How much blame was his, and how much was the fault of Kali's aunt or of Kali herself?

During Joyner's closing argument, he pointed out that Kali had already outlived the average life span of someone with her diagnosis, thereby implying that the pH Miracle had in fact helped extend her life.

But to Fell, that was the wrong framing. "It's not just, did she get a few more years," she said later. "That's not part of the equation. She should have survived, with the surgery."

After just three hours, the jury filed back into the courtroom. The unread verdict in the hand of the foreperson created unbearable levels of suspense for both Kali and Young. Conventional wisdom is that a deliberation of less than four hours is a bad sign for the plaintiff, often indicating an impasse or a fatal flaw in the case. But as Kali watched, one of the men in the jury caught her eye and threw her a wink.

That's when she knew she had won.

The jury found that Young was at fault for Kali's medical state, but they disagreed with Fell's request of $33.8 million for her anticipated loss of life. Instead, they awarded her $84.5 million for that category of damages.

In all, the judgment against Young totaled a staggering $105,356,000. Among those staggered was Young, who told reporters that it was "totally outrageous" and "appalling."

"It's one-tenth of a billion," he said, as if still trying to wrap his hirsute head around it.

A colleague of Fell's told the press that he hoped the verdict would "have an effect on the miracle, cure-all cancer industry."

But not only did the verdict fail to have a discernible impact on the One True Cure industry; it failed to have a discernible impact on Young, at least in terms of his accepting any moral responsibility for Kali's health.

After the trial Young posted an online rebuttal, "The Truth About Dawn Kali," in which he noted that (1) an Italian doctor (who had been stripped of his license) also gave baking soda IVs; (2) people die while on chemo, and no one is blaming chemo; and (3) he had actually been very generous with Kali, not only giving her free treatments but actually paying her (for her work). Young estimated that from 2010 to 2013 he gave Dawn Kali more than $450,000 in services and money. Apparently he threw in the cancer for free.

"No good deed," he wrote, "goes unpunished!"

Joyner said the jury had improperly awarded damages as if Young were acting maliciously. "No matter if you believe in the pH Miracle or disbelieve it, it's clear that Robert believes it," Joyner said. "He sincerely believes what he is doing."

After Young appealed, a trial court found that Kali could be paid for suffering only for the years she was expected to live, not the years in which she would be dead. They reduced the damages significantly.

Still, she wound up with a $26 million judgment.

Among Young's many defenses is a libertarian position that holds that when a person is led to bad decisions, the fault lies with the decision maker, who is ultimately the individual. Philosophically, it is the opposite of terrain theory. Instead of the root cause lying within the confusing conditions of a fact-muddling atmosphere, Young says the cause of a flawed decision lies with the individual who has come to that decision.

In other words, don't blame the water. Blame the fish.

After Kali's victory, the main operation at the Miracle Ranch—the treating of "clients" with IVs and other exorbitantly priced treatments—was, at last, closed. But, admissions about hair transplants aside, Young said he still believed in himself. And he was about to find others who also believed in him. Soon he was putting the FDA on trial before the members of a judiciary assemblage who were the highest authorities in the world.

According to them.

.•.:`

DAWN KALI TOLD ME THAT FOR YEARS AFTER THE TRIAL, SHE GOT EMAILS from Young's supporters. From their perspective she'd committed the worst kind of treachery: he gave her everything, and then she turned on him.

But everything he gave her—money, employment, even hope—was ephemeral. Only the cancer remained. In 2014, when she decided to abandon the pH Miracle in favor of established science-based treatments, she found the medical establishment difficult to love.

It certainly didn't seem to love her. The streets surrounding the hospitals were jammed with traffic. Each potential parking spot was occupied by a stranger, someone with their own problems, their own incipient tragedy, whether that meant a terminal illness or an infected toenail.

Once inside the hospital, she felt tiny and lost, caught on the back of an uncaring beast. There was no wheedling her way into a trip to Thailand. There was no impromptu karaoke with her medical provider. She walked down long hospital hallways, alone in the crowds. It was always a different nurse with a needle in hand, poking her wrong, or overpoking her. The staff who administered her chemo practically wore hazmat suits.

Sometimes she cried.

"Even with everything I knew, it was so overwhelming," she said. "How many times do I have to say my name and my birth date over and over?"

She tried to get to know the staff, but it was impossible. When she got mad at them, they didn't seem to care about that either. She was just a patient. A bit of work to do, indistinguishable from the next. Spiritually, there was nothing positive about the experience, no sustenance, no warmth, no humanity.

But there was something. At the ranch, she told me, her cancer was out of control.

"It was raging," she said. But enduring the indignities of the hospital changed things. "Now I'm getting it tamed. I'm managing it."

Over time, she learned the ins and outs of the hospital. She figured out where the parking spots were. Once she understood the layout, the hallways seemed to shrink to a less imposing size. Kali even began to see an upside to the hospital's enforced anonymity. It became a form of independence. A form of freedom.

"Now I don't want to know anyone," she said. She was a survivor. "Everyone at the ranch, they're all dead. Now the impersonality is okay."

.· : ·

IN LATE 2019 FIVE COMMISSIONERS SAT AT A LONG CONFERENCE TABLE on a dais in Bali, Indonesia. They were dressed in black. The table was draped in dark fabric, and a black cloth covered the wall behind them.

This was a proceeding of the International Tribunal for Natural Justice, "a judicial organ of the free and sovereign peoples of the world";

though, as organs go, it was quite modest. It was founded to hold a global conspiracy of secret world leaders accountable for their crimes against humanity. Then they will no doubt address the typos on their website. But first, justice!

The ITNJ had been doing its work for about six years. In that time, it closed just a single case, one involving the National Child Protection Alliance. The NCPA sought an ITNJ ruling that the Commonwealth of Australia was in breach of the United Nations' Convention on the Rights of the Child. But after applying for its case to be heard, and paying roughly $1,400 in application fees, the NCPA wound up filing a complaint against the ITNJ members themselves, accusing them of misrepresenting the ITNJ's credentials to induce the NCPA's application. In fact, the NCPA complained, the ITNJ had no recognition or standing in Australia. Or, really, in any country on the planet.

The NCPA's complaints against the commissioners of the ITNJ were heard by the commissioners of the ITNJ. Not surprisingly they denied all charges, bringing their first case to a speedy resolution. Justice!

Among the dark-robed commissioners sitting at the table in Bali was Sacha Stone. He'd pursued a brief, failed career as a rocker in the 1990s and still had a bit of Russell Brand appeal to him—long black hair, beguiling British accent, shirts often worn open to the midriff, and a free-flowing eloquence that struck the right balance between personal warmth and intellectual argot.

Stone was the primary promoter of a product called the 5GBioShield, a "wearable holographic nano-layer catalyser" intended to protect one from 5G mobile phone network emissions. It retailed for $465, but according to a London antifraud organization, it is nothing more than a USB drive with a light embedded in a bit of glass, available for five dollars from Chinese suppliers.

But Stone hadn't come to Bali to sell BioShields. He addressed his fellow commissioners.

"Among the 7.5 billion-odd souls that inhabit the surface of the world," Stone said, the next witness was "probably one of the dozen top-targeted individuals, targeted by the global corporatocracy, the global pharmaceutical enterprise, that element of the global pharmaceutical enterprise which appears . . . to have been weaponized against humanity."

The person Stone introduced sat at an adjacent black-swathed table and had followed the color lead of the commissioners by wearing a black jacket with a gold disk on the lapel.

It was triple-PhD (unaccredited), research scientist (uncertified), Eagle Scout (certified), grower of avocados (certified), and grower of hair (uncertified) Robert Young.

Young had, since his legal troubles, broadened his scientific understanding. He'd written a paper that attributed the success of his alkaline One True Cure to cosmic energies, his own version of Lytle's universal healing light.

"The microzyma," he wrote, "may be seen as an early, if not the primary, transmutation from the fine vibrations of the Cosmic Life Force into a denser form or pattern of life. . . . During formation, or once formed, they may be stimulated by cosmic energy, . . . which is ionizing, and which has been interpreted as carrying part of the holographic human archetypal information. Is the microzyma Colloidal Intelligence, or a modus of the Creative Intelligence—a living transducer for the Idea in Consciousness, which it translates into the cellular anatomy?"

It was a good question. The microzyma could indeed be either a Colloidal Intelligence or a modus of the Creative Intelligence. It was hard to be sure if you didn't have a quality Creative Intelligence modus finder, which most people don't.

In the medical establishment Young had to scrap to get the least bit of attention, but the ITNJ welcomed him, as it had welcomed various pillars of the medical-freedom movement. The commission had collected evidence from Joseph Mercola, Andrew Wakefield, and even the alien in Jim Humble's skin, who told them that MMS "kills irradiation poisoning too. But the official people don't like you to know about it."

Unlike when Young was on the stand in the American judicial system, here his testimony was unfettered by any sort of rules of engagement. He spoke uninterrupted for more than an hour.

Early on, he addressed the Dawn Kali lawsuit. He claimed that witnesses had been offered six-figure bribes to bring false testimony against him. He said his attorney had failed to attack the perjured testimony of his opponents, for fear of defying the shadowy controllers of the system. He said that Kali's PET scans showed that, three months after undergoing his treatments, she was cancer free.

"She for some reason decided to move from what she believed in, that literally saved her life, and become a witness for the district attorney," Young said.

The ITNJ commissioners did not publicly ask him to produce specifics about the bribes, evidence of his attorney's corruption, or, actually, any facts or documentation at all.

Young's testimony also showed that he, and many other alternative practitioners in the medical-freedom movement, had become so radicalized that they believed their literal lives were on the line. He said practitioners of alternative medicine were being actively assassinated, with the deaths covered up as heart attacks and suicides. In a two-month period, he claimed, "eleven of my associates have lost their lives."

Although Young said he himself was a primary target, he had no specific knowledge of the would-be assassins' identity.

"I haven't met these Luciferian people, wherever they may be," Young said. "They hide because they fear the light which I represent." Though Young believed his life was still in danger, he said he would not be quieted. It was a matter of faith. Not the kind you might be thinking of. A different thing, called F.A.I.T.H.

"This is mine," he said modestly. He meant the acronym. It was just a little something he had come up with.

It stood for "First Attribute In Thinking Healthy."

"When you have F.A.I.T.H. in the powers of the angels and those protecting angels and God in his majesty, I will not die any sooner or any later until I have finished my mission," he said.

"As I saw my friends and colleagues being taken out one by one by assassination, I saw I had my life at risk. And I also realized—because I'm very, very sensitive because I love my family, I love my children, I love my grandchildren—that if they can't get you, then they take out those who you love," Young said tearily, without naming the supposed murder victims.

During his criminal trial, Young said, part of him wanted not to accept a plea deal. He would have fought against the system to the bitter end. But his children convinced him not to.

"'Dad,'" they said. "'Let it go. You are not your titles. You are not your research.'" Young was once again nearly overcome with emotion, but he pushed through. "'We love you, who you are,'" he said his kids had said to him. "'Your work stands for itself. We know who you are. The world will know who you are.'"

"And now," he said, voice husky and quavering, hands in a pose of supplication. "You all know who I am."

Young's presentation was complete. During a brief Q&A with the commissioners, Sacha Stone returned to the idea that alternative healers were in a life-and-death situation.

"Underpinning the imperative of this commission of inquiry is the recent apparent murders, assassinations of multiple natural practitioners and advocates of natural cures," Stone said. "Are you happy to hear that, that this commission, that is an imperative underpinning this?"

"You're making me cry," said Young, who was sort of crying.

Young's testimony was a hit, racking up roughly 290,000 views on YouTube. Within days, Young was himself sworn in as a commissioner of the ITNJ.

Young had gone down the ladder. He'd descended from a promising young missionary to a health guru pimping smoothies on talk shows, to an asserter of unaccepted science, to an outlaw profiting from the cures he espoused, and now he claimed he was being persecuted by evil forces threatening to kill him and his family.

There was only one more rung at the bottom. The zed rung. The zombie rung. Young had not yet touched it. But he was getting awfully—and I do mean awfully—close.

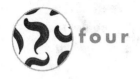four

ALICJA KOLYSZKO'S LEECHES' SUCK-CESS

"How do you feel, Miss Baedeker?"

The girl addressed was trying, unsuccessfully, to slump against my shoulder. At this inquiry she sat up and opened her eyes.

"Wha'?" . . .

"We heard you yelling, so I said to Doc Civet here: 'There's somebody that needs your help, Doc.'"

"She's much obliged, I'm sure," said another friend, without gratitude, "but you got her dress all wet when you stuck her head in the pool."

"Anything I hate is to get my head stuck in a pool," mumbled Miss Baedeker. "They almost drowned me once over in New Jersey."

"Then you ought to leave it alone," countered Doctor Civet.

"Speak for yourself!" cried Miss Baedeker violently. "Your hand shakes. I wouldn't let you operate on me!"

It was like that.

—F. Scott Fitzgerald, *The Great Gatsby*, 1925

HOURS PASSED. ALICJA KOLYSZKO SPOKE FASTER AND FASTER. IT was the only time we had together, and there was so much to teach me about leeches.

Teaching comes naturally to Alicja; back when she taught Polish high school students how to speak Russian, there was a certain formality to her approach, one that paid the utmost respect to both an ancient way of speaking and the vibrant young minds before her.

That same drive for dignity had her putting adult forks and spoons into the hands of her infant children and speaking to them seriously, without any denigrating baby babble. This was how her father, Vasili, had done it, back when she was a baby. And this was how it should be done.

Alicja had high expectations of everyone. When they worked hard, humans had the potential for grace. There was a right way and a wrong way.

It was the same with leeches.

And that was what led her to embark on her most ambitious project: in 2011 she founded the Academy of Hirudotherapy, whose doors opened in Las Vegas.

At the academy, students learned about a One True Cure that sucked. They learned that when the leech is done sucking, it becomes a potential disease vector and must be disposed of—the right way.

"Never in the toilet, neither alive nor dead, leeches," she told me, firmly. "You do not put them in the sewer. It's not allowed."

The fate of the creatures makes the leech queenpin a bit sad. "That's the worst part of my profession," she said, referring to them as she would a family pet, "because we have to put them to sleep."

She urges her students not to make the same mistake as Angela, whose clumsy leech killing had caused blood to explode from their bodies, covering Alicja in her own blood. That was not dignified. It was not respectful, to patient or leech.

"They have to be submerged in the isopropyl alcohol. Usually less than 70 percent [concentration]," Alicja said. "They do not make the leech suffer. If you do lower, 50 percent, the leech will be struggling and fighting and moving, etcetera. It won't die."

Once the submerged leeches have stopped moving, they get a sort of ritual funeral. They turn into black clots, which Alicja gently, respectfully wraps in cotton and medical dressings, then triple-bags.

Once dead, the leeches become medical waste, which also has to be handled properly. She instructs her students to use a sharps container, of the sort diabetics use for their syringes, and then to follow the legal requirements that apply to the state they are in. This sort of treatment, she says, maintains the spiritual benefit that comes when a practitioner, patient, and small slithy animal engage in a joint sanguinary effort.

"It's about fire and energy in the circle," she told me, "the close circle between the leech and the host and the hirudotherapist."

Unlike the other One True Cure practitioners I spoke with, Alicja has accepted the responsibility of ensuring that her operation is within the scope of the law. The academy is powered by a curriculum designed to keep patients safe and practitioners out of regulatory trouble. To do this, Alicja drew on her experience working as a dialysis technician within the US health care system. She is well versed in how to create and maintain a sterile working environment, and she studied applicable regulations in various states to make sure she was legal.

This is trickier for students who are already licensed medical practitioners, because legally, "it's nothing to do with health care," she said. "They can lose their license if they commingle with the medical side any way."

One student, a gynecologist, ran a hirudotherapy practice out of a separate office. Alicja certified similar arrangements for a nurse and even for a veterinarian who wanted to use leeches to treat his animal wards.

Because of Alicja's approach, the academy's certification process was accepted by various international organizations, including the British Hirudotherapy Association. She turned out dozens of certified hirudotherapists, who went on to carry her methods of leeching to their own practices in fifteen states around the country.

For the entire time we talked, her phone was lighting up. She didn't give it even a fraction of her attention when we were speaking—that is not the proper way to be interviewed—but the moment there was a break in our discussion, she consulted it and gave me a glimpse into the world of America's leading hirudotherapist. She scrolled through pictures of limbs blackened, or purple, or red, some thin and withered like vacuum-packed bones, others blown up like pufferfish. There were messages from patients setting appointments, seeking advice. She knew the names of most of them. She has visited their homes, drunk their tea, held their hands, calloohed and callayed over their promotions and achievements. This, she said, is healing with dignity. It is something the FDA and the medical establishment will never match, for patient or leech.

"It's so different from what I represent," she told me, "and because of that, we are not a part of the health care."

But nearly as bad as the FDA are those on the other end of the spectrum, those whose interest in leeching is governed by neither regulation nor a sense of personal responsibility and therefore has the potential to hurt the hirudotherapy brand.

"There are many," she confided to me, "underground people who do it."

.·:·

A BEAGLE NAMED KELSEY PROWLED THE ARRIVAL GATES AND BAGGAGE areas of Toronto's Pearson International Airport on Wednesday, October 17, 2018, striking fear into the hearts of pork smugglers and other ne'er-do-wells. In an effort to tamp down the flow of contraband into the country, the Canadian border patrol was relying on the hardware inside Kelsey's nose, which is literally beyond human comprehension—minuscule side corridors that trap inhaled scent so it doesn't get exhaled, a bean-sized organ that analyzes trace chemical signals, a massive lobe of the brain devoted to smell, and 225 million scent receptors, all of which combine to give beagles a sniffing capacity that is as much as a hundred thousand times better than a human's.

Beagles can determine whether the person standing in front of them has lung cancer. They can find a mouse in a one-acre field in less than a minute—blindfolded. Unlike almost any other creature on the planet, when trailing a person they can distinguish between the amount of scent in the first footstep and the fifth footstep.

Kelsey is an excellent border patrol agent. And a good dog.

Some detector dogs bark, jump, and scratch at offending baggage, but Kelsey was trained in "passive detection," an approach that is a bit subtler and much, much cuter. In the baggage hall she approached a man whose carry-on was an innocent-looking cloth grocery bag; she sat next to the unsuspecting suspect and turned her liquid brown eyes on her partner, parting her jaws in a grin.

The grocery bag belonged to Ippolit Bodounov, whose paper ticket indicated he'd just gotten off an eight-hour flight from Moscow; he was probably headed to his home in Niagara Falls. His E311 customs card indicated that he had "nothing to declare."

Bodounov was directed to a secondary examination area, where he surrendered the grocery bag to an Officer Young (not the pH Miracle guy). Inside were ten packages, each the size and shape of a large burrito, wrapped in cloth and closed with elastic bands. The first package was unpleasantly wet and yielding to the touch.

Leeches.

The second bag? Leeches.

Bags three through ten? Leeches as well.

In all, Ippolit Bodounov's reusable grocery bag held 4,788 leeches, enough to drain, in one feeding, every ounce of blood from the boy bands BTS and One Direction (plus two Backstreet Boys for good measure).

Bodounov's explanation for the contraband was as brief as it was unbelievable: "personal use," he said. (The record is unclear on whether he spoke with an icy Russian accent. Or, alternatively, a chummy Canadian one.) When pressed, he claimed that he intended to keep the leeches in tanks so his wife could use their wastewater to fertilize her orchids.

Soon, media outlets across the world were reporting on the largest leech-smuggling bust in history. Canadian authorities basked in the glory.

"Our dogs are adorable and effective," Judith Gadbois-St-Cyr, a spokesperson for the Canada Border Services Agency, told me. She said the leech bust was a record for that species but unremarkable in many ways.

"People with turtles wrapped around their bodies. Animals hidden"—she added darkly—"in all sorts of places. They've seen it all."

Russia is home to Udelnaya, a town whose biggest employer, the International Medical Leech Center, churns out millions of leeches for the alternative-wellness industry (including for use as an ingredient in a cosmetics line sold by its owner, a Dr. Nikonov). This close to the source, leeches are cheap—people exit the building's lobby with jars of leeches for as little as sixty cents per animal.

If Bodounov bought the leeches there, they would have cost roughly US$3,000. But on the open market they had a street value of as much as $67,032—the equivalent of fourteen pounds of marijuana or four pounds of cocaine.

In truth, the value of a leech had been climbing ever since the FDA's approval of leeches had boosted interest. People were paying more on average for giant buffalo leeches ($700) than for border collie puppies ($550), and the leeches don't even play fetch. Actresses Miranda Kerr and Demi Moore admitted using "leech facials" to keep their skin looking young.

Bodounov was one of many unscrupulous leech dealers who capitalized on all this interest. Since 2012 he'd posed as a law-abiding leech guy, registered as a domestic Canadian breeder with tens of thousands of leeches he was supposedly raising domestically. The Canadian government had signed off on Bodounov exporting leeches on fifty-three different occasions.

Investigators soon found he'd gotten the leeches even more cheaply than he would have if he'd bought them in Udelnaya. By testing the DNA of the blood in the stomachs of the leeches, they realized that Bodounov's leeches had grown up in the wild, feeding on frogs, birds, and freshwater fishes of considerable variety. It eventually came out that Bodounov was acting as a bagman for his wife, Dianova Svetlana Evgenievna, who had bought the eight pounds of leeches for 21,582 rubles—about CAN$425.

If the illegal wildlife harvesting in the leeches' past was troubling, their future was downright bananas. His wife was associated with the website www.leeches.biz, which sold them for eight dollars apiece (about a hundred times what she'd paid for them).

All across America, people were taking advantage of a renewed climate of health freedom to treat themselves with leeches. The flavor of the underground leech scene is apparent in the Q&A forum of the US-based retailer leech.com (which seems to be a much larger operation than the site associated with Evgenievna).

"Is it possible to order too many leeches? I need around one metric ton."

"Will these leeches be safe inside my body? My husband and I are experimenting with fetishes. . . ."

"can u eat leeches?"

"Which type of leaches works the best for Psoriasis?"

"Would you have a retail shop in Jayapura that do sell your Indonesian Leech Oil for Penis Enlargement?"

"Will reusing the leeches on someone else transfer the disease if they have sucked HIV positive blood?"

If the questions are troubling, the answers provided by the retailers provide little reassurance.

"The results will last as long as you need perform in bed."

"There is no risk of receiving blood borne diseases from our leeches."

"Leeches are not known to transfer deceases."

"If you want the fish blinded, than you would put the fish in with the leech. Since the leech can not bite the fish on the scales, it only has one place left to bite: on the eyes. This means your fish's eyes will be gone before you know it."

They also advise one questioner to buy a collection of leeches and use them to seed the lake or pond of their choice, an act that would be illegal—and potentially disastrous for the local ecosystem.

Bodounov eventually pleaded guilty to unlawfully importing southern medicinal leeches (*Hirudo verbana*). In May 2019, the Ontario Superior Court fined him a measly $11,000, about a sixth of the value of the leeches he tried to bring into the country in that particular shipment.

The website leeches.biz soon raised its prices to ten dollars per leech, which I imagine more than covered the cost of occasional legal fees and court fines.

five

THE NEUMANNS' PRAYERS
RAISED HELL

"I just sat and held it softly till Mrs. Hummel came with the doctor.
He said it was dead, and looked at Heinrich and Minna, who
have sore throats. 'Scarlet fever, ma'am. Ought to have called
me before,' he said crossly. Mrs. Hummel told him she was poor,
and had tried to cure baby herself, but now it was too late."

—Louisa May Alcott, *Little Women*, 1868

LEILANI.

Dale.

She keened. He mourned.

Leilani felt numb. Dale's sadness swelled. Her daughter was dead.
He'd lost his youngest. Her sleep turned dark, troubling. Dale listened
to her dreams.

She distrusted the ongoing police investigation; he steeled himself
for criminal charges. Leilani felt misunderstood by a judgmental world;
Dale agreed to a joint public statement. "We are just a normal family,"
she said; Dale was not ready to give up God. In Leilani's recurring dream,
state troopers targeted her family; Dale and the other kids were in the
dream too, fleeing.

Awake, Leilani learned her brother and Ariel Neff were separating,
while Dale's sister Susan asked police to protect Luke, Hamilton, Ariel.

Together, they were embraced only by Eells and other supportive
faith healers, who sent them cash donations for their legal defense.

Four days after Kara's death, Eells still suggested she might return to
life. "We are sure Kara does not want to come back [from Heaven]," he

wrote, "but we have asked God to send her for her parents' sake and as a testimony of His love for us."

Unsurprisingly, Eells said little about the effectiveness of prayer as a One True Cure and much about the right to religious freedom. Failing to defend the Neumanns, he wrote, paved the way for the government to install microchips in the hands and foreheads of all Christians.

Medicine was, in his view, one of two totally equivalent dark arts. "Witchcraft can heal also," he said. (Big if true!) "Should Christians also seek witches?"

. : :

BUT OUTSIDE THIS VERY NARROW SLICE OF THE RELIGIOUS COMMUNITY, Kara's death had every bit the impact one might expect. Atheists and mainstream Christians set aside their antagonism, differing only in whether the Neumanns should rot in the ground or in Hell.

The media circulated a photograph of Kara in the sunshine, head cocked, smile bright, long brown braid dangling past a gold earring to rest on a green T-shirt.

"She was the sweetest friend I ever had. Her smile would melt your heart. I don't even remember one thing she ever did wrong," Anna Rose, a childhood friend, wrote from California. "When I found out she died . . . my heart got ripped out and I broke into tears."

How had an earnest desire to worship God led to this?

Some argued that the Neumanns did nothing to save their daughter, but this isn't true. The nonstop frantic activity that surrounded Kara in the days leading to her death show that they did, in fact, do a lot—exhausting themselves by mustering Herculean levels of communal prayer, swallowing their pride to mend fences with antagonists. But what they were doing was completely, hopelessly ineffective.

What killed Kara Neumann?

It was, in one sense, the ketones overwhelming her blood. The ketones were allowed to do their deadly work by Dale and Leilani. But Dale and Leilani were *allowed* to allow the ketones to do their work by something else, something bigger.

In a very real sense, religious freedom—or at least, the extreme notion that religious freedom should be so absolute as to inure parents
from consequences for child abuse—killed Kara Neumann.

It began in 1974, when lobbyists with the Christian Science Church
convinced the federal Department of Health, Education, and Welfare
to withhold federal funding from social service agencies that interfered
with the right to rely on prayer as medicine for their children. The number of states with religious exemptions to their child abuse codes quickly
jumped from eleven to thirty-four. By 1988 it was legal to forgo medical
care for children in forty-four states.

In Wisconsin, state legislators amended child abuse laws to read, "A
person is not guilty of an offense . . . solely because he or she provides a
child with treatment by spiritual means through prayer alone for healing
in accordance with the religious method of healing . . . in lieu of medical
or surgical treatment."

With that legal cover in place, it's little wonder that a community
of faith healers was emboldened to publicly normalize the Neumanns'
outlook.

After all, when Kara fell ill, Dale and Leilani didn't act furtively, like
child-abusing criminals. They broadcast their intentions to a deep bench
of like-minded people. Their actions were actively endorsed by Eells and
Unleavened Bread Ministries. They were also tacitly endorsed by everyone in the Neumanns' Bible study group and extended family. Everyone
knew that Kara was in crisis, and everyone (except Ariel Neff) trusted
Dale and Leilani's spiritual solution—or at least did not intervene to stop
them.

Once such a culture has been established, how should society
respond?

.∴

ALMOST FROM THE MOMENT IN 2009 WHEN THE NEUMANNS ENTERED THE
courtroom (holding hands, he in a bulky leather jacket, she in a white,
knee-length, open sweater), it became clear they were not there to ask
forgiveness.

Dale, Bible in hand, took the stand, sporting a pencil-thin mustache and chin beard so subtle they looked like skin tones. His testimony often took on the pitch of a preacher's fiery sermon; he quoted scripture and made lots of eye contact with the jury, repeating the narrative he told about himself—of an unhappy young man who had been born again.

"That's the day," he said, "when Dale R. Neumann died, and he was buried in baptism."

He shared the evidence of his own experiences, the miraculous cures he said he'd witnessed. He put Kara's death in the context of the faith-healing community.

"If I go to any other source, that's idolatry. I'm putting something else in the place of God," he said. "That is idolatry. That is sin."

Near the beginning of Leilani's trial, she suffered what her attorney called "a total mental and emotional breakdown." She lost all feeling in her arms and legs and slumped onto the defense table, requiring medical attention and the temporary use of a wheelchair. Later, she read from her Bible and circled the defense and prosecution tables several times in prayer.

She told the jury that taking Kara to the doctor would have been "complete disobedience to what we believe."

In the whole sorry affair, the only person who could be held blameless was Ariel Neff. And she was miserable.

"I knew that if nothing was done, that little girl was going to die," she sobbed during her courtroom testimony. "I knew that she hadn't gotten food for a couple of days. I could not let the little girl just sit there and die."

Despite the religious exemption to child abuse, the juries found the Neumanns guilty of reckless homicide. During sentencing, the judge essentially gave the Neumanns a moral pass. The evidence showed that the Neumanns were sincere. Just deluded.

"This was really about two good people," he said, "who made a bad decision, a reckless decision."

Dale and Leilani were each sentenced to 180 days in jail and ten years of probation. They served thirty-day increments, one parent each March, the other each September, for six years.

After being interviewed and physically examined, Kara's three siblings were placed in the home of a relative. Child Protective Services soon determined that the other kids were not being subjected to abuse or neglect, and they were returned under a mandatory "Safety Plan" that included medical exams.

For the five Neumanns who had survived the One True Cure of faith healing, life would go on.

.·:·'

COULD FAITH HEALING BE DONE WITHOUT HARMING INNOCENT VICTIMS?

It seemed to me that a morally responsible religious leader could help followers enjoy the benefits of praying for health while also sharing guidelines about the need for medical care for children in unexplained comas.

I wondered whether the Neumanns had gone rogue and come by their extreme form of faith healing independently, or whether they were— maybe not brainwashed, but strongly encouraged to do what they did. In other words, did the leaders and influencers within the faith-healing community kill Kara by accident? Or was it on purpose?

Those questions were in my mind when I went to Torben Søndergaard's faith-healing training session near Miami. But they exited my mind as soon as Søndergaard announced to the congregation that everyone—including, presumably, journalists who wished to be anonymous observers—would now learn how to heal.

Torben was joined onstage by a woman who complained of five years of back pain. He role-played with her.

"Hey, hi, hi," he said, holding his hand up in an adorably exaggerated greeting. "Are you a Christian?"

She replied that she was.

"That," Torben told the crowd, to hearty laughter, "means nothing in America!"

He explained how to lay hands on the afflicted person. "Just keep it simple," he said. "You lay the hands, then you pray, and then you get them to test it."

He put his hands lightly on her back as she closed her eyes.

"Okay, speaking right now in the name of Jesus I command all pain to go right now," he said, quickly and without drama. Then he immediately asked her to assess her back.

"Just test it," he said. "How is it? How does it feel now?"

The healing was so lightning quick that for a blink of an eye the woman seemed unsure of what she should say. Tentatively, she answered that it seemed better. When he urged her to test it, she walked ten feet across the stage with exaggerated and hammy movements, indicating by broad mugging to the crowd that she was now pain free.

Everyone cheered and laughed.

Torben then offered help to another woman, who also had back pain. In short order, he was standing in her personal space, hand on her back, speaking directly to the demon inside her, his microphone broadcasting the interaction to everyone.

"Freedom," Torben said to the demon. "Freedom. Holy Spirit, fill her up. More."

His speaking grew more rapid and more intense. "More. More. More."

What he said to the demon next surprised me. He began to speak in tongues. I didn't recognize the language, so I transcribe it here phonetically.

"Bacala geeyes," Torben said to the demon. "Geeyes sahlahdahdahdah. Geeyes geeyes sahlahdahdahdah."

When his patter quieted a moment, the woman's voice became audible. She said, "Dahdahdahdahdah."

"Geeyes geeyes sahlahdahdahdah geeyes geeyes sahlahdahdahdah dahdahdahdahdahdahdadada geeyes geeyes sahlahdahdahdahdahdahdahdada," Torben said to the demon inside the woman.

"Dahdahdahdahdadada," said the woman.

"Sheilah bahdahdahdahdahdahda geeyes guess sahlahdahdahdada," said Torben before shifting to a higher energy level and announcing, with a triumphant tone, "Sheilahbahdada dAH-AAHHH AHHHH!"

He then yelled as if he had just scored the game-winning goal: "Come ONNNNNNN!"

She opened her eyes, and they looked at one another.

"How was it?" Torben asked, expectantly.

She nodded emphatically. "Awesome," she said.

"Awesome!" he shouted to the crowd.

Torben announced an open season on demons in the room. Those who wanted to be healed should gather in one half of the church, and those who wanted to try healing should stand in the other half. People seeking healing should raise a hand to attract a healer.

Just as I was trying to figure out how to handle this wrinkle, Torben, to my great relief, said, "If you don't want to, this is fine. Just stay sitting."

But as the room rearranged itself around me, I saw how isolated I was becoming. Including me, roughly 4 of about 150 people were still seated. And one of them was in a wheelchair, hand raised.

As the healing commenced all around me, a few young people took the stage with instruments and began to sing a long, looping refrain about Jesus. The room abuzz with conversation, a man in a buttoned-down shirt asked me if I would like to be healed of anything, casually, as if he were offering me a can of Coke.

"No, thank you," I said. And he moved on.

That was a pretty easy deflection, I reflected. The noise in the room grew louder and more energetic. People had by now progressed to the active praying stage, and I could see prayees and prayers, joined by healing hands and delusion.

It was like orchestral jazz healing, a hundred different riffs on Torben's original tongues-laden tune all going at once. Torben's demonstration had been relaxed and light, but most of the healers were intense and serious, an appropriate demeanor for demon battling.

Then I heard the scream. It was really more of a full-bodied, anguished wail, so upsetting that a jolt of adrenaline flowed through me. The wail, which went on and on, emanated from a woman in a pale yellow skirt who had fallen to her knees and was now, as an 1800s doctor sawing off a leg might say, experiencing something really intense. It must have been a big-boss demon, because the healer hunched over her was joined by another, with still others hurrying toward the commotion, laying on hands, issuing stern commands to the dark spirit.

As her cries grew louder and more guttural, I heard another loud cry, from my left, indicating another boss demon, perhaps unhappy with the amount of attention being given to the first demon. Within minutes, other demons were clamoring for attention by sending their human hosts, howling, to the ground. Torben's students rushed about eagerly, clustering around screaming people on their knees or lying prone. It was without a doubt the most fantastic and earnest LARPing session I had ever seen.

As silly as it was, I could also see how alive and in the moment everyone felt. They were each the center of an exciting drama, heroically throttling demons in the name of Jesus. It was clear that the rush of casting out evil was far more engaging than the long, drudgery-filled work of designing a society in which pain is lessened and curative resources are equitably distributed among rich and poor.

The medical establishment thinks that science-based evidence will carry the day, but there is nothing in their arsenal that matches the ecstasy of healing and being healed. (One tangible measure of Torben Søndergaard's power would come in July 2022, when he would tell his followers that he had been detained by US immigration officials; his crowd-funded "legal defense fund" quickly raised $194,000 toward a $250,000 goal.)

The noise in the room was now deafening, which is why I almost didn't hear the words.

"How's it going, brother?"

It was a young man making direct eye contact. Worse, he was smiling. I knew this was trouble. I smiled back.

.•.:

HIS NAME WAS REGGIE, AND HE ASKED ME ABOUT MY RELATIONSHIP WITH God.

I was vague, saying things that were technically true, without mentioning my actual purpose.

I told him that it was my first time there, that I had heard about the meeting from a follower of Torben, and that I saw a lot of positive energy in the room. Trying to forestall further questions, I bombarded him with my own.

"Do you think when someone is healed in this way, does the healing last as long as they keep faith? Or does it last for less time than that?" I asked. "How long before you think that woman's back pain comes back, or do you think it's never going to hurt her again?"

"God heals us. Like brother was saying," Reggie said, referring to Jeremy, the earlier speaker who had told the audience to chuck their medicine in the trash bin. "He threw all his prescription pills away."

"So as long as his faith is strong, he'll be free?" I asked.

"Yes," said Reggie. "Yeah."

I asked Reggie about his life, but by now there were so many screaming demons that I caught only snatches. "I came from a street life . . . hard drugs. . . . That took a toll on me . . . had to hustle to help my family. . . . Salvation, I never really had that. . . . I was in and out of jail . . . two times. . . . I know the court system. . . . That's my life, three times. . . . The only thing I had was a gun. . . . My own . . . tried to set me up. And he was calling me, bro! I accepted the call."

I couldn't tell whether the person calling him was God or the person who had set him up, as part of some sort of sting operation. But then Reggie wrapped up, saying, "The Holy Spirit just fell on me and I started crying. It was over."

"That was it for you?" I asked.

"Yeah," Reggie said. He then shifted the conversation back into uncomfortable waters. "And it's the same with you, man. God wants you. He wants you to come back."

He asked for more details about my own religious journey and status. I continued to pursue my pointless, stupid path of giving a false impression while making only true statements. I didn't want to lie.

"I just started, uh, you know, paying attention a little bit," I said lamely. "And paying a little more attention, and like that, you know."

I knew I sounded like an idiot. So I threw more questions at him. I asked about Leilani Neumann.

"One of the things that gave me doubt was, I knew a woman who, her child was very sick," I told Reggie. "And she tried to heal her child through prayer, and the child died. She actually got in a lot of trouble. There were news articles about her because she didn't seek medical attention, you know? So that kind of made me feel like that doesn't make sense. So that made me kind of question whether that was really the way to go."

Would Reggie see the clear lunacy in withholding medical care from a child who had actually died?

"Why do you think that would happen?" I asked. "Her child died."

Reggie told me there was only one possible explanation. "A lack of faith." He said Kara's death proved their faith wasn't strong enough. After all, he said, "Jesus called Lazarus back. He was four days dead."

It was a staggeringly brutal take on Kara's death. A lack of faith. Stinking thinking. Negative energy. It held leaders like Torben blameless, instead shifting responsibility onto an eleven-year-old girl who couldn't defend herself because she was dead, even though she prayed for health right up to the moment she lost consciousness.

I knew then that inside this particular bubble of society, allowing a child to die for want of medical care was not just accepted. It was expected.

Within three feet of me one of the women that Torben had already healed on stage collapsed, apparently infested with new demonic spirits that demanded more attention. The possessed shrieked, their voices punctuating the droning Jesus song blasting through the amps.

Reggie was done with pleasantries.

"Matt," he said to me. "Want to pray?"

I had been prayed over before, while hitchhiking through a rural and God-fearing land of midwestern cornfields. A guy in his pickup truck preached to me for the duration of a thirty-minute drive, marveling at how the mere speaking of God's name—Yahweh—had caused armies to be defeated. Just before I left his truck, he clutched my hands in his and asked God to look over me, as a traveler far from home. I had no faith, but I didn't mind. I knew it was an expression of good intentions. Expecting Reggie's prayer would be similar, I reluctantly agreed.

Reggie's agenda was to infuse me with spiritual fervor. My agenda was to end the prayer process as quickly and quietly as possible so Reggie would let me blend back into the crowd.

We were both disappointed.

He started by asking me if there was anything I wanted to release.

There was not, I said.

Did I have any pain?

No, I didn't, I told him, looking for the quick, no-frills version.

He asked me to stand up and bow my head, so I did. He told me to repeat his words, and so I parroted them, as well as I could hear them. Together we asked Jesus to set me free, and we welcomed the Holy Spirit.

I smiled and made as if to turn away, sure that we were done.

But then Reggie sneak-attacked me. I'd told him I had no pain, but he started speaking in tongues over me.

"Out right now. Out right now. Out of here in the name of Jesus Christ," said Reggie, speaking to the demons he sensed were inside me.

I stood mute, awkwardly waiting for him to run out of steam. My demons remained rooted. Or maybe they left. Or maybe—and this seemed to me the most likely option—maybe demons don't exist as malevolent ephemeral beings outside of human intent.

"Leave right now. Out in the name of Jesus. You have no power. You have no authority. I'm coming to you now in Jesus's name. Take your hands off him."

Around us, the bedlam continued. The woman on the floor behind me had attracted a team of healers, who knelt around her like paramedics, praying, occasionally bumping into me inadvertently.

Finally, Reggie took his hands off me and looked me in the eyes.

"How are you feeling?" he asked, all optimism and expectation.

Well, I was relieved to be done.

"I feel good," I said, technically truthfully. Again I started to turn away, but Reggie had affixed himself to my shoulder, leaning into my personal space to be heard above the noise.

"What God wants to do," Reggie bawled into my ear, "he wants to encourage everyone to repent and be baptized. You have the opportunity to make that happen tonight."

I missed some of what he said next, but I did make out "The next step is, I will talk to one of the brothers here and let them know that you are ready."

I had terrifying visions of alligators and cheering Pentecostals. My inner demons and I agreed there was no way in Heaven we were submitting to that.

"Maybe tomorrow," I said.

"If you want to get baptized tonight, you can," Reggie said. I could see he would continue the discussion all night, if that was what it would take.

"I'm gonna do it tomorrow," I promised firmly.

I walked out of the church with a Cheshire Cat smile on my face, thinking of the lunacy I had just witnessed. I wondered whether the public would be more likely to prevent the deaths of innocent victims by confronting faith healers at every turn? Or would understanding and empathy be more effective?

My smile faded.

I had done neither. Perhaps that's how One True Cures get out of hand in the first place.

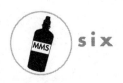 **s i x**

THE ALIEN'S DRINK BLEACHES THE PRESIDENT

> Those who maintain the ridiculous idea that individuals are endowed with supernatural gifts and knowledge, and become skilful physicians without education or study, betray a pitiful credulity, equalled only by the conceits of those who believe in ghosts and spectres, haunting the dwellings of the dead.
>
> —James Thacher, *An Essay on Demonology, Ghosts and Apparitions, and Popular Superstitions*, 1831

ON JANUARY 22, 2020, THE FORMER GAME SHOW HOST TURNED American president took a break from an economic summit in Switzerland to sit down with Joe Kernen, a journalist with CNBC. A few hours earlier the president had tweeted a message to the public congratulating an MMA fighter whose recent cage match had drawn huge ratings.

The main topic of the interview was supposed to be the economy, but Kernen opened the interview with another topic, one that seemed more pressing.

"The CDC has identified a case of coronavirus in Washington state," Kernen said. Cases had been identified in Thailand, Taiwan, and Japan. The American media had been reporting on it for about two weeks. Kernen said he was unsure as to whether the president had been briefed about the coronavirus by the CDC. The president indicated that he had. Kernen asked his question.

"Are there worries about a pandemic at this point?"

"No. Not at all," the president said. "And we're—we have it totally under control. It's one person coming in from China, and we have it under control. It's going to be just fine."

That's when people knew for sure. It was going to be a disaster.

Over the coming weeks, twin viruses—COVID-19 and panic—began to sweep through the American populace.

The following month, the former game show host used the awesome power of the presidency to commute the sentence of his former *Celebrity Apprentice* castmate. Blago walked free.

.⁚.

IN BILLINGS, MONTANA, TOBY MCADAM KNEW HE HAD TO HELP.

In March, he told his tiny following on social media that he expected the virus to subside within a month.

"The politicians need to step aside and let us big boys handle this," he said. In this, he was echoing the assurances of both the game show host and emerging medical-freedom advocate Elon Musk, who tweeted in March, "Based on current trends, probably close to zero new cases in US . . . by end of April."

The pandemic did not subside. It grew, and kept growing.

COVID's dominance of America's headspace allowed for the perfect intersection of the alternative-health industry, antivaccine activists, and the medical-freedom movement. Thousands of people peddling false coronavirus cures flooded digital communication channels, completely overwhelming enforcement officers. The FDA identified seven hundred groups that were promoting fake COVID cures.

In March, Congress passed a massive coronavirus relief package; after signing it into law, the game show host's administration approved $850,000 of the money in loans to five different antivaccine groups. Joseph Mercola, who was later identified as the chief spreader of coronavirus misinformation online, received $335,000 in loans.

Later in the year, as case counts grew, Toby adopted a new position.

"Areas with cold weather, I think they're going to find that the cold will just about wipe the virus out," he said, shortly before the start of a long, dark winter in which infection rates rose to an all-time high, killing nearly a quarter million Americans.

.∙∵

In Valley Center, California, secret assassination target, cosmic-life-force aficionado, and ITNJ commissioner Robert Young knew he had to help.

He made a round of appearances on the media outlets that accepted him as a guest—a constellation of extremely conservative networks that dealt in theories of both the conspiratorial and pseudoscientific persuasions.

In April of 2020 he appeared on *Let's Talk America*, a talk show hosted by Alan Keyes, the former presidential candidate and a spokesman for the supplement Prevennia. Keyes also had legitimate credentials that ranged from a Harvard PhD to state department appointments during the Reagan administration. Keyes addressed his national audience through shows like *Let's Talk America* on his web-based digital platform, IAMtv.

Young explained to Keyes the true cause of coronavirus. It was the same thing that caused cancer. It was the same thing that caused AIDS. As explained by Antoine Béchamp's theory of pleomorphism, the body's own cells were turning against their host. People who were walking around with too much acid in their system were susceptible to environmental triggers that could cause symptoms.

"What can tip this thing off could be, you know, radiation from your, from, from a cell tower," Young said. "It could be a vaccine. It could be a drug that you took that was not proper."

Young advised that an alkaline diet was the key to riding out the pandemic, and he actively advertised his supplements as effective coronavirus treatments or preventives. Keyes said Young's plan seemed like a promising long-term approach.

Young made similar claims during a two-hour interview with Joseph Mercola (who was himself selling various supplements to combat coronavirus), and again during a two-hour roundtable that included antivaccine activist Judy Mikovits. Mikovits was the creative force behind the documentary *Plandemic*, which attributed the pandemic to a secret conspiracy carried out by Big Pharma, the CDC, and Google.

.∴·

IN WISCONSIN, DALE AND LEILANI NEUMANN KNEW THEY HAD TO HELP.

Their old church in Turlock, California—the New Life Christian Center—followed the recommendations of public health officials and pitched in by shifting to online services, hosting vaccine clinics, and encouraging their members to make masks for those in need.

But the Neumanns were no longer into that sort of church.

In the summer months of 2020, Dale and Leilani asked God for guidance.

God told them they needed to be on "active duty" and led them to a faith healer: Torben Søndergaard, whose followers had told me that Kara Neumann died because Leilani lacked faith.

The Last Reformation was ambivalent about masks and social-distancing measures; its events were big, germ-passing gatherings of as large a fervent clump of religiosity as the market would bear.

In Florida, Dale and Leilani enjoyed the Last Reformation crowd. They followed Torben's teachings and preached in the street, learning how to heal people who were potentially infected with coronavirus by a laying on of hands. (This same dynamic became famous in Sierra Leone in the 2014 Ebola outbreak, during which a traditional faith healer was believed to have caused three hundred cases and was mocked globally for scientific ignorance.)

Dale and Leilani made friends with another attractive Pentecostal couple, Starr and Scott, and walked the beach with them, trolling for seashells. Starr taught them how to make little towers out of the stones.

I had actually met Starr and Scott briefly, when I was in Margate, Florida. At that time, Starr wore a nice floor-length dress and Scott was showing off his biceps in a T-shirt, his red baseball cap proclaiming that we should "Get America Born Again." They took the stage to deliver a half-hour testimony in which they described a weekend-long training exercise that happened during their Last Reformation schooling at an old hotel in North Carolina. It is a long and wacky story—the briefest summary is that they brainstormed on a whiteboard to see what thoughts God might cause to pop into their heads ("Fruit!" "A moose!" "A blue house with white shutters on a hill!"), and then drove around rural North Carolina for many hours, following those signs like Scooby-Doo clues, until they found a woman who embraced them and allowed them to baptize her, all of which offered irrefutable evidence of God's something-or-other.

By the time the pandemic hit, Leilani, too, had adopted the language of the medical-freedom movement: she said on social media that the pandemic was a plot to infect people so that money could be made selling vaccines. To support the game show host's reelection bid, she wrote vituperatively about his opponents' stance on abortion rights.

"So much spiritual blindness in this world. America needs to repent. There's so much blood on people's hands," said the woman convicted of manslaughtering her own child. "We must be the voice for these murdered babies. Continue to pray evil is exposed."

.∴.

IN NAPLES, FLORIDA, ALICJA KOLYSZKO KNEW SHE HAD TO HELP.

She took to social media and began spreading information that she thought would be relevant to those worried about coronavirus.

"Home remedies and proven evidence based remedies could do more than any conventional medication and methods," she wrote in one post. She shared articles that were a pastiche of the alternative-health view of the pandemic. One bore the headline "No Disease Can Exist in an Alkaline Environment."

Her own remedies for coronavirus included gargling with Listerine and oregano oil, and, of course, hirudotherapy.

To Alicja, it was no longer simply an academic debate about whether leeches provided a valid health benefit. It was something bigger. Her medical activism veered into unrelated issues. She shared information about the medical-freedom agenda from the American Institute for Economic Research. She circulated a petition to reopen Florida beaches in Miami-Dade County (the public pressure campaign worked, and the beaches were opened amid protests from public health officials).

The Polish native even attacked illegal immigrants, writing, "Love It Or Leave It! America for Americans! Americans for America!"

This all made me really sad. Because I like her. I wasn't sad because she had different political opinions from my own. I was sad that a loving woman who had, until a few years earlier, used Facebook primarily to spread warm thoughts about Christmas and Easter had come to parrot a constellation of extreme political positions against immigrants, social justice activists, voting by mail, and public health recommendations on mask wearing. She had been utterly radicalized.

America had been radicalized too. Not against foreign powers, or demons, or the threats posed by a warming climate. America was radicalized against itself.

To the detriment of everyone.

One night, Alicja fell into a sleep, one that was longer and deeper than she was usually able to enjoy. But she found herself in a nightmarish dream. Joe Biden stood at her bedside, staring at her with a fiendish grin on his face; beside him was White House pandemic adviser Dr. Anthony Fauci, Democratic Party leaders Nancy Pelosi and Chuck Schumer, and other members of what she had come to think of as the "swamp horde." All stared at her with ghastly Joker smiles.

How was it, she wondered, that none of them were ever touched by COVID?

"Are they chosen by Lucifer or God?" she wondered. Hollywood, too, seemed to be mysteriously unaffected. Did the masks protect them? Or had they been given some sort of secret government immunity?

"I don't want to join their secrets," she wrote later on Facebook. She urged people to work on their own immune systems so that they could survive "without their poison."

.∴.

IN HIS COMPOUND IN SANTA MARTA, COLOMBIA, MARK GRENON KNEW HE had to help.

He had already treated some coronavirus victims with MMS and reported that "people recovered fast." (Of course, given that the virus kills only 1 percent or so of its victims, that's like pointing out that swinging a dead cat in the light of a full moon has a 99 percent effective track record.)

He had also been laying tracks for MMS to make deeper inroads into the Republican establishment. He and his son Jonathan had dinner with Alan Keyes, after which the IAMtv digital channel became one of MMS's biggest supporters, occasionally mentioning the One True Cure on its various shows. Keyes spoke to a woman who claimed that MMS reversed her child's autism, and he broadcast another episode with two bottles of MMS sitting on his desk.

This sort of support kited MMS's fortunes higher and higher. By then, the Genesis II Church of Health and Healing claimed to have more than three thousand active members and to have given MMS to more than five million people.

And now the pandemic was causing sales of MMS to explode, from $30,000 each month to $120,000 in March 2020. But in early April Grenon got a letter from the FDA; the church was one of seven hundred groups identified as promoting fake COVID cures. A week later the church was slapped with a court injunction from US District Judge Kathleen Williams to halt distribution of MMS immediately.

The Grenons penned a belligerent thirty-five-page response that asserted their right to distribute healing sacraments. In a series of podcasts heard by tens of thousands of people, Mark Grenon began hinting at violence—and by hinting at, I mean threatening.

"When Congress does immoral things, passes immoral laws, that's when you pick up guns, right?" he asked, adding later, "You could be taken out, Miss Williams."

That's when he had a great idea. He should get MMS into the hands of the former game show host.

"Dear Mr. President," his letter began.

He wrote that he knew the game show host listened to antivaccine activists. He name-dropped Alan Keyes and noted that he would appear on Keyes's show that very day. He laid out the scientific case for MMS. "There is so much evidence proving it is a wonderful detox through

238 - IF IT SOUNDS LIKE A QUACK . . .

oxidation that can kill 99 percent of the pathogens in the human body," he wrote.

He told the president that he was doing a good job of draining the swamp that included the FDA, the CDC, and the FTC. But mostly he framed the right to distribute MMS as a matter of medical freedom.

"All we want is the right to choose, sir," he said. "We will not tolerate our rights, to keep our temples clean by our sacraments, to be taken from us. This is not preference to us, but a conviction. A conviction is something you will die for sir."

Then he added, almost as an afterthought, "Please get rid of Dr. Fauci and Gates" (Gates being billionaire Bill Gates, who was not employed by the government and thus could not be "got rid of" except by unsavory means).

.•:˙

THE WHITE HOUSE WAS BY THEN HOSTING FREQUENT NEWS BRIEFINGS ON the coronavirus pandemic. The briefings were, according to the game show host, a tremendous success.

In 2015 *Celebrity Apprentice* had drawn an average audience of 7.6 million (thanks in part to the star power of Beverly Hills Real Housewife Brandi Glanville), while a rival gameshow, *The Bachelor*, had had an average audience of 8.02 million, counting live and same-day viewing. But now, 8.5 million cable television viewers were tuning in each day to hear him speak about the pandemic.

So, you know, all things considered, the coronavirus press conferences were doing very well.

"Because the 'Ratings' of my News Conferences etc. are so high, 'Bachelor finale, Monday Night Football type numbers' . . . the Lamestream Media is going CRAZY," the president tweeted as the American death toll from COVID-19 approached twenty-five hundred.

And the April 24 press conference was shaping up to be one of the best yet.

The game show host stood respectfully while Bill Bryan, acting undersecretary for the Department of Homeland Security Science and Technology Directorate, explained to the press that scientific tests had yielded some new information in the battle against the mysterious virus. Solar light killed it in the air and on "non-porous surfaces," reducing the half life from six hours to two minutes.

"We're also testing disinfectants, readily available," said Bryan. "I can tell you that bleach will kill the virus in five minutes, isopropyl alcohol will kill the virus in thirty seconds, and that's with no manipulation, no rubbing."

This was positive news, both because it hinted at steps people could take to protect themselves and because it demonstrated that the little-understood coronavirus was vulnerable. It also seemed to remind the former game show host of something.

"I asked Bill a question that some of you are probably thinking of if you're totally into that world, which I find to be very interesting," he began. "So, supposing we hit the body with a tremendous—whether it's ultraviolet or just very powerful—light. And I think you said"—he turned to Bryan, who looked like he wished that either one of the two of them was not present—"that hasn't been checked, but you're going to test it."

The former game show host turned back to the throng of reporters hanging on his every word.

"And then I said, supposing you brought the light inside the body, which you can do either through the skin or some other way, and I think you said you're going to test that too. Sounds interesting."

The president was not done.

"And then I see the disinfectant knocks it out in a minute. One minute. And is there a way you can do something like that by injection inside, or, or almost a cleaning," he said. "Because you see it gets in the lungs and it does a tremendous number on the lung, so it would be interesting to check that. So you're going to have to use medical doctors. That sounds interesting to me."

The former game show host roped Deborah Birx—a medical doctor, an Army colonel, and the White House coronavirus response coordinator—into the conversation.

"I would like you to speak to the medical doctors to see if there's any way that you can apply light and heat to cure," the game show host told the medical doctor. "Maybe you can, maybe you can't. . . . Deborah, have you ever heard of that? The heat and the light?"

Birx, who undoubtedly had heard of both heat and light, offered a noncommittal set of gestures in response.

The event touched off a firestorm in the media. Whatever message Bryan was trying to communicate was completely lost in the idea that the president had, perhaps, suggested that the deadly virus could be expunged from the human body by somehow disinfecting the lungs and other interior organs with some combination of injection and "cleaning" with disinfectant. Also, bombarding the body with light.

.∙ ∶ ˙

THE PRESIDENT'S PERFORMANCE DREW RAVE REVIEWS FROM AT LEAST ONE group: sellers of MMS.

A few hours after the press conference, Grenon posted on Facebook that the president "has got the MMS and all the info!!! Things are happening folks! Lord help others to see the Truth!"

During an interview, Grenon told Zakariya Adeel (author of *Secrets of the Combined Astrology*) that he had delivered bottles of MMS to the White House through a personal relation and that the president had actually consumed it.

"We were able to give, through a contact . . . a family member, the bottles in my book," Grenon told Adeel. "And he mentioned it on TV: 'I found this disinfectant.' He was drinking it. On a press conference. And they started mocking him, saying he was drinking bleach."

He posted on Facebook that the FDA's efforts to stop his distribution of MMS were a trampling of the Genesis II Church's religious rights. "We pray that we will see the end of the FDA and we will thank the Lord that He used us to be apart [*sic*] of it and bring 'Health Freedom' to the world!"

The alien's plan to bring disease-killing MMS to the world kicked into high gear.

Marketers of MMS incorporated the game show host's statements into their promotions, and sales spiked in Latin America, where hundreds of buyers lined up outside hastily erected MMS distribution centers. There were ten reports of poisoning in Bolivia. Argentina opened a criminal investigation into two poisoning deaths associated with a member of the Genesis II Church.

In Illinois, soon after the game show host's remarks, the state's poison control center received a call from a person who had tried to kill the coronavirus by gargling with a mixture of mouthwash and bleach. There was another call about someone trying to rinse their sinuses with a detergent-based solution. A man turned to the Kansas Poison Control center, where reports of poisoning cases shot up 40 percent, after drinking unspecified cleaning chemicals in "a product because of advice he received," according to a public official.

In New York City, the poison control center fielded calls about 30 cases of poisoning in the eighteen-hour period after the game show host made his comments. The Maryland Emergency Management Agency received more than 100 calls about people who tried to treat COVID by ingesting disinfectants. Calls were also up in Michigan. In all, there were 9,348 cases of bleach or disinfectant poisoning reported to US poison control centers in April of 2020 (as compared to 4,870 in April of 2019).

It was really, really tremendous.

A COUPLE OF DAYS LATER THE PRESIDENT WAS ASKED ABOUT HIS DISINfectant comments by reporters while sitting at the Resolute Desk in the White House. The president expressed a barely contained outrage at the stupidity. Not of his own words but of those who had misconstrued the masterful comedic bit that he had unfurled during the news conference. The reporters, he said, had been pwned.

"I was asking a question sarcastically to reporters like you, just to see what would happen," said the former game show host. He then seemed to immediately go back to suggesting that perhaps the basic idea contained in his supposedly sarcastic comment had been sound.

"Now, disinfectant, maybe on the hands like this, maybe that would work. I was asking the question to the gentleman, Bill," he said.

He then shifted back to the sarcasm line.

"I was asking a sarcastic question, a very sarcastic question to the reporters. That was done in the form of a sarcastic question to the reporters," he said, ending the debate. Though, he added, "I do think that disinfectant on the hands could have a very good effect. Now Bill has gone back to check that in the laboratory. It's a very amazing laboratory by the way. . . . I said, 'Well, how do we do it inside the body or even outside the body with the hands?' And disinfectant I think would work, he thinks would work. But you do it when you're doing your hands."

A reporter, clearly wanting desperately to report that the American president had definitively debunked the idea of disinfecting the lungs with bleach injections or other cleaners, practically begged him to say words to that effect.

"Just to clarify, sir," said the reporter. "You're not encouraging Americans to—"

"No. Of course not," said the president. "It was put in a question to a group of extraordinarily hostile people, namely the fake news media."

The reporter, submissively giving the impression that of course he himself understood the game show host's intentions, said timidly that some doctors—not the reporter, mind you, just the doctors—thought the president should clarify the statement.

"Well of course," said the president, as if the doctors in question were persecuting him. He looked directly at the reporter. "*You* know the way it was asked," the former game show host said irritably. "I was looking at *you*."

"Sir," said the reporter, miserably, "I wasn't there yesterday."

"I know," said the president. "I know."

The subject was changed.

.∵˙

THE DISCUSSION IN THE WHITE HOUSE WAS AN EXTRAORDINARY ACCOMplishment for Grenon and the shadow health empire in general. For them to get there so many things had to go wrong. Or, from their perspective, right.

They needed a weak-enough enforcement environment to enable them to distribute MMS over a period of years with minimal interference. They needed a rogue media network on which prominent national politicians and media personalities would be willing to hawk their wares to large audiences. And they needed a network of social and political connections that allowed them to get bottles—let's assume they contained

MMS, but they could have contained literally anything—to the most powerful man in the free world so that he could try it with a whole rotten pyramid of supporters urging him on. And then they needed the president to talk about it on national television, preferably to the tremendous-sized audiences like the ones that were being drawn to shows like *The Bachelor* finale.

This was not the only victory of the increasingly sophisticated network of quacks. As the year 2020 ground painfully on, the former game show host's response to the pandemic was suffused with messaging put out by those who had discovered the One True Cure.

In July, after the FDA revoked authorization of the unproven drug hydroxychloroquine as a coronavirus treatment, the game show host tweeted a video of Stella Immanuel, a Houston doctor and church leader, touting hydroxychloroquine as the answer to coronavirus. Immanuel, a featured speaker at events supporting the game show host's political career, had a vision of American health care that included acknowledging the true causes of disease, including astrally projected female demons and alien DNA (she, like the alien in Jim Humble's skin, believed that extraterrestrials were controlling the US government).

A few weeks later, the game show host held a huge rally, without mask or social-distancing provisions, in Oklahoma. It was attended by Herman Cain, who as a Republican presidential candidate had himself sold his supporters on alternative medicines. Cain died of coronavirus soon after.

A wealthy pillow salesman named Mike Lindell pushed the game show host to back an herbal oleander extract as a coronavirus treatment. Lindell sits on the board of Phoenix Biotechnology, a Texas-based firm that claims its oleandrin treats not only coronavirus but also erectile dysfunction–causing infections. Both the FDA and the US Army invested valuable resources to study the poisonous plant as a treatment, but each soon concluded that it showed no promise. That November Ben Carson declined to wear a mask at public functions, caught coronavirus, and took oleander extract.

The president's political opponents criticized his handling of the pandemic. "Really sad," the game show host responded via tweet, "but even 'sadder', watch flunky @Lawrence CRY when I whipped his mind & he was FORCED to apologize to me over Apprentice fees. Even Psycho Cold Case Joe Scarborough (bad ratings) beat him up, on air, unmercifully."

In all, the game show host had by then tweeted about ratings 384 times and *The Apprentice* 465 times. He had used the word "health" about 100 times.

One vaccine researcher, Peter Hotez, maintained that the president's administration had actively conspired with the medical-freedom, anti-vaccine movement to undercut public health messaging about masks and social distancing.

"This was deliberately done by the White House," Hotez told the *New Yorker*. "And the only way to disentangle it was that I had to call it out and say, 'Look, this is a disinformation campaign coming out of the White House.' There was no other way to discuss it."

But there were other ways to discuss it. For example, a supporter of the game show host asked in an interview whether it was really a coincidence that public health officials were telling people to wear masks and stand six feet apart when attendees of Satan-worshiping rituals *also* wore masks and stood six feet apart?

Pwned.

.∵.

To Mark Grenon, now Bishop Mark Grenon, healing was a means to an end, a by-product of his mission to save souls.

"They'll listen to you if you heal them of cancer," he said.

Even as he was spreading MMS around the world, Grenon was writing a book that tied together the myths of the Bible and actual history. For research, he traveled to Israel and Gomorrah, taking soil samples containing sulfur that he said demonstrated they were once biblical cities that had been set aflame. He went to Saudi Arabia. He took a chip of wood from a five-thousand-year-old tree that Abraham reportedly had sat under. He visited an altar at the mountain where Moses was said to have received the Ten Commandments.

"All the things that they talked about, the wells, everything's still there," Grenon said.

He began to map out a visit to Egypt to see the Red Sea crossing. You could supposedly find chariot wheels from biblical times there. He began to coordinate the visit with the ambassador to Egypt.

And that's when the federal agents kicked in his door.

On August 10, 2020, the day after Grenon's birthday, he was in his Colombian compound, reading the Bible at about six a.m. and drinking coffee with his wife.

"Boom. I hear a smash." He thought there had been an accident outside.

When there was a second smashing sound, he knew his compound was being stormed. They broke in through the back door. It was a full SWAT team, a dozen armed agents with "machine guns in my face."

Working to carry out FDA-initiated directives, they also arrested his son Joe in Colombia, and Jonathan and Jordan in Bradenton, Florida, where authorities seized fifty gallons of hydrochloric acid and eighty-three hundred pounds of sodium chlorite, the raw materials of MMS, from a steel warehouse. They took computers and cell phones. They closed out his bank accounts with Wells Fargo, Chase, and ClickBank, and confiscated $80,000 from a safe. The family members lost their YouTube account, their domain address with GoDaddy, and their Face-book pages. Grenon was flown to Bogotá on a police plane.

The immortal being who had introduced Grenon to MMS was no-where to be found.

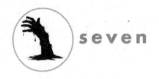

seven

AMERICAN HEALTH CARE
A REFUGE FOR ZOMBIES

The Doctor fed, but talk'd the while,
Of gastric juice and flowing bile;
Of kidneys and o'ergrowing liver,
As of sore eyes now cur'd for ever;
What his fam'd Nostrum had perform'd,
And how it had the bowels storm'd
Of guttling Gourmand with such force,
That it a passage made of course,
Which three great Doctors tried in vain,
With all their boasted skill to gain.
Besides our hero did not know
How cookery went on below,
And he might think, poor dainty sinner,
That the same hands had dress'd the dinner,
Which were entrusted with the care
Each daily med'cine to prepare;
To melt the salves and spread anon
The cerates and diacolon;
That did the drugs or grind or pound,
And dress the sore leg's running wound:
But so it was, a sick sensation
Check'd all his powers of mastication,
And caus'd his stomach to resent
The very taste of nutriment:
Nay his sad appetite approv'd
When all the dishes were remov'd.

—William Combe, *The History of Johnny Quae Genus,*
the Little Foundling of the Late Doctor Syntax, 1822

EVEN BEYOND CONSOLIDATING RADICALIZED AMERICANS INTO A political bloc and lining the pockets of people promoting alternative treatments, the medical-freedom movement had an impact on the health of America.

The antivax sentiment represented a deep self-wounding as millions of Americans, mostly in the South and West and mostly in rural counties that had voted for the former game show host in his presidential campaign, flouted social-distancing, mask, and vaccine recommendations during the COVID-19 pandemic, leading to more cases and more deaths from the virus in those regions.

When 2020 finally came to a close, the US had suffered more coronavirus deaths per capita than any other country. That death toll was a by-product of the massive though largely invisible transformation of how health care worked in America and of the medical establishment's hemorrhaging of both patients and trust. Millions of individuals responded to perceived flaws in medical doctors by simply abandoning them. Nationally, fewer than one in three Republicans said they trusted medical scientists to act in the public's interests. Rates of people who lacked health insurance were higher in red states, topping 20 percent in the deep-red South by 2018. A 2020 survey found that 105 million Americans—roughly a third of the country—had opted out of all professional medical care during the preceding twelve months.

They weren't opting out of health care, mind you—just *professional* health care.

They were defecting to forms of health care that had less regulation, less science, and less transparency. A 2017 Pew Research poll showed that 20 percent of Americans had rejected conventional medicine and exclusively used alternative medicine. The National Association of Boards of Pharmacy, which counted 400 online pharmacies in 1999 and 11,000 in 2005, estimated that there were now 35,000 active online pharmacies, of which roughly 33,250 were not in compliance with the law. By 2027, analysts predicted, the global alternative-medicine market would be worth $296.3 billion, a tenfold increase over 1998. (At the same time, global spending on health care as a whole doubled between

1998 and 2020 to $8.5 trillion and is expected to decline in future years as coronavirus-related spending is stepped down.)

By partnering with the medical-freedom movement, alternative healers were not merely competing with the medical establishment. They were breaking it.

The game show host elevated two members of the congressional "Dietary Supplement Caucus," Mick Mulvaney and Mike Pompeo, to White House chief of staff and secretary of state, respectively.

At the FDA, agents who had once showed up on the doorsteps of hucksters now found representatives of those hucksters in the corner offices of their headquarters. Political appointees fell on the agency like a corrosive acid rain. The game show host's new cadre, which was cheered by the supplements industry, included FDA commissioner Stephen Hahn, medical-freedom advocate David Gortler as senior advisor to the commissioner, and top spokesperson for the agency Emily Miller, a recent talking head on the hard-right, supplement-infused media channel One America News Network and author of *Emily Gets Her Gun: But Obama Wants to Take Yours*.

Antivaxxer Andrew Wakefield had said the establishment was in for a shakeup. Under the new regime, it was not only shaken up but shaken sideways, shaken violently, and shaken down, leaving its data-loving bureaucrats visibly shaken.

For example, the game show host successfully pressured the CDC to revise COVID testing recommendations so that those who came in close contact with coronavirus patients no longer received a recommendation to be tested. At the same time, the science that underpinned the FDA's authority was being undermined, as in August 2020, when the FDA obtained the results of a study indicating that roughly 8 percent of hospitalized coronavirus patients who received blood plasma within three days died, versus roughly 11 percent who died after receiving blood plasma on day four or later. It was a pretty ho-hum finding, but the White House was eager to inflate any shred of good news. So FDA spokeswoman Miller and Commissioner Hahn completely misrepresented the study as a supposed major breakthrough, inaccurately saying that it showed blood plasma infusions would save the lives of thirty-five out of one hundred hospitalized coronavirus patients.

Meanwhile, the FDA *Operations Manual*'s 567 pages of directives were being referenced much less often because its enforcement wing was taking far fewer actions against One True Cures. The agency secured injunctions—its most powerful enforcement tool—against half as many criminal violators as it had during its Obama-era peak. Its hyper-capitalized warning letters also decreased by half (thereby saving lots of money on uppercase *W*s and *L*s), while those targeting medical devices, like fraudulently marketed lasers, dropped even more steeply, by two-thirds.

For FDA staffers, efforts to cling to science became perilous. After the agency rejected the use of oleandrin (the poisonous plant extract championed as a coronavirus treatment by the pillow salesman who holds a spot on the board of an oleandrin-selling company) as a dietary supplement, the game show host attacked both the FDA and the National Institutes of Health as "Deep State."

The overall picture was clear. The FDA was in tatters. And the One True Cures had won.

⠄⠒⠈

As the first days of January 2021 rolled by, much of the country—and certainly those in the medical establishment—breathed sighs of relief. The nation had resoundingly rejected the game show host's re-election bid, and people were eager to turn the page.

But on January 6, as Congress met to certify the election results, the game show host held a rally just outside the US Capitol building. Thousands of supporters showed up; some gathered around a "health-freedom" stage to hear speakers like Denise Aguilar, head of an all-female militia group that taught members natural medicine and its seemingly distant cousin, firearms use. On the main stage, immediately after the game show host's speech ended, the crowd marched on Congress, pushing past blockades and a small number of Capitol police officers who got in their way.

Over the course of the next few hours, as members of the crowd expressed vehement support of the president (who neither addressed the throng nor allowed for the deployment of the National Guard to control them), they grew increasingly—well, afterward they strongly objected to being described as violent, so let's just say they grew increasingly animated. They also didn't like the mainstream media's characterization of the event as a riot, but even they wouldn't deny that it was a five-alarm kerfuffle.

As the crowd began to break doors and windows in an effort to hunt down members of Congress, there were signs of the health-freedom movement everywhere. A New Jersey antivaccine and medical-freedom organizer named Stephanie Hazelton used her pink phone to record herself urging people into the building. Aguilar was in the crowd, as were Tennessean activists Ty and Charlene Bollinger, founders of a PAC called United Medical Freedom. The Bollingers, who helped to organize rallies in advance of the animation, made tens of millions of dollars selling video series called *The Truth About Cancer* and *The Truth About Vaccines* for up to $500 each.

The crowd began to flow into the federal building; some wore animal pelts, some wore bulletproof vests, and some wore both. There was face paint and campaign swag. Someone carried a spear.

Inside, Simone Gold, head of the antivax group America's Frontline Doctors, gave an impromptu, shouty speech to some of the kerfufflers and at another time was part of a crowd that animatedly pushed and pulled Capitol police officers out of the way. Gold, who had received roughly $150,000 in federally funded COVID relief grants, had organized a rally earlier that day for health freedom.

Police officers defending the Capitol were repeatedly taunted and beaten. Someone used a tomahawk axe against them. Others used flagpoles, a fire extinguisher, and a wooden plank. Few people had ever seen such an animated kerfuffle.

As the crowd broke through the glass of a locked hallway door inside the Capitol building, police shot and killed libertarian activist Ashli Babbitt. Three other kerfufflers died in the commotion.

About 150 Capitol police officers were injured, one officer died from a series of strokes that were induced by the injuries and trauma of the day, and several others committed suicide in the following days and weeks.

Many felt that America had hit rock bottom.

The medical-freedom movement, which had a great deal of practice disagreeing with people, disagreed.

Mainstream America had a blind spot: it tended to allocate attention to an idea in direct proportion to that idea's relevance to reality. This meant that when people heard about something ridiculous—a secessionist drive in Texas, a game show host seeking the presidency, a plan to derail a legitimate election by storming the Capitol—they either discounted it or discussed it as an entertaining trifle.

Every time public officials sank to a new low by embracing an undemocratic, preposterous, or even dangerous idea, mainstream America thought the country had, this time, hit bottom. It was unable to see the next ridiculous idea, the next potential low, as a serious possibility. One cannot *see* through the looking glass; one can only *go* through it.

As I researched this book, I found the actual bottom. It is becoming a reality. And it is so ludicrous that it has, to date, been utterly dismissed.

A prime example of this blind spot came when a team of academic researchers documenting the pandemic's effect on dream imagery found that zombies were turning up more frequently, which they understood to represent the threat of the pandemic.

I'll put forth an alternate theory: the zombies represented zombies.

HAMILTON NEUMANN, THE YOUNGEST SON OF DALE AND LEILANI NEUmann, maintained his passion for filmmaking and cameras into adulthood. In August 2015, at the age of twenty, he landed a gig as a cameraman for one of the best-known televangelists of the 1980s: Jim Bakker, whose *PTL Club* was once the largest religious-themed TV show in America. Tall and lean, Hamilton would eventually become Bakker's director of video production, and he sometimes traveled with members of Bakker's family to film segments for the show.

Bakker's ratings weren't what they had been in his heyday, but he was doing well enough. The show earned money by selling a variety of branded and affiliated products—including the "silver solution," Bakker's One True Cure for COVID-19—to his followers, many of whom were actively preparing for the end of days. Bakker also regularly hawked an array of survival products, including large buckets of "Cheesy Broccoli Rice" and "Creamy Potato Soup," which could cost up to $4,500.

In April of 2021, soon after sitting down to film another episode, Bakker introduced his guest, a radio host named Steve Quayle, who sold a handheld device that detected EMF (electromagnetic field) frequencies in food for just $279.

Quayle had Black friends. And he had Mexican friends. I know this because after mentioning Hillary Clinton, he interrupted himself to say, "I have Black friends. I have Mexican friends."

But Quayle wasn't there to discuss the finer points of Black-and-Mexican-friend-having. He had an important message for Bakker's apocalypse-indulgent audience.

Quayle told Bakker that COVID variants were in fact biological weapons designed to depopulate the Earth, and that nasal-swab COVID tests were efforts to collect, en masse, genetic material. And "now they want to take our South-end swabs," he added, referring to people's butts in politer terms than he had used to refer to genocide.

Quayle moved on, getting all the way down to the brass tacks embedded within the set's cushily upholstered chairs. He referenced a new COVID variant emerging in Brazil, which he said was a prophetic signal. Why? Because Brazil was also a known habitat for zombies.

"A zombie is literally a life form that has—how should I say this—animation. But if you've seen them, they're not all there. They may have missing parts. But they have a taste for human flesh."

The zombies, he said, were "coming up from under the Earth" to invade the "dimensional reality" of the world, creating "a supernatural battle for our very existence."

Quayle, a longtime believer in zombies, had become a sort of hub for news of the undead. And lately, he said, his email inbox was blowing up with firsthand accounts of zombie encounters, some of them from people in the military and law enforcement.

"I have a friend that was in Iraq who sent me the account, actually coming into an entire camp of zombies. He said, 'Steve, they were dragging one leg like in a movie. One of them only had half a body.'"

Quayle added that he was not trying to freak people out. And in the spirit of not freaking people out, he also added that certain diseases could initiate cannibalism in human beings.

Jim Bakker broke in. "I know my audience [members] are having a hard time with 'zombies,'" he said, trying to keep the discussion in a world that was—well, sensible isn't the right word, but in that narrow range of insensibility in which people might shell out $4,500 for buckets of soup.

Bakker gave Quayle a chance to step it back, just a bit. "Do you believe in zombies?"

"Absolutely," said Quayle.

Bakker seemed a bit taken aback. This was, perhaps, a matter of semantics. He suggested that maybe Quayle was calling a real-life, transmissible disease by the inflammatory name of zombieism.

"Is that right, Steve? Zombies that are on the Earth are a disease like any other disease that affects people and they become like zombies," Bakker said. "Is that right?"

"Forgive me," Quayle said. "But that's only part of the story."

Quayle explained that vaccines could indeed induce zombieism, like a disease. But zombies were also possessed by demonic entities imbued with the sole purpose of destroying humanity. And because the vaccine-induced disease rewrote the victim's DNA, the zombies were literally inhuman beasts.

"The whole subject of zombies could be just boiled down at one end to a genetically modified human that is no longer a human on the level that you and I or a living being is," said Quayle.

He offered some rock-solid evidence to back up his assertions. "If this is all wild stuff," he asked rhetorically, "why does the military have a manual about it, when it happens? Why does the CDC?"

Quayle believes that the presence of walking dead is proof of the resurrection, which denotes biblical end times. In Quayle's version of world history, zombies overran the original inhabitants of Easter Island; they annihilated Indigenous Americans and the lost colony of Roanoke; thousands of zombified supporters of the Confederacy were put down by victorious Union soldiers during the Civil War; in 1935, infected rats spread zombieism through a population of hurricane survivors on an island in the Florida Keys.

Quayle is not the only person who believes in zombies. America was suddenly, somehow, full of them. Believers in zombies vary in their specific viewpoints, but they return to the same cultural touchstones: The Miami attack. Ali Khan's zombie-apocalypse instructions on the CDC website. A shadowy conspiracy behind it all.

David Eells of Unleavened Bread Ministries, who joined with the Neumanns in treating their dying, totally treatable eleven-year-old daughter with prayer, told his ministry that "a demon possession of people who actually devour others came to pass." It was, per the CDC zombie-training plan, an act of the Deep State government.

"The government," Eells told his followers in one online missive, "has been joking about this Zombie apocalypse for some time in accordance with the powers that be's habit of telling us beforehand what they are planning to do."

"Remember," he said in another, "those who partook of the bath salts began to physically devour one another."

A preacher named Lance Wallnau warned that the media was using mind control and witchcraft to whip up the left against the game show host. "Many of them are so zombified that they're taken captive by a spirit," he said.

A woman named Jillian Epperly (whose One True Cure, Jilly Juice, is a drink of fermented cabbage and salt that she says can regenerate lost limbs, eliminate cancer, and "cure" homosexuality) told her viewers that zombies were an extreme example of a body compromised by poor nutrition and susceptible to violent "glitching" when exposed to triggers like electromagnetic frequencies.

A 2019 poll showed that 14 percent of Americans had an active plan in mind should the zombie apocalypse happen. Among those with a plan, 26 percent intended to get their hands on guns, 6 percent planned to actively kill zombies or survivors, and 12 percent, even more disturbingly, refused to say what their plans were.

Followers of Quayle and Bakker might have rejected the notion of zombies had they not already been primed to accept conspiracy theories about a global ring of Satan-worshiping pedophiles. The idea was established by QAnon, a grassroots community built around conspiracy theories that were released by a public official who used the pseudonym "Q." The impact of the idea became national news in late 2016, when North Carolinian Edgar Maddison Welch fired an assault rifle inside a DC pizza restaurant that he believed was a front for a Democratic-controlled child sex-trafficking ring. When the criminal case against him was adjudicated, District Judge Ketanji Brown Jackson sentenced Welch to four years in prison. But the false ideas that had inspired him continued to grow. In 2019, an anonymously authored QAnon book claiming that Democrats eat children became an Amazon best seller, peaking in a group of the seventy-five most popular books in the country. A poll revealed that a majority of Republicans thought the Deep State pedophile-ring story was either "mostly true" (33 percent) or true in "some parts" (23 percent), while another found that half the people who supported the game show host's reelection campaign believed he was fighting against a child sex-trafficking ring run by Democrats.

In 2022, five years after Jackson sentenced Welch for storming the pizzeria, she was nominated to serve on the US Supreme Court. During her confirmation hearings, her incarceration of a QAnon believer boomeranged back on her in the form of QAnon-based criticism from top-level Republicans that held, or pandered to, these beliefs. Senators Josh Hawley and Lindsey Graham accused Jackson of being unreasonably lenient on crimes related to child pornography, false accusations that quickly echoed through far-right QAnon-friendly media channels.

And so it was only natural that when Bakker and Quayle were chatting, they reminded their audience that the very crazy idea of zombies roaming the Earth was just an extension of other crazy ideas that audience members already believed.

"What about these left-wing dinner parties?" Bakker asked Quayle, referencing a conspiracy theory that the Clintons eat babies. "They eat crazy things. I don't even like to talk about it because it's so, so weird."

"It's an absolute occult ritual," Quayle agreed. "Spirit cooking means you're providing the sustenance for evil spirits."

"The lady," said Bakker, "the famous one, I won't even say her name, you see the bloody ghost head. . . . Even a famous politico had a picture in his house of two men sitting over a cadaver, eating it."

"I'll be blunt," said Quayle, who had apparently not been blunt yet. Hollywood, Quayle said, was in on it.

"Two of the most famous, wealthy pop singers have said they are serving Satan and have talked about the taste of human flesh," he said.

The medical-freedom movement starts with a perfectly reasonable desire not to have Big Brother breathing down your neck, takes a hard right when it is monetized in the poorly regulated internet marketplace, and ends with fears that zombies will overrun your bomb shelter.

It's bizarre. It's wacky. It's almost laughable.

But it's not laughable. Here's why: The Americans who believe in zombies don't think they're equally spread throughout the population. They believe that the zombies are Democrats. Or liberals. Or liberal Democrats. Or the shadowy cartel of elite puppet masters behind the Demoncrats.

And once you've convinced yourself that those with opposing political views are literally undead monsters, it can be difficult to sit down with them for Thanksgiving dinner.

Zombie credence showed that even an absurdity like the QAnon satanist narrative was not the bottom. It was just another gateway down a slippery slope that ended in a deep, shit-steeped rabbit hole with a dehumanizing narrative as powerful as those deployed in Nazi Germany against the so-called "inferior races."

Democrats were zombies.

The show wrapped. It was another great episode, the kind that would be sure to sell a lot of soup.

.∙:˙

QUAYLE'S APPEARANCE ON THE BAKKER SHOW WAS JUST ONE EXAMPLE OF how the idea that Democrats were literal flesh-eating zombies was sweeping through segments of the American public.

On the website Infowars (where for $562.30 one can buy six hundred pills containing "DNA Force Plus"), Alex Jones told his large audience that liberals "want to get you in a dungeon. They want to strap you down and take a buzz saw and cut the top of your head off like a pumpkin and pull it off and get a little spoon and go . . . 'I'm going to eat your brain now.'"

Conspiracy theorist Sherry Shriner's bread and butter was the sale of pricy "Orgone Blasters" (containing the imaginary substance orgone), which protected one from the shape-shifting alien reptiles that were replacing humans. Though Shriner supported the game show host and the game show host admired Katy Perry, Shriner's followers had identified Perry as a secret reptilian, along with Justin Bieber and Taylor Swift. Shriner announced that her orgone products would also protect her followers from government-created zombies, which were totally real.

The video game *Covid: Survive the Plandemic* invited players to shoot people who have been turned into flesh-eating zombies by vaccinations. Another video game, in which players shoot "Democratic zombies," was in development but was put on hold when its designer, Jack Jesse Griffith, was arrested for participating in the Capitol kerfuffle. The point of the game, Griffith posted on Facebook, was to "raise awareness."

To me, the idea of dead-eyed mobs with not-quite-human gaits had been most memorably brought to life by the motion-capture special effects of the detestably saccharine holiday movie *The Polar Express*, but the sinister tone of the zombie propaganda I heard showed that I was very much behind the times.

Conservative radio host Tom Horn (whose book of conspiracy theories was available in Walmart for $15.77), told his audience to actively prepare for the coming apocalypse—but to hide their beliefs and preparations from their own adult children and other nonbelievers within the family.

"Assume you will be betrayed. . . . Keep your survival and prep plans private. I know that sounds harsh to some people, but you cannot entrust to people who think you're crazy," Horn said. "There are some people listening that need to hear this. You cannot entrust to people who think, 'Oh, Mom's a little off, Dad's wacky.' You can't trust them at that point. . . . It applies to spouses too."

Scott Lively, president of Abiding Truth Ministries (an anti-LGBTQ group) and a failed two-time candidate for governor of Massachusetts, held an online Bible study in which he said violence would likely be needed to stop the "emerging Beast government."

"If at all possible, you disarm the zombies trying to kill you without hurting them," said Lively. "But if it's not possible, you do whatever is necessary to stop them. . . . That, I believe, is the duty of an American."

With this sort of zombie buzz happening at the street level, savvy political operatives began slipping zombie references into their rhetoric. If you didn't believe in zombies, it sounded like a mere metaphorical insult; if you did, it was a rallying cry against the literal undead.

In 2020, Jo Rae Perkins, the GOP's Senate nominee in Oregon, said mask mandates and social-distancing guidelines were part of a plot to turn the public into zombies. She knew this "based on what I have read on some of the Marxist theories." Five days after she lost, she announced that she would be running again, and in 2022 she once again secured her party's nomination.

The reelection campaign of the game show host aired an ad in 2020 in which viewers were told to prevent "a zombie" from entering the White House.

"Look for someone with a corpse-like appearance, exhibits aggressive behavior, craves human flesh, and utters incoherent moans and groans," the voice-over noted while distorted footage of Democratic presidential nominee Joe Biden doing all the above played in the background. "With your help we can prevent the zombie uprising," the short ad concluded.

One of the most unsettling scenes in Romero's canon of genre-defining zombie movies comes late in his 1990 remake of *Night of the Living Dead*, after the humans had nearly eradicated the zombie threat. As they mopped up the few remaining undead, vigilante yahoo whooped and hollered, knocking the helpless zombies down and torturing them. It was disturbing because it focused not on the capacity of zombies to eat brains but on the capacity of Americans to lose theirs.

Mainstream media outlets and Democratic political leaders responded to the zombie narrative in their way.

A *USA Today* fact check wearily responded to a viral video that amassed ten thousand interactions on Facebook: "Vaccination will not turn vaccine recipients into zombies; the CDC website on 'Zombie Preparedness' was created in 2011 as a vehicle for spreading information on emergency preparedness."

When film provocateur Sascha Baron Cohen caught two men on video telling his Borat character that the Clintons tortured children, removed their adrenal glands, and drank their blood, Hillary Clinton called the idea "hurtful."

In July 2021, during a CNN town hall, President Biden pleaded for reason. "The idea," Biden said, "that the Democrats or that Biden is hiding people and sucking the blood of children. I'm serious. Now you may not like me, and that's your right. . . . But the kinds of things that are being said of late. . . . Do you ever remember a time like this before, in our entire history, whether a Democrat or a Republican?"

Fact checks, expressions of hurt, denials, calls for reason.

Establishment politicians were bringing a brilliantly annotated and painstakingly highlighted copy of *Robert's Rules of Order* to a gunfight.

.ᐧ:ᐧ

WHEN QUAYLE WAS SELLING THE IDEA OF DEMONIC FLESH-EATING zombies to Jim Bakker, he relied mostly on a spiritual explanation. But he did have a scientific one as well, tied to vaccines.

"It's important that people understand . . . the digital insertion of nanobot technology," he said.

The digital insertion of nanobot technology. To the mainstream scientific community it sounded pretty thin, but in fact the scientific evidence behind the notion came from an authoritative source. Someone who many people felt was among the best research scientists in the world. An ITNJ commissioner. An Eagle Scout. A certified avocado grower.

In the past—2015—Robert Young had referred to zombies in a metaphorical sense, writing, "Acidic religions, governments, politics, businesses, lifestyles and diets have turned the majority of earthlings into Zombies!"

But in 2020, his teachings evoked zombies in the context of the coronavirus. Young's theory of the vaccine was simple. The shots supposedly contained a nefarious brew of ingredients, including "fragmented genetic matter from a 14 week old male aborted fetus," various acidic substances, "luciferase dye," and "aluminum oxide."

The metallic nanoparticles in the vaccine could be activated by an electromagnetic network (of the sort used in cell phone towers) to assert total control over people's bodies, thereby turning them into mind-controlled slaves.

This didn't really square with the biblical notion of zombies put forth by Quayle, but that's the beauty of the One True Cure worldview: squaring is a mathematical function, and the medical-freedom crowd abandoned the Numbers Junkies long ago.

After raising the issue in a blog, Young explained the science of the vaccine/zombie connection on a show hosted by "Dr." Charlie Ward (not a doctor, and he sells thirty-dollar "holographic disks" that purport to protect against 5G cellular networks). Ward in turn explained to Young that the COVID crisis was perhaps a smokescreen to clear the way for a reset of the world's financial structures to the "quantum financial system," which is being installed by benevolent extraterrestrials to foil the evil cabal that rules us all.

Young's message blew up. He received wide coverage in various disreputable media outlets and talk shows, including that of Stew Peters, a bounty hunter with a freedom-themed radio broadcast. Young told anti-vaxxer Del Bigtree (who spoke to the crowds at the January 6 kerfuffle) that the graphene oxide in the COVID vaccine allowed a supercomputer to mind-control people. "This is why they need boosters," Young said. "In order to make that human a transhuman."

Before It's News, a junk news website sometimes cited by the game show host during rallies, quickly picked up on Young's rhetoric and was soon awash in articles explaining that the "Covid Depop Shot Will . . . Turn You Into a Zombie Without A Spirit or Soul! Must See Interview!" And that those zombies would be used in a coming genocide.

The site celebrated Young as the expert who proved that vaccines contain nanobot technology: "Absolutely bombshell and major reveals on what is in the vaccines, with use of electron and other kinds of microscopy from original research by Dr. Robert Young and his team."

Dr. Young. Bombshell. Major reveals. Microscopy. Original research.

It was the sort of adulatory validation that Young had pursued for so much of his "scientific" career. The fact that it came in relation not to pleomorphism but to zombieism didn't seem to phase him at all.

.∙∴∙

BY 2021, A NATIONAL SURVEY OF AMERICAN FEARS FOUND THAT 9.3 PERcent of adults—about thirty-one million people—actively feared zombies. Predictably, those fears led some fringe leaders to call for action against the zombies. Also predictably, those calls for action resulted in a select group of (mostly mentally ill) people taking action against zombies.

In East Liverpool, Ohio, a member of ZORT (the just-for-fun Zombie Outbreak Response Team, whose members decked out their vehicles in antizombie swag) was arrested by police and tagged as an "apocalyptic hunter" after someone reported that he'd been searching through an abandoned florist's building with "a very large knife" in his hand. A search of the vehicle, which had a fake skull mounted on the hood, yielded "a loaded handgun with multiple loaded magazines of ammunition, a plethora of knives, multiple crossbows and arrows."

In August 2021 alone, a variety of headlines showed just how deeply a belief in zombies was warping reality. The *New York Times* described a woman working at an eyewear store who said she wouldn't get vaccinated because the movie *I Am Legend* featured people who were turned into zombies by a vaccination campaign. (Incidentally, although the fictional *I Am Legend* does feature zombies, the culprit is a lab-engineered virus and has nothing to do with vaccines.)

A woman named Lori Vallow was found to be incompetent to stand trial in a case involving the murder of her children Tylee Ryan, seventeen, and Joshua "JJ" Vallow, seven. Vallow and her new husband, a fringe Pentecostal leader named Chad Daybell, were part of a small doomsday cult headed by Daybell, who was also involved in various Armageddon-centric religious circles. Vallow and Daybell were convinced that Vallow's children were zombies possessed by dark spirits and could be released only through death. Police were investigating a string of other suspicious deaths in the family.

A Santa Barbara high school teacher named Matthew Coleman loaded his two-year-old son and ten-month-old daughter into the family car and drove them to Rosarito, Mexico, where he shot each child in the chest with a spearfishing gun. He told the FBI that he had learned through QAnon that his wife had passed some of her inhuman DNA on to the kids and that killing them would save the world from monsters.

Foiling an imaginary cult of Democratic, zombie, child-eating, pedophile serpents by shooting a real child in the chest with a spearfishing gun.

Scale that up. That's the bottom.

Epilogue

Whenever a doctor cannot do good, he must be kept
from doing harm.

> —Hippocrates, c. 400 BC

I hasten to wish that you may take a dose of your own poison
by mistake, and enter swiftly into the damnation which you
and all other patent medicine assassins have so remorselessly
earned and do so richly deserve.

> —Mark Twain, letter responding to a man who sold the
> "Elixir of Life," a One True Cure that he promised could
> heal meningitis and diphtheria, the diseases that killed
> Twain's two young children, 1905

DURING LARRY LYTLE'S LENGTHY PRISON TERM, HIS VISION WAS deteriorating. It dropped to 20/50 in his right eye and 20/400 in his left, which meant he couldn't read emails, use a telephone, read a computer monitor, or recognize the faces of those standing near him.

As he awaited a decision on his application for compassionate release, he sometimes had to rely on his fellow inmates for help to get to the bathroom. He learned that Fredretta, now his wife, could no longer visit. She suffered from the onset of dementia, which caused her to move to another part of the country, where she could be cared for by her sons. Lytle felt isolated and depressed. In part because of his decreased mobility and in part because of his age, he suffered from incontinence and wore prison-issued adult briefs to help manage it.

Still, government prosecutors argued that he should not be released. They said that if an ailing Lytle at eighty-one years old had insisted so vehemently on breaking the law, an even more ailing Lytle at eighty-five could not be trusted to abstain from the same. He had never shown remorse.

Outside the prison walls, in the world that Larry Lytle wanted to rejoin, the laser industry he'd worked so hard to promote was still going strong. Websites trolled potential franchisee investors with offers of QLaser-based businesses. His patent was used as the basis for other questionable laser treatments. Hundreds or thousands of people, some of whom cited him as an expert in the field, offered fraudulent laser treatments to victims of Lyme disease, hair loss, cancer, coronavirus, and smoking addictions, overwhelming the ability of consumer and public health protection agencies to regulate them.

More broadly, the America outside the prison seemed to be suffering its own age-related dysfunction, though analysts disagreed on the root cause: partisan polarization, or digital dehumanization, or social media siloing, or a culture of selfishness and helplessness, or corporate exploitation, or perhaps simply the fact that the richest nation on Earth was creaking under the weight of a capitalist system that blends godlike corporate powers with an outlook that is blind to everything but short-term profits.

The societal malaise was marked by a sour national mood and bizarre, depressing behaviors on the part of individuals and companies. A teenage boy went blind after years of living almost exclusively on Pringles, white bread, processed ham, and french fries. A four-foot-tall hairball amassed by an Ohio barber went on a public tour. Two million people signed up for a Facebook event to storm Area 51 in search of aliens, leading concerned event organizers to cancel it lest they be accused of fomenting a violent antigovernmental mob. The makers of Crocs footwear began selling fanny packs designed to hang from the shoes' ankle straps. An umbrella fell against the door of a Washington, DC, WeWork office, locking the employees out for three days. Heinz released Kranch, a mixture of ketchup and ranch dressing. Someone advertised a five-bedroom, six-bathroom underground bomb shelter in Las Vegas, complete with pool, for $18 million. The creator of a "free speech" web forum called 8chan asked that it be shut down after it was overrun by QAnon conspiracists and was connected to three mass shootings over a span of months. The personal information of hundreds of millions of Americans was compromised in a series of massive corporate data breaches. The two biggest operators of dollar stores, notorious for hurting mom-and-pop shops in low-income neighborhoods, surpassed thirty thousand locations, with twenty-four thousand more planned.

America was suffering.

These situations all led to calls for fixes in the form of public policies from the democratically elected government. The FDA was by then trying new methods—it had hired Amazon coordinators and eBay coordinators who trolled listings, looking for home gastric bypass kits or human organs up for bidding, after which they could contact the retailers and request to have the listings removed. But overall America's political institutions were, like the country they served, awash in signs of strain and dysfunction. The federal government shut down for a month over the game show host's demands that public funds be used to construct a wall along the Mexican border. The CIA joined Instagram. The federal deficit was approaching a trillion dollars. The US Supreme Court ruled that people could take hovercrafts moose-hunting on the rivers of national conservation lands. The game show host was impeached but not removed from office.

And the authorities concluded that having an elderly laser salesman on the loose would not help society any. Lytle's request for compassionate release was denied.

He sat in his wheelchair, awaiting what came next.

I KNEW IT WAS UNLIKELY THAT COLOMBIAN PRISON AUTHORITIES WOULD allow me to speak to a prisoner who was awaiting extradition to the United States. But fortunately, he had use of a cell phone that let him engage in back channel conversations.

"They're evil geniuses, bro," he told me from his prison cell in La Picota penitentiary in Bogotá. "Evil geniuses. They want to depopulate the world."

Someone in the background called out to him in Spanish.

"Yeah?" he said to them. "Better. *Blando. Ahorita, ahorita!*"

Then he came back to me and explained that although he was awaiting extradition, he hadn't hired any lawyers.

"You're not going to pay lawyers to sign you into jail. They literally make a deal to sign you into jail. It's like a bank," he said. "Me and my boys knew better. We didn't sign anything. They just lock you up to shut you up." Grenon fully expected to be vindicated and released.

"We're not worried about winning. We're just upset they just can lock you up as an accusation without any evidence whatsoever," he said. "Cause they have the keys. They have the Department of Justice judges. They have the guns. If I had the guns and an army waiting when they came to get me, they wouldn't have gotten me."

In some ways prison life was hard.

"I'm living in a little cubicle, in bunk beds. Three bunk beds in each room. Six guys. It's very small. The food was really bad when I first got here."

But despite those hardships Mark Grenon actually seemed to be doing quite well. He spent some of his time collecting material for volume four of his book series on MMS. He was also getting along well with his fellow prisoners, including the South American drug dealers.

"They're just trying to make some money. They're just guys that saw a way to make some money. Somebody said 'cocaine' to them. What's the difference between that and pharmaceutical companies?" he asked. "Think about it."

The drug dealers were actually making life in prison a lot more bearable.

"There's rough guys, but they're all our friends. We're all in this together, you know what I'm saying?"

The drug dealers had ample financial resources, which kept contraband like drugs and prostitutes flowing into the prison. And because they were friendly with Grenon, it was easy for the guards to overlook Grenon's cell phone, which was pretty small potatoes.

But not entirely easy.

"Hang on—I gotta." He suddenly sounded a bit tense. "There's a guard here. Hang on."

He hung up.

But we were able to have more conversations. By the last time I spoke to him, I was beginning to appreciate just how difficult it was for society to stop people who were disseminating One True Cures that endangered the public. A short jail term or a massive civil judgment, like Robert Young received, did little to deter. Life in prison, as Lytle saw, seemed sad. On a spectrum that began with administrative warning letters, prison in a foreign country was about the most extreme deterrent the government had to employ against someone like Grenon.

So would locking him up prevent him from distributing MMS on his release?

Actually, it didn't even prevent him from distributing MMS in prison. He told me he was treating the drug dealers, other inmates, and even some guards. In all, he'd treated sixty-five individuals so far, with new ones coming to him every day.

"We have friends here," he said. "The work continues."

.•:

So if locking up the One True Cure crowd isn't the answer, what is?

In 2001, the Office of Inspector General for the Department of Health and Human Services suggested creating a national federal registry for dietary supplements, which "would allow FDA to instantly access a list of all the ingredients in a particular product and determine the product manufacturer's name as soon as it receives an adverse event report." Having a digital Rolodex of the eighty thousand products on offer is a common-sense solution that would undoubtedly help, but for more than twenty years the move has been fended off by various supplement makers and their political allies. And even if it were enacted, the root problem is much larger.

Various experts are working to untangle and fix this whole mess—a mess resulting in a society in which the public is harmed by rogue alternative healers, medical misinformation, and the political operatives who want to profit off of them.

They've got different ideas.

Perhaps the answer is battling misinformation with a task force that targets organized groups and does more to remove dangerous falsehoods from the internet, as has been suggested by Peter Hotez, the vaccine scientist.

Or perhaps a good start would be for public health authorities to acknowledge what everybody knows: that efforts to protect the health of the many can impinge on the freedom of the few. This is the position of Ronald Bayer, a professor of the history and ethics of public health at Columbia University.

"It would be more honest—and in the long term more protective of public health—to acknowledge that intervention is sometimes necessary to protect individuals from their own foolish or dangerous behaviour because such efforts can have a broad and enormous impact at a population level," Bayer wrote in a paper on the topic. "An explicit acknowledgement would also help to understand the trade-offs involved. Ironically, the use of the social impact argument can, in the end, be more subversive of rights than the explicit embrace of paternalism. After all, everything can be shown to have a social impact."

Or maybe it's like Benjamin Mazer, a doctor at Johns Hopkins University, says—that "alt-med" (the health sector version of the alt-right) has thrived because the medical establishment forced doctors to shift away from doctor-patient relations in favor of serving corporate interests.

"When the alt-med community discusses these problems, it isn't wrong, though the facts are often exaggerated beyond recognition," he wrote. He suggested that more doctors should acknowledge and vocally fight against the kernels of truth: physician kickbacks, diseases invented to sell pills, and drugs priced to maximize profit rather than achieve public good.

The solutions proposed by the FDA, Hotez, Bayer, and Mazer are each, in their way, a One True Cure for a real societal ill. But if I've learned anything from researching this book, it's that, appropriately, there is no One True Cure for the One True Cure.

Harsh action may be needed to address critical and urgent threats to the public. But the real problem can only be solved in the long game.

In 1811, French philosopher Joseph de Maistre famously said, *"Toute nation a le gouvernement qu'elle mérite,"* or "Every nation gets the government it deserves." De Maistre, who lived through the French Revolution of 1789, spent most of his life wrestling with the need for a government that could maintain order. He concluded that people must believe in a government as an expression of divine rule; to employ reason in the evaluation of the sensibility of a government would result in a lack of faith that would invariably give rise to chaos and revolution.

And clearly, in America, a lack of faith in government is weakening the social fabric in ways that threaten its very viability. But in this case I think the popular interpretation of de Maistre's aphorism is misleading. Instead, it seems to me that it also works the other way around: every government gets the nation it deserves. I see the evolution of One True Cure peddlers—from lone outlaws, to swarms of scofflaws and organized freedom fighters, to organizers of a near-dominant paradigm that led to a revolution-minded storming of the nation's capital—as the embodiment of the flaws of the medical establishment and governmental institutions.

I wish I could rewind time and reach out to the self-appointed healers before they became deeply committed to paths that caused so much pain to others—and to themselves and their families.

There was a time when Toby McAdam was just a sad sack grappling with his mother's terminal illness; when Robert Young was a Mormon missionary singing about the importance of family; when Larry Lytle was a dentist and civic leader; when Alicja Kolyszko was an immigrant looking for a taste of the American Dream; when Dale and Leilani Neumann were ordinary churchgoers falling in love; when Jim Humble was—okay, that guy was going to be wacky no matter what; and when Mark Grenon's message of natural living, peace, and brotherhood had not been so completely overshadowed by conspiracy theories.

That time is long gone, and nothing can bring it back. Never can then be now.

But somewhere out there, everywhere out there, is a new generation of people who want to live a dream—to find personal fulfillment by

270 - IF IT SOUNDS LIKE A QUACK . . .

fighting against the ills of humanity. And if those people mature in an America that is this dysfunctional, this toxic, their paths to success will become similarly disfigured.

In other words—to borrow a phrase—if we want to treat the people, we have to change the water.

.·.·

THE ALIEN IN JIM HUMBLE'S SKIN WOUND UP MOVING TO MEXICO. IT WAS for the most part a quiet life.

Sometimes he looked up at the sky; his frail human eyes did not allow him to see the space stations, but he knew they were there, overlooking Earth on behalf of various alien civilizations.

"We have to get free of this prison planet," he said.

The alien had survived a lot. One day he was on a ladder when, he said, "all of a sudden the scene switched, it just changed."

The alien in Humble's skin found himself in the presence of other extraterrestrials. They were not of the alien's benevolent race; it was "a couple of these aliens that they talk about who have big heads."

The big-headed aliens strapped him to a chair and inserted some sort of conductor wires into his chest. They didn't use any painkillers, so it hurt like hell. But that pain was nothing compared to the electric shocks they zapped him with. They did it "many, many times . . . and they did that for quite some time and it was very painful," the alien in Humble's skin recalled.

Eventually, the big-headed aliens sent him back to his terrestrial home. Spooked, he hopped in his car and began to drive away from the spot, but it turned out the big-headed aliens had done something to trigger a cardiac episode inside him. It was an intergalactic assassination attempt.

"But I had released the tension so that couldn't happen, so that was the reason I lived through that, I think," said the alien in Humble's skin.

All things considered, the human body he inhabited had shown amazing resilience. He had nearly dropped an eyeball out of its socket, broken the back, broken the neck. He had injected it with MMS. But the body had not rebelled against him; it withstood everything, like a patient ass enduring a multitude of leeches, serving its master well.

But for all that, the human form was nearly worn out, turning ninety earthly years old. Soon it would be time for the alien to discard this body like a snakeskin.

But the alien would come back in a new skin, in a new generation—if not to promote MMS then to come up with some other One True Cure to benefit humanity. With the FDA being what it was, and American society structured the way it was, that was a near certainty.

.∙:∙'

IN THE YEARS AFTER HIS RELEASE, WHEN HE WASN'T MAKING SOUP OR being sued by purchasers of his inventions, Toby McAdam continued his fight to sell supplements. But this time he tried to do it legally, by exercising his actual rights as a citizen in a democratic society. He called his congressmen constantly. He also called the FDA ombudsman two or three times a week.

"I was worse than a rash," he said.

Every call had the same purpose: to get him back into business as a manufacturer of herbal supplements.

They put him off. His labels were all wrong, they said.

So he hired a certified label expert, who devised a legal label for one of his products, Lugol's Iodine. In Toby's heyday, Lugol's had been a terrific seller, even when there wasn't irrational panic about nuclear radiation traveling from Japan to Montana. He felt that, if he could get it back on the shelves, his other products would be close behind.

Toby sent the label to the FDA and asked officials to allow him to resume manufacturing Lugol's Iodine. They said the labeling wasn't the only problem. He would have to be certified to be in compliance with Current Good Manufacturing Practices.

He asked what that meant, exactly.

They told him he would have to revamp his workspace to remove all the metal, because Lugol's Iodine corrodes metal. So Toby got disposable glass and plastic containers and implements. They told him he had to be able to safely neutralize and dispose of any inadvertent iodine spills. So he got baking soda and placed it in FDA-approved containers.

They put him off. He would have to be audited by a certified third party at his own expense, they said, before they would even consider the matter further. In 2018, he convinced a certified expert associated with Montana State University to audit him. After he followed the expert's feedback, the expert found that he was eligible for further evaluation by the FDA.

They put him off. He didn't have an approved Manual for Standard Operating Procedures, they said. He spent months writing a thirty-page proposed manual for their review.

It was rejected.

He revised it. It was rejected again, so he revised it again.

He was in a whole new universe of mimsy nitpickery. Toby suspected that Big Pharma was behind it all. But really it was just the same Numbers Junkie spirit that infused the FDA's bureaucracy. Toby made a log where he could record the changing of each light bulb in the space. He agreed to track the manufacturing lots of the printer ink cartridges he used to print his labels. Every time, as he tried to accommodate their feedback, his manual grew longer. Soon it was fifty pages long, then ninety.

In October of 2019, the FDA officials said his manual was in compliance. They were running out of excuses, and so in November they sent investigators to visit his facility. They spent three days going over everything with a fine-toothed comb. They asked where the raw materials for his iodine crystals came from. He showed them documentation; he imported potassium iodide from an FDA-approved seller in South America.

The FDA investigators left. Then they went silent.

Toby kept calling. He asked how the inspection had gone.

Really, he knew how the inspection had gone. He just wanted to hear the FDA say it.

And finally, in spring of 2020, the FDA made a grudging admission with regard to Toby's desire to sell Lugol's Iodine at 5 percent and

2.2 percent solutions. It contained the seven magic words he had been pushing for.

"You appear to be in sufficient compliance."

And with that, RisingSun became the only company in the country to have been shut down by a court-ordered consent decree and then allowed to reopen.

Toby sent a multipart tweet to the man who had made all this possible.

"I explained I tried everything and contacted Senator Baucus whom was at the summit," he tweeted to Elon Musk. "You advised to keep pushing the issue and continue. I took your advise, I was fined $80K and sent to prison for contempt for 120 days. On March 27, 2020 the FDA approved me to resume operations. It took close to 10 years. Your advice worked, it cost me but it was well worth it. Sometimes sacrifice is important. Thank you."

Musk didn't respond, but Toby didn't mind. His purpose was restored.

He made as much Lugol's as he could, as quickly as he could. In the midst of a national pandemic-fueled mask shortage, he argued that sanitizing masks with Lugol's Iodine could help extend the life of an existing mask.

This was true.

Soon, he was selling a thousand bottles a month.

Toby McAdam has come to a different understanding of the role the government should play in his industry. Now that he was following the rules, he wanted the FDA to rein in the bad actors he saw selling counterfeit Lugol's Iodine on Amazon. Some products labeled Lugol's, he complained, were actually povidone-iodine, which he said should not be ingested.

"I did not know the industry was this bad," he told me. "I thought everybody was following the rules like I did. But that's not true. It's wide open."

Herbal supplements, he said, "should be held to a higher standard. Herbal supplements need to be manufactured like pharmaceuticals."

And that's why his website has gone from touting unfounded health claims to trumpeting how "RisingSun Iodine Is Different" from its competitors: "Labels reviewed by FDA. GMP Certified facility. FDA inspected facility."

Those statements mean that even if the seller is an ex-con, the bottle contains what it says it does. And to the American consumer, all that really matters is what's in the bottle.

It's the sort of claim one can have faith in.

IN THE SWELTERING 2021 MIDSUMMER OF FLORIDA, ALICJA KOLYSZKO PRE-pared to leave the Baleen restaurant to continue her lonely leech work, straddling the line between an FDA that is too restrictive and an amateur leech community that is far too lax.

She was considering expanding the curriculum of the Academy of Hirudotherapy to include acupuncture and other established alternative practices that could help shore up support for her One True Cure.

At any given time, Alicja has a couple of hundred leeches in her home; she uses a select few on herself once every two weeks. The leeches give her energy, she said. And she needs energy.

"Demand is incredible." In Europe, she told me, so many people are using leeches that breeders can't keep up. "It's demand like in the nineteenth century."

Though she is in her seventies, she is constantly on the move, hopping from one patient to the next in a never-ending circuit from Miami to Ventura to Naples and all points in between. She is like a jolly, Slavic, female Santa Claus, off to visit homes with a sack of bandages, rolled gauze, cotton balls, feminine napkins, alcohol pads, gloves, syringes of different sizes, and sometimes an aftercare cream to help patients with characteristic itching. And, of course, leeches.

Often she winds up working twelve sessions in a single day, napping in her car before beginning the next day's marathon. The schedule is taxing, but not a word of complaint escapes her lips. Once a penniless immigrant, she has treated thousands of patients with hundreds of thousands of leeches. This is her American Dream in the tangible, turgid flesh, and every day she glows with pride.

"I will never give up," she told me. "Of course. That's my mission. That's why I am here in this world."

.•: ·

OUR BLIND SPOT, OUR INABILITY TO IMAGINE THE NEXT DESCENT WITHOUT actually stepping through the looking glass, breeds complacency. We have institutions with billions of dollars and tens of thousands of employees working to protect the public health. This gives us a false sense of security, a comforting delusion that however many cracks might appear, the foundation will never crumble.

People who hold that belief may be interested to learn about an oft-forgotten chapter of American history. In the early 1800s, at the urging of medical doctors, an itinerant and illiterate quack herbalist named Samuel Thomson was thrown into a rancid, freezing dungeon for having challenged the medical establishment. Thomson believed that all disease was the result of too much cold in the body, and so his One True Cure was heat applied in various ways, including cayenne pepper enemas and the inducement of vomiting through a poisonous herb named lobelia. His most famous treatment involved enclosing a patient into a small space that was pumped with hot steam; accordingly, his Thomsonian followers were derisively called steam doctors.

Thomson dedicated his life to bringing the medical establishment down. After months of imprisonment he emerged from his dungeon with a dragon's thirst for vengeance, seeking to play a vital role in a game of propaganda; he pitted the strength of his country wisdom and rough charisma against the licensed medical doctors' bookish intelligence and skin-snipping dexterity—eventually, Thomson would even claim an ally in the US Constitution.

Beneath the banner of medical freedom, Thomson turned to the uneducated herbalists who scrapped for a living on the fringes of society, plying their trade in farmhouse kitchens, covered wagons, and freestanding shacks in the woods. Thomson spent several years welding hundreds of these isolated fragments into a single, united front of Thomsonian herbalists. Together they joined with other unscientific schools of quackery. They seized on a Jacksonian spirit that fomented riots in the streets against regular doctors, with mobs whipped into a killing frenzy. In the 1830s the Thomsonians successfully lobbied every state in the country to abolish its medical-licensing laws.

In the absence of state licensing standards, untrained quacks competed in a pure free market against doctors who had gone to medical school. The result was horrific; across the country reports began surfacing of people being steamed literally to death. The medical establishment regrouped only due to the urgent need for real medicine that arose during the Civil War.

Thomson's story is a chilling reminder that the authority of science-based medicine ultimately relies on the belief and trust of the patient being treated.

For those who have grown up in the age of science-dominated institutions—every person living—it can be hard to imagine a world without the Numbers Junkies running the show. We scorn them for their lack of people skills and their impersonality and their objectification. But deep down we also secretly love and admire them for their dedication to finding the objective scientific truths that remain relevant and precious in the modern flood of misinformation. Now, however, their rule may be nearing its end.

Between 2000 and 2020, cries that the medical establishment was not trustworthy became a sort of self-fulfilling prophecy; efforts to regain trust resulted in an abandonment of the science-driven judgment that had merited the public trust in the first place.

One sign of this was when hospitals built on a foundation of medical science began incorporating bunk treatments into new wellness centers offering spa-like services. A 2017 study by a team of journalists at *Stat* news documented the use of alternative therapies at hospitals affiliated with fifteen top medical research centers, including Duke, the University of Florida, Johns Hopkins, and Yale. Duke marketed a pediatric program that embraced botanical medicines and detoxification remedies for kids suffering autism, asthma, and ADHD. The team also found plugs for spiritual healing, a public forum promoting acupuncture for infertility, homeopathic bee venom to treat fibromyalgia, herbal therapy to reverse Alzheimer's, and energy healing for multiple sclerosis. By compromising the science, these institutions have capitulated to the forces of irrationality that lie at the heart of One True Cures.

The article quoted a Yale neurology professor, who sounded resigned.

"We've become witch doctors," he said.

.•:'

IN 2022, THE LAST TIME I SPEAK WITH DAWN KALI, SHE TELLS ME HER life has become defined by a pattern: the doctors knock the cancer back with something, and then the cancer becomes resistant and reasserts itself, over and over. She hops from treatment to treatment as if they're hummocks in a swamp, never knowing which hummock will be her last.

But she is alive.

As we speak, she realizes that her youngest son, Jonathan, age eleven, forgot to take his lunch to his Waldorf school. While talking with me she limps out to her car, phone in one hand and lunch in the other.

Her favorite aunt never accepted that the lump in her own neck was actually a tumor. The aunt continued to seek alternative treatments, reading about various miracle cures and paying for unlicensed therapies. The cancer ate away at her neck until she could barely move. "It was pretty gruesome," Kali says. "She died of it."

I listen on the phone as she hands her boy his lunch.

"Thanks," he says, unbidden.

"I love you," he says, unbidden.

Then he is gone.

"I deal with the fear of that sweet little boy losing his mother," Kali says. "I never know. I don't know if this is my last year."

She still hasn't seen a penny of the judgment against Young and says her hopes of receiving any court-awarded money rest on the sale of the ranch. Young initially listed it at $3.9 million, but now, at $2.5 million, it still has no takers. The lawsuit's original award was $105 million; she says she expects to get $100,000 or so after legal fees.

Cancer aside, her life has, in many ways, gotten better.

"It was like I was in a cult in my family, and then in a cult with Young," she says. "I was able to get away from that and get sober and therapy, and out blossomed this new me."

As she learned to live with her disease, Kali began to take a renewed interest in herself. She rediscovered a love of fashion and began buying scarves and fabrics. Soon she opened an Etsy shop selling her designs— caftan dresses, robes, face masks, and pajamas. Her bohemian aesthetic caught the attention of the celebrity Nicole Richie, who bought Kali out and then commissioned a signature collection from her.

"I was going to be a career waitress," she says. "I'm now a designer. The light has returned. I found myself in the midst of all this chaos. I'm shining again."

This appreciation of Kali's talents and skills were a form of validation that she'd never received before. Not as a waitress. Not at the pH Miracle Ranch, which she now calls a death camp. Not anywhere.

Before we hang up, I ask her something I've been wondering about. She spent years in Young's inner circle, watching him tell patients about the One True Cure.

Does Kali think he believes in his own science? Or is he merely trying to enrich himself with bunk?

She tells me that even now she isn't sure. But one memory sticks in her mind.

"He once said to me, 'When you can't go through the door, you go through the window. If you can't go through the window, you go through the garage. If you can't go through the garage, you find another way.'"

Kali thinks that Young is caught in a hyperaggressive loop of acting on the business maxim "Fake it till you make it." Her impression is that he believes he is always one step away from irrefutable proof of the One True Cure, and that he will employ any means to get to that end.

Ultimately, Kali says, whether Young is deceiving himself along with his victims is immaterial. Her cancer is just as deadly either way.

.∵

WHEN I SAT DOWN FOR A ZOOM INTERVIEW WITH ROBERT YOUNG, I KNEW him only as an alternative healer who had encountered trouble with the government. I didn't know about the tragic story of Dawn Kali, let alone that he had discovered the relationship between vaccines and zombieism. And neither of us knew that Kali's court case against him would prompt another victim to come forward, resulting in Young being slapped with a fresh slate of five felony charges in San Diego Superior Court in 2022.

When he appeared on my computer screen, I could see that he was older and had a slight paunch (and by slight, I mean you could fit four or five of his paunches inside my own paunch). He looked more casual than I thought he would. Young was still selling alkaline supplements and advertising consultations for $300, but he was in reduced circumstances.

"I ran out of money, and I'm still out of money," he said, "from fighting this."

Much of what he said during our conversation would, to someone who has read this book, seem pretty old hat: his legal troubles were the result of being targeted by evil Luciferians; two hundred alternative healers had been assassinated by Big Pharma; to abandon his mission to heal the sick would be against his moral code ("That's who I am. I can't change who I am. What, do I see someone bleeding out or someone suffering or someone in need of help and do nothing?").

The patient, he says, is ultimately responsible for whether they choose a treatment that works for them. "I believe in agency," he told me. "I believe in free choice."

Though zombies seemed like the lowest rung of the ladder, he—and maybe America—was already stretching his foot downward to see if there were even lower depths to dip his toe into. Soon after our conversation he would "discover" that COVID vaccines included graphene hydroxide, which contains six each of protons, neutrons, and electrons. "The Plan today of Luciferians is clear," he wrote: to inject the satanic triple-six into people, marring their God-given genetic code with the mark of the beast.

When we spoke, he didn't mention any of this to me, and it would have been hard for me to connect the dark and bizarre conspiracy theories to the friendly, affable, and completely sane-sounding person I was talking to. But after we hung up I watched a particular video he'd posted—it was chilling, yes, and in hindsight it seemed to speak to the broader picture of what I'd learned.

YOUNG POSTED THE VIDEO WHILE THE NATION WAS SPLITTING ITS ATTENtion between the coronavirus and the holiday season. He recorded it wearing big clunky headphones and standing behind a professional-grade mike. A guitar leaned against the wall. Amp cords were coiled and hanging on designated hooks.

"I hope you will enjoy one of my favorite Christmas songs," he wrote in the video description.

It began with a close-up of his face as gentle music played in the background.

"Children sleeping," Young sang. The camera panned slowly around his face, which was poised in a mask of earnestness. "Snow is softly falling / Dreams are calling."

It was from the movie *The Polar Express*. Young swayed to the music, threw open his arms, tilted his head back in song. His performance didn't quite reach *American Idol* quality, but he hit the high notes without slipping into full falsetto.

The video, which had been nicely edited, began to cut in scenes from *The Polar Express*, with its hideous motion-capture animation. A zombie-looking boy sleeping beneath a blanket embellished with the stripes of the American flag. A zombie with Tom Hanks's voice pointing to the Northern Lights. Zombie children of different races embracing in a performative and artificial show of racial amity.

"We were dreamers / Not so long ago," Young sang. "But one by one / We all had to grow up / When it seems the magic slipped away."

On the wall behind him was a framed certificate of one of his many achievements. It hung beneath a black-and-white photo of what I think was Young in England, holding a guitar and posing with three other young men with instruments, proud and happy and full of the confidence that they could build any future they chose.

"If you just believe! If you just believe!" he sang, full-throated now, vocal cords straining. "If you just believe! If you just believe!"

Images of zombie children awash in brightly decorated presents. A horde of zombie elves throwing their hats into the air in triumph and then lurching in inhuman, irregular strides alongside the train.

Somewhere, Dawn Kali was dying of cancer because she had believed in pH Miracles. She would one day lie beneath the ground, one more potential recruit in an undead army of believers, waiting to rise and avenge themselves. Genia Vanderhaeghen was dead. Kim Tinkham was dead. Vicki Felix was dead. Dan Barkin was dead. Naima Houder-Mohammed was dead. Kara Neumann was dead. The laser-using mother of a fifteen-year-old girl was dead. A woman in Washington State was dead from measles. All had their fates handed down because they believed. They believed in Young, in faith healing, in other True Cures, in conspiracies, in lasers, in aliens, in medical freedom, in political leaders and hucksters who themselves believed in votes and money and power at any cost. All these things fused together at the far side of the looking glass, where a terrible, zombie-plagued dreamworld was spilling into reality. Whether Young was living *the* dream or living *a* dream, I couldn't tell.

"Just believe! Just believe!"

His song went on and on.

Acknowledgments

THIS BOOK STARTED AS A DISORGANIZED HEAP OF RAMBLINGS AND HALF-baked ideas (plus some bad jokes). Thanks to a lot of hard work on the part of lots of good people, the book has become a tidy stack of narratives and ideas that have been three-quarters baked (plus some bad jokes). And so, my deepest gratitude goes to PublicAffairs editor extraordinaire Benjamin Adams, who helped shape the book's original conception and then expertly guided me through crises by suggesting a title, pruning characters, instilling structure, and telling me what to expect when my first child's first tooth arrived. Throughout it all, Ben oozed kindness and expertise like a zombie oozes pus and bile. Also at PublicAffairs, Melissa Veronesi held my hand through the various steps of production with un-diluted good cheer and patience; Kelley Blewster's impressively brainy copy editing preserved my quirks and saved untold trees by trimming ten pages off the book in commas alone; and Chris Nolan undertook the legal review with a wisdom and humanity that provided me a master class in lawful snark. Thank you to my wonderful longtime agent, Ross Harris, who shortly before publication moved on to a different career, and to my short-time (but also wonderful) agent, David Patterson, who is already guiding me on to bigger and better things. I also owe a huge debt of gratitude to Martin Frank, the first person to read the first draft, and whose insights helped me see the book's strengths and flaws when I could still do something about them. Also many thanks to those who granted me interviews and then spoke to me thoughtfully and honestly about some difficult subjects—Robert Young, Alicja Kolyszko, Mark Grenon, Toby McAdam, Dawn Kali, and many others who appear less prominently in these pages.

Of course, no one has suffered for this book more than my dear and darling partner Kimberly Hongoltz-Hetling, who did everything in her power to give me the time to write before, during, and in the immediate aftermath of her pregnancy. Because of her superhuman sacrifices, she can take much more credit for this book than I can for our beautiful, bouncing baby boy. She is, quite simply, the best there ever was. And the best there ever will be.

Bibliography

ABC News. "Dale and Leilani Neumann Did Not Get Medical Help for Their Daughter's Diabetes." April 28, 2008. https://abcnews.go.com/Health /DiabetesNews/story?id=4741392&page=1.

Adalian, Josef. "The Celebrity Apprentice Ratings Haven't Been Great for a Long, Long Time." *Vulture*, January 6, 2017. www.vulture.com/2017/01 /celebrity-apprentice-ratings-were-down-for-years.html.

Adams, Jon, David Sibbritt, and Chi-Wai Lui. "The Urban-Rural Divide in Complementary and Alternative Medicine Use: A Longitudinal Study of 10,638 Women." *BMC Complementary Medicine and Therapies* 11, no. 2 (2011). https://doi.org/10.1186/1472-6882-11-2.

Adeel, Zakariya. "The Zakariya Adeel Podcast—Mark Grenon—Imprisoned for Healing the World—from Colombian Prison." Video, YouTube, June 17, 2021. www.youtube.com/watch?v=axogxXSoXfA.

Adler, Ben. "Why Is Herman Cain Trying to Cure Your Erectile Dysfunction?" *New Republic*, January 26, 2014. https://newrepublic.com/article/116237 /newt-gingrich-herman-cain-are-now-making-money-spam.

Ahmadiani, Saeed, and Shekoufeh Nikfar. "Challenges of Access to Medicine and the Responsibility of Pharmaceutical Companies: A Legal Perspective." *DARU Journal of Pharmaceutical Sciences* 24, no. 1 (2016): 13. https://doi .org/10.1186/s40199-016-0151-z.

Allen, Arthur. "How the Anti-Vaccine Movement Crept into the GOP Mainstream." *Politico*, May 27, 2019. www.politico.com/story/2019/05/27/anti -vaccine-republican-mainstream-1344955.

Allen-Ebrahimian, Bethany. "Some Chinese Netizens Actually Think Ebola Creates Zombies." *Foreign Policy*, August 14, 2014. https://foreignpolicy .com/2014/08/14/some-chinese-netizens-actually-think-ebola-creates -zombies/.

Altonen, Brian. "Thomsonian Timeline." Accessed March 20, 2022. https:// brianaltonenmph.com/6-history-of-medicine-and-pharmacy/hudson

-valley-medical-history/early-thomsonianism/the-essentials-of-thomsonianism
/thomsonian-timeline/.

Amadeo, Kimberly. "Historical Gold Prices: 30 BCE to Today." *The Balance*,
November 23, 2021. www.thebalance.com/gold-price-history-3305646.

Amadi, Cecilia Nwadiuto, and Orish Ebere Orisakwe. "Herb-Induced Liver
Injuries in Developing Nations: An Update." *Toxics* 6, no. 2 (2018): 24.
https://doi.org/10.3390/toxics6020024.

American Academy of Pediatrics Committee on Bioethics. "Religious Exemptions from Child Abuse Statutes." *Pediatrics* 81, no. 1 (1988): 169–171.

American College of Healthcare Sciences. "The Hidden Dangers in Your Dietary Supplements." December 2, 2016. https://achs.edu/blog/2016/12/02
/dangerous-supplement-ingredients/.

American Diabetes Association. "The History of a Wonderful Thing We Call
Insulin." July 1, 2019. www.diabetes.org/blog/history-wonderful-thing-we
-call-insulin.

Amodio, David M., and Chris Frith. "Meeting of Minds: The Medial Frontal
Cortex and Social Cognition." *Nature Reviews Neuroscience*, April 1, 2006.
www.nature.com/articles/nrn1884.

"Anatomy of an Insurrection." *Yale Medical Magazine*, Spring 2002. https://
medicine.yale.edu/news/yale-medicine-magazine/article/anatomy-of-an
-insurrection/.

Andersson, Atle. "Gold for Green Forests." Forest Peoples Programme, July
9, 2015. www.forestpeoples.org/en/topics/mining/news/2015/07/guyana
-article-gold-green-forests.

Andrade, Chittaranjan, and Rajiv Radhakrishnan. "Prayer and Healing: A Medical and Scientific Perspective on Randomized Controlled Trials." *Indian
Journal of Psychiatry* 51, no. 4 (2009): 247–253. https://doi.org/10.4103/0019
-5545.58288.

Appel, Toby A. "The Thomsonian Movement, the Regular Profession, and the
State in Antebellum Connecticut: A Case Study of the Repeal of Early
Medical Licensing Laws." *Journal of the History of Medicine and Allied
Sciences* 65, no. 2 (2010): 153–186. www.jstor.org/stable/24632012.

"Arrest of a Steam Doctor." *Adams Sentinel*, May 14, 1849. http://genealogytrails
.com/penn/monroe/newspaper.html.

Associated Press. "Food Stamps for Flood Area." *New York Times*, June 12,
1972. www.nytimes.com/1972/06/12/archives/food-stamps-for-flood-area
.html.

Associated Press. "Parents Who Prayed as Child Died Face Charges." NBC
News, April 28, 2008. www.nbcnews.com/health/health-news/parents-who
-prayed-child-died-face-charges-flna1c9459626.

Associated Press. "Rapid City Man Ordered to Stop Selling Medical Devices."
Mitchell Republic, October 9, 2015. www.mitchellrepublic.com/news
/crime-and-courts/3857553-rapid-city-man-ordered-stop-selling-medical
-devices.

Associated Press. "Relative: Mother Knew Daughter Was Gravely Ill." NBC News, May 18, 2009. www.nbcnews.com/id/wbna30811786.

Associated Press. "V.F.W. Aids Flood Victims." *New York Times*, June 14, 1972. www.nytimes.com/1972/06/14/archives/vfw-aids-flood-victims.html.

Associated Press. "Woman Charged After Allegedly Throwing Blood at California Senators." KCRA 3, January 10, 2020. www.kcra.com/article/woman-charged-after-allegedly-throwing-blood-at-california-senators/30473443.

Associated Press. "Woman Pleads Guilty in Alleged Bogus Medical Device Scheme." *Washington Times*, January 12, 2018. www.washingtontimes.com/news/2018/jan/12/woman-pleads-guilty-in-alleged-bogus-medical-devic/.

Ayres, B. Drummond, Jr. "Survivors of Dakota Flood Vow to 'Get On with It.'" *New York Times*, June 13, 1972. www.nytimes.com/1972/06/16/archives/officials-in-dakota-ask-nation-to-give-cash-as-flood-aid.html.

Barrett, Stephen. "A Critical Look at 'Dr.' Robert Young's Theories and Credentials." Quackwatch, July 3, 2017. https://quackwatch.org/11ind/young3/.

Barrett, Stephen. "'Dr.' Robert O. Young Arrested." Quackwatch, February 4, 2014. https://quackwatch.org/cases/crim/ro_young/complaint/.

Barrie, Leslie. "Herbal Remedies and Your Liver: 7 Safety Tips to Follow." *Everyday Health*, April 16, 2021. www.everydayhealth.com/news/toxic-not-healthy-surprising-liver-dangers-herbal-products/.

Baumgaertner, Bert, Juliet E. Carlisle, and Florian Justwan. "The Influence of Political Ideology and Trust on Willingness to Vaccinate." *PLoS One* 13, no. 1 (2018). https://doi.org/10.1371/journal.pone.0191728.

Bayer, Ronald. "The Continuing Tensions Between Individual Rights and Public Health: Talking Point on Public Health Versus Civil Liberties." *EMBO Reports* 8, no. 12 (2007): 1099–1103. https://doi.org/10.1038/sj.embor.7401134.

Before It's News. "Dr. Zev Zelenko & Dr. Robert Young Both Confirm That All the Clot Shots Have Tracking Nanoparticle Technology in Them! Fauxi Should Hang for This!! Top Scientists/Doctors Confirm Covid Jab Causing Brain Damage and Blood Clots! Must See!" September 12, 2021. https://beforeitsnews.com/christian-news/2021/09/dr-zev-zelenko-dr-robert-young-both-confirm-that-all-the-clot-shots-have-tracking-nanoparticle-technology-in-them-fauxi-should-hang-for-this-top-scientistsdoctors-confirm-covid-jab-causing-2601304.html.

Before It's News. "Operation Crimson Mist & the Coming Genocide by Vaxxed Mind-Controlled Zombies." June 5, 2021. https://beforeitsnews.com/christian-news/2021/06/operation-crimson-mist-the-coming-genocide-by-vaxxed-mind-controlled-zombies-ny-mom-fights-back-against-teaching-critical-race-theory-the-great-reset-exposed-covid-vaxx-shedding-hurting-unva-2598599.html.

Before It's News. "Proof That the Covid Depop Shot Will Change Your DNA and Either Kill You, Give You a Serious Injury or Turn You into a Zombie

Without a Spirit or Soul! Must See Interview!" April 22, 2021. https://
beforeitsnews.com/eu/2021/04/proof-that-the-covid-depop-shot-will
-change-your-dna-and-either-kill-you-give-you-a-serious-injury-or-turn-you
-into-a-zombie-without-a-spirit-or-soul-must-see-interview-2671165.html.

Benton, Joel. "A Dead Medical System." *New York Times*, September 22, 1901.
https://timesmachine.nytimes.com/timesmachine/1901/09/22/issue.html.

Bernstein, Nina. "Chefs, Butlers, Marble Baths: Hospitals Vie for the Afflu-
ent." *New York Times*, January 21, 2012. www.nytimes.com/2012/01/22
/nyregion/chefs-butlers-and-marble-baths-not-your-average-hospital-room
.html.

Blackstone, Erwin A., Joseph P. Fuhr, and Steve Poiask. "The Health and Economic Effects of Counterfeit Drugs." *American Health and Drug Benefits* 7,
no. 4 (2014): 216–224.

Blakinger, Keri, and Joseph Neff. "31,000 Prisoners Sought Compassionate Release During COVID-19. The Bureau of Prisons Approved 36." Marshall
Project, June 11, 2021. www.themarshallproject.org/2021/06/11/31-000
-prisoners-sought-compassionate-release-during-covid-19-the-bureau-of
-prisons-approved-36.

Boone, Rebecca. "Police Detail Cultish Beliefs of Mom Charged in Kids' Deaths."
ABC News, October 8, 2021. https://abcnews.go.com/US/wireStory/police
-detail-cultish-beliefs-mom-charged-kids-deaths-80478440.

Bor, Jonathan, and Frank D. Roylance. "Solomon Stripped of License: Doctor Admits Sex with Patients over Last 20 Years." *Baltimore Sun*, October
28, 1993. www.baltimoresun.com/news/bs-xpm-1993-10-28-1993301186
-story.html.

Bor, Jonathan, and Frank D. Roylance. "Solomon's Patients: Trust Betrayed,
Lives Ruined. Other Doubts Arise About His Ethics, Medical Practices.
The Rise and Fall of Dr. Neil Solomon." *Baltimore Sun*, October 31, 1993.
www.baltimoresun.com/news/bs-xpm-1993-10-31-1993304005-story.html.

Boseley, Sarah. "How Disgraced Anti-Vaxxer Andrew Wakefield Was Embraced
by Trump's America." *The Guardian*, July 28, 2018. www.theguardian.com
/society/2018/jul/18/how-disgraced-anti-vaxxer-andrew-wakefield-was
-embraced-by-trumps-america.

Boyle, Alan. "The Science of Bloodsuckers." NBC News, October 31, 2008. www
.nbcnews.com/science/cosmic-log/science-bloodsuckers-flna6c10404754.

Branich, Lauren. "Memorial Walk Commemorating Rapid City 1972 Flood."
Newscenter 1, June 11, 2018. www.newscenter1.tv/memorial-walk
-commemorating-rapid-city-1972-flood/.

Brantley, Kayla. "Jury Awards Terminally-Ill Mother-of-Four $105 Million After
the pH Miracle Author Duped Her into Thinking He Was a Doctor and Persuaded Her to Get Baking Soda Infusions Instead of Chemotherapy." *Daily
Mail*, November 4, 2018. www.dailymail.co.uk/news/article-6351723/Jury
-awards-terminally-ill-mother-four-105million-pH-Miracle-author-duped
-her.html.

Brown, Erin. "How the Dietary Supplement Industry Keeps Regulation at Bay." Open Secrets, June 21, 2019. www.opensecrets.org/news/2019/06/dietary-supplements-industry-keeps-regulation/.

Bruneau, Emile, and Nour Kteily. "The Enemy as Animal: Symmetric Dehumanization During Asymmetric Warfare." PLoS One 12, no. 7 (2017). https://doi.org/10.1371/journal.pone.0181422.

Butler, Kiera. "The Anti-Vax Movement's Radical Shift from Crunchy Granola Purists to Far-Right Crusaders." Mother Jones, June 18, 2020. www.motherjones.com/politics/2020/06/the-anti-vax-movements-radical-shift-from-crunchy-granola-purists-to-far-right-crusaders/.

"California in Brief: Woman Held in Bite Attack on Mother." Los Angeles Times, November 7, 1991. www.latimes.com/archives/la-xpm-1991-11-07-me-1333-story.html.

Cameron, Chris. "These Are the People Who Died in Connection with the Capitol Riot." New York Times, January 5, 2022. www.nytimes.com/2022/01/05/us/politics/jan-6-capitol-deaths.html.

Canham, Matt. "Feds Plow New Ground in Spiked Supplement Case." Salt Lake Tribune, October 1, 2011. https://archive.sltrib.com/article.php?id=52657684&itype=CMSID.

Carey, Benedict. "Long-Awaited Medical Study Questions the Power of Prayer." New York Times, March 31, 2006. www.nytimes.com/2006/03/31/health/longawaited-medical-study-questions-the-power-of-prayer.html.

Cavallo, Christian. "Top Private Label Supplement Manufacturers in the USA." Thomas website, accessed March 20, 2022. www.thomasnet.com/articles/top-suppliers/private-label-supplement-manufacturers/.

CDC. "CDC.gov and Social Media Metrics: May 2012." www.cdc.gov/metrics/reports/2012/oadc-metrics-report-05-2012.pdf.

Cecil G. Sheps Center for Health Services Research, University of North Carolina at Chapel Hill. "181 Rural Hospital Closures Since January 2005." Accessed June 7, 2022. www.shepscenter.unc.edu/programs-projects/rural-health/rural-hospital-closures/.

Chastain, James. "Streets of Paris." Encyclopedia of 1848 Revolutions, accessed March 20, 2022. www.ohio.edu/chastain/rz/parisstr.htm.

Cheney, Jillian. "After Falling from Grace, Televangelist Jim Bakker Is Still on the Air." Religion Unplugged, October 8, 2021. https://religionunplugged.com/news/2021/10/7/vxke0h70taaio670r9dggy8haxl9zj.

Chotiner, Isaac. "The Influence of the Anti-Vaccine Movement." New Yorker, December 18, 2020. www.newyorker.com/news/q-and-a/the-influence-of-the-anti-vaccine-movement.

CNBC. "CNBC Transcript: President Donald Trump Sits Down with CNBC's Joe Kernen at the World Economic Forum in Davos, Switzerland." News release, January 22, 2020. www.cnbc.com/2020/01/22/cnbc-transcript-president-donald-trump-sits-down-with-cnbcs-joe-kernen-at-the-world-economic-forum-in-davos-switzerland.html.

CNN. "Many Americans Use Alternative Medicine to Feel Better." February 26, 2015. www.cnn.com/2015/02/10/health/gallery/alternative-medicine /index.html.

CNN. "Parents Pick Prayer over Medical Care." March 31, 2008. http:// transcripts.cnn.com/TRANSCRIPTS/0803/31/ng.01.html.

CNN. "Parents Pray Instead of Visiting Doctor—Daughter Dies." Video, Videosift, March 30, 2008. https://videosift.com/video/Parents-Pray-Instead-of -Visiting-Doctor-Daughter-Dies.

Cohen, Pieter A. "The FDA and Adulterated Supplements—Dereliction of Duty." *JAMA Network Open* 1, no. 6 (2018). https://jamanetwork.com /journals/jamanetworkopen/fullarticle/2706489.

Cohen, Pieter A., et al. "Presence of Banned Drugs in Dietary Supplements Following FDA Recalls." *JAMA* 312, no. 16 (2014): 1691–1693. https:// jamanetwork.com/journals/jama/fullarticle/1917421.

Collins, Laura. "Exclusive: How Doomsday Cult Author Chad Daybell's Lie About Shooting a Raccoon in Broad Daylight Led Cops to the Bodies of Lori Vallow's Two 'Zombie' Children Buried in His Backyard." *Daily Mail*, January 12, 2022. www.dailymail.co.uk/news/article-10390639/Chad-Daybell -unwittingly-caused-Lori-Vallows-downfall-text-message-book-reveals.html.

"Confirmed, Massive West Coast Fires Set by Zombie Army of Leftists." *Alex Jones Show*, September 15, 2020. https://banned.video/watch?id=5f6145d7 dc50dc07a1ffcc91.

Connor, Jennifer H. "Thomsonian Medical Books and the Culture of Dissent in Upper Canada." *Canadian Bulletin of Medical History* 12 (1995): 289–311. www.utpjournals.press/doi/pdf/10.3138/cbmh.12.2.289.

Cook, Tena L. "Lytle Families Honored with Family Tree Award." *Chadron State College News*, October 10, 2016. www.csc.edu/news/story.csc?article=11403.

Cooke, Richard. "Right Brain." *New Republic*, September 3, 2019. https://new republic.com/article/154629/right-brain-ben-shapiro-alex-jones-conservatives -love-affair-nootropics.

CorvetteReport. "Dr Larry Lytle, Laser Therapy Expert-Enhancing Learning & Memory FarOutRadio 6.17.14." Video, YouTube, June 30, 2014. www .youtube.com/watch?v=RKFZKBCJ844.

CorvetteReport. "Dr Larry Lytle QLaser Therapy-Dental Alignment for Vitality FarOutRadio 4.22.14." Video, YouTube, April 26, 2014. www.youtube .com/watch?v=-qRXVxleBa4.

Cowell, Annie N. "Mapping the Malaria Parasite Druggable Genome by Using in Vitro Evolution and Chemogenomics." *Science*, January 12, 2018. https:// science.sciencemag.org/content/359/6372/191.

Crawford, Cindy C., Andrew G. Sparber, and Wayne B. Jonas. "A Systematic Review of the Quality of Research on Hands-On and Distance Healing: Clinical and Laboratory Studies." *Alternative Therapies in Health and Medicine* 9, no. 3 suppl. (2003): A96–A104. https://pubmed.ncbi.nlm.nih.gov /12776468/.

Crockett, Zachary, and Javier Zarracina. "How the Zombie Represents America's Deepest Fears: A Sociopolitical History of Zombies, from Haiti to *The Walking Dead*." *Vox*, October 31, 2016. www.vox.com/policy-and-politics/2016/10/31/13440402/zombie-political-history.

Cronin, Jeff. "FDA and FTC Urged to Bring Enforcement Proceedings Against Joseph Mercola for False COVID-19 Health Claims." Center for Science in the Public Interest, July 1, 2020. https://cspinet.org/news/fda-and-ftc-urged-bring-enforcement-proceedings-against-joseph-mercola-false-covid-19-health.

Cuddy, Amy J. C., Mindi S. Rock, and Michael I. Norton. "Aid in the Aftermath of Hurricane Katrina: Inferences of Secondary Emotions and Intergroup Helping. Group Processes and Intergroup Relations." *SAGE Publications* 10, no. 1 (2007): 107–118. https://doi.org/10.1177/1368430207071344.

Cummings, William. "'This Is Not a Reality TV Show': Trump Criticized for Tweets on TV Ratings as Coronavirus Death Toll Rises." *USA Today*, March 29, 2020. www.usatoday.com/story/news/politics/2020/03/29/trump-tweets-touting-tv-ratings-coronavirus-briefings/2936761001/.

Daily, Stephen. "A Brief History of the FDA." *Cataract and Refractive Surgery Today*, October 2011. https://crstoday.com/articles/2011-oct/a-brief-history-of-the-fda/.

Dalen, James E., and Joseph S. Alpert. "Medical Tourists: Incoming and Outgoing." *American Journal of Medicine* 132, no. 1 (2019): 9–10. https://doi.org/10.1016/j.amjmed.2018.06.022.

Daley, Beth. "Why It's Grim, but Unsurprising, That the U.S. Capitol Attack Looked Like It Was Out of a 'Zombie Movie.'" *The Conversation*, January 4, 2022. https://theconversation.com/why-its-grim-but-unsurprising-that-the-u-s-capitol-attack-looked-like-it-was-out-of-a-zombie-movie-174038.

Daly, Dan. "State Wins Claim Against Former Dentist." *Rapid City Journal*, August 28, 2001. https://rapidcityjournal.com/state-wins-claim-against-former-dentist/article_4b919a98-c5ab-5533-97a3-355c1fdb8864.html.

D'Ambrosio, Amanda. "Simone Gold Arrested for Role in Capitol Insurrection." *MedPage Today*, January 20, 2021. www.medpagetoday.com/washington-watch/washington-watch/90778.

Dapcevich, Madison. "Did Cirsten Weldon Say Hillary Clinton Died of Disease Associated with Cannibalism?" Snopes, May 9, 2021. www.snopes.com/fact-check/cirsten-weldon-hillary-cannibalism/.

Davis, Jeanie Lerche. "Can Prayer Heal?" WebMD, March 26, 2004. www.webmd.com/balance/features/can-prayer-heal.

Davis, S. Peter. "6 Mind-Blowing Ways Zombies and Vampires Explain America." *Cracked*, September 6, 2011. www.cracked.com/article_19402_6-mind-blowing-ways-zombies-vampires-explain-america.html.

Dawn Kali v. Robert O. Young. No. D076121 (Cal. Ct. App. Feb. 8, 2021).

Dawn Kali v. Robert O. Young, pH Miracle Living, Ben Johnson, case no. 37-2015-00043052-CU-P0-CTL, December 28, 2015. Reproduced on

Quackwatch. https://quackwatch.org/wp-content/uploads/sites/33/quack
watch/casewatch/civil/young/complaint.pdf.

De Salazar, Pablo M., et al. "The Association Between Gold Mining and Malaria
in Guyana: A Statistical Inference and Time-Series Analysis." *Lancet Plan-
etary Health* 5, no. 10 (October 1, 2021): 731–738. https://doi.org/10.1016
/S2542-5196(21)00203-5.

"Defend Your Right to Know and Freedom to Choose What's Best for You and
Your Family's Wellbeing." *Good News NY*, updated September 24, 2021.
www.thegoodnewsny.org/post/defend-your-right-to-know-and-freedom-to
-choose-what-s-best-for-you-and-your-family-s-wellbeing-1.

Delka, R. K. *Democrat Zombies from Space: A Wall Won't Keep These Aliens
Out.* New York: Belliam Books, 2016.

Department of Environmental and Engineering Services of the City of Margate,
Florida. *Comprehensive Plan, Conservation Element.* January 2010. www
.margatefl.com/DocumentCenter/View/190/Element-VII—Conservation.

Devine, Shauna. "Health Care and the American Medical Profession,
1830–1880." *Journal of the Civil War Era*, July 6, 2017. www.journalof
thecivilwarera.org/2017/07/health-care-american-medical-profession-1830
-1880/.

Dickson, E. J. "Wellness Influencers Are Calling Out QAnon Conspiracy
Theorists for Spreading Lies." *Rolling Stone*, September 15, 2020. www
.rollingstone.com/culture/culture-news/qanon-wellness-influencers-seane
-corn-yoga-1059856/.

Diehl, Phil. "Sentencing Delayed for pH Miracle Author." *Baltimore Sun*, May
1, 2017. www.baltimoresun.com/sd-no-ph-miracle-sentencing-20170501
-story.html.

Divett, Robert T. "Medicine and the Mormons: A Historical Perspective." *Di-
alogue: A Journal of Mormon Thought* 12, no. 3 (1979): 16–25. www.jstor
.org/stable/45224796.

Dogwood School of Botanical Medicine. "History of Physiomedicalism." Accessed March 20, 2022. https://dogwoodbotanical.com/history-of-physio
medicalism/.

Dr. Clark Store. "Zappers & Accessories." Accessed March 19, 2022. https://
drclarkstore.com/collections/zappers-accessories.

Dr. Larry Lytle v. U.S. Department of Health and Human Services. CIV. 13-
5083-JLV (US Dis. Ct. D.S.D. Western Div., January 7, 2014). www
.casemine.com/judgement/us/5914f043add7b04934973baf.

Drezner, Daniel W. "Metaphor of the Living Dead: Or, the Effect of the Zombie
Apocalypse on Public Policy Discourse." *Social Research* 81, no. 4 (2014):
825–849. www.jstor.org/stable/26549655.

Drinkard, Jim. "Drugmakers Go Furthest to Sway Congress." *USA Today*,
April 26, 2005. https://usatoday30.usatoday.com/money/industries/health
/drugs/2005-04-25-drug-lobby-cover_x.htm.

Dube, Tendai. "Discredited US Naturopath Makes False Claims About Gates." *AFP South Africa*, January 19, 2021. https://factcheck.afp.com /discredited-us-naturopath-makes-false-claims-about-gates.

Dushman, Amber. "Ads and Labels from Early 20th-Century Health Fraud Promotions." *AMA Journal of Ethics* 20, no. 11 (2018): E1082–1093. https:// doi.org/10.1001/amajethics.2018.1082.

Earthlink, Inc. v. Pope. Civil Action No. 1:03-CV-2559-JOF (N.D. Ga. Aug. 31, 2006). https://casetext.com/case/earthlink-2/?PHONE_NUMBER _GROUP=P.

Edwards, Linden F. "Resurrection Riots During the Heroic Age of Anatomy in America." *Bulletin of the History of Medicine* 25, no. 2 (1951): 178–184. www.jstor.org/stable/44443608.

Eells, David. "Press Release from Unleavened Bread Ministries Regarding the Death of 11-Year-Old Madeline Kara Neumann and Our Experience with Her Parents, Dale and Leilani." Unleavened Bread Ministries, March 27, 2008. Archived at Wayback Machine. https://web.archive.org/web/20080426231758 /http://www.unleavenedbreadministries.org/?page=pressrelease.

Eells, David. "Second Press Release from Unleavened Bread Ministries Regarding the Death of 11-Year-Old Madeline Kara Neumann." Unleavened Bread Ministries, March 31, 2008. Archived at Wayback Machine. https://web.archive.org/web/20080401232301/http://www.unleavened breadministries.org/?page=pressrelease2.

Eells, David. "Third Press Release from Unleavened Bread Ministries Regarding the Death of 11-Year-Old Madeline Kara Neumann." Unleavened Bread Ministries, April 2, 2008. Archived at Wayback Machine. https://web .archive.org/web/20080413180627/http://www.unleavenedbreadministries .org/?page=pressrelease3.

Eler, Alicia. "Conspiracy Theories of QAnon Find Fertile Ground in an Unexpected Place—the Yoga World." *StarTribune*, February 9, 2021. www .startribune.com/conspiracy-theories-of-qanon-find-fertile-ground-in-an -unexpected-place-the-yoga-world/600020902/?refresh=true.

EmCeeBT. "Fiddler on the Roof—L'Chaim—To Life!" Video, YouTube, August 28, 2011. www.youtube.com/watch?v=B0IhKS47Ijc.

Essley Whyte, Liz, Joe Yerardi, and Alison Fitzgerald Kodjak. "How Drugmakers Sway States to Profit Off of Medicaid." Center for Public Integrity, July 18, 2018. https://publicintegrity.org/politics/state-politics /how-drugmakers-sway-states-to-profit-off-of-medicaid/.

Facher, Lev. "More than Two-Thirds of Congress Cashed a Pharma Campaign Check in 2020, New STAT Analysis Shows." *Stat*, June 9, 2021. www.statnews .com/feature/prescription-politics/federal-full-data-set/.

Facher, Lev. "Pharma Is Showering Congress with Cash, Even as Drug Makers Race to Fight the Coronavirus." *Stat*, August 10, 2020. www.statnews.com /feature/prescription-politics/prescription-politics/.

Facher, Lev. "Trump Has Launched an All-Out Attack on the FDA. Will Its Scientific Integrity Survive?" *Stat*, August 27, 2020. www.statnews.com/2020 /08/27/trump-has-launched-an-all-out-attack-on-the-fda-will-its-scientific -integrity-survive/.

Factor, Janet L. "The Ties That Bind." *Free Inquiry*, October/November 2009. https://secularhumanism.org/wp-content/uploads/sites/26/2018/08/FI-ON -09-1.pdf.

Faulders, Katherine. "Ben Carson Says It's Premature to Promote Latest Unproven Coronavirus Treatment." ABC News, August 19, 2020. https://abcnews .go.com/Politics/ben-carson-premature-promote-latest-unproven-coronavirus -treatment/story?id=72476046.

Federal Trade Commission. "FTC and FDA Crack Down on Internet Marketers of Bogus SARS Prevention Products." News release, May 9, 2003. www.ftc.gov/news-events/news/press-releases/2003/05/ftc-fda-crack-down -internet-marketers-bogus-sars-prevention-products.

Federal Trade Commission. "FTC Permanently Stops Six Operators from Using Fake News Sites That Allegedly Deceived Consumers About Acai Berry Weight-Loss Products." News release, January 25, 2012. www.ftc.gov /news-events/news/press-releases/2012/01/ftc-permanently-stops-six-operators -using-fake-news-sites-allegedly-deceived-consumers-about-acai.

Fell, Bibi. "*Kali v. Young, et al.*" Interview by Steve Lowry and Yvonne Godfrey. *Great Trials Podcast*, March 1, 2022. www.greattrialspodcast.com/podcast /bibi-fell-kali-v-young-et-al-105-million-verdict.

Figueroa, Teri. "Jury Awards $105 Million to Terminal Cancer Patient in Suit Against 'pH Miracle' Author." *Los Angeles Times*, November 2, 2018. www .latimes.com/la-me-ln-san-diego-ph-miracle-lawsuit-20181102-story .html.

Figueroa, Teri. "Split Verdict for 'pH Miracle' Author." *San Diego Union-Tribune*, February 3, 2016. www.sandiegouniontribune.com/sdut-criminal -trial-robert-young-ph-miracle-2016feb03-story.html.

FiveThirtyEight. "Are Republicans or Democrats More Likely to Survive the Apocalypse?" March 5, 2015. https://fivethirtyeight.com/features/are -republicans-or-democrats-more-likely-to-survive-the-apocalypse/.

Flagg, Anna. "Survey of the Incarcerated." Marshall Project, March 5, 2020. https://github.com/themarshallproject/incarcerated_survey.

Flannery, M. "The Early Botanical Medical Movement as a Reflection of Life, Liberty, and Literacy in Jacksonian America." *Journal of the Medical Library Association* 90, no. 4 (2002): 442–454. www.ncbi.nlm.nih.gov/pmc/articles /PMC128961/.

"Flow Rate in Creek Flood Was 10 Times Old Record." *New York Times*, June 12, 1972. www.nytimes.com/1972/06/12/archives/flow-rate-in-creek-flood -was-10-times-old-record.html.

Forer, Arthur Hanan. "Evidence for Two Spindle Fiber Components." 1964. Digital by Dartmouth Library. https://doi.org/10.1349/ddlp.2726.

Forer, Arthur, Rozhan Sheykhani, and Michael W. Berns. "Anaphase Chromosomes in Crane-Fly Spermatocytes Treated with Taxol (Paclitaxel) Accelerate when Their Kinetochore Microtubules Are Cut: Evidence for Spindle Matrix Involvement with Spindle Forces." *Frontiers in Cell and Developmental Biology* 6 (2018). https://doi.org/10.3389/fcell.2018.00077.

Forman, Jonathan. "Dr. Alva Curtis in Columbus, the Thomsonian Recorder and Columbus' First Medical School." *Ohio Archaeological and Historical Quarterly* 51, no. 4 (1942): 332–340.

Franchise Help. "QLaser Franchise." Accessed March 19, 2022. www.franchise help.com/franchises/qlaser/.

French, Shannon E., and Anthony I. Jack. "Dehumanizing the Enemy: The Intersection of Neuroethics and Military Ethics." In *Responsibilities to Protect Perspectives in Theory and Practice*, edited by Bradley J. Strawser and David Whetham, 169–196. Boston: Brill Nijhoff, 2015.

Frith, Chris D., and Uta Frith. "Social Cognition in Humans." *Current Biology* 17, no. 16 (August 21, 2007): 724–732. https://doi.org/10.1016/j .cub.2007.05.068.

Galli, Cindy, et al. "Husband Says Fringe Church's 'Miracle Cure' Killed His Wife." ABC News, October 27, 2016. https://abcnews.go.com/US /husband-fringe-churchs-miracle-cure-killed-wife/story?id=43081647.

Ganguli, Ishani, et al. "Declining Use of Primary Care Among Commercially Insured Adults in the United States, 2008–2016." *Annals of Internal Medicine* 172, no. 4 (2020): 240–247. https://doi.org/10.7326/M19-1834.

Gerson Institute. "FAQS." Accessed March 19, 2022. https://gerson.org /faqs/.

Gibson, Joel. "How Disgust Explains Everything." *Sydney Morning Herald*, January 9, 2010. www.smh.com.au/national/death-in-paradise-20100109-lz8e .html.

Good, Chris. "Why Did the CDC Develop a Plan for a Zombie Apocalypse?" *The Atlantic*, May 20, 2011. www.theatlantic.com/politics/archive/2011/05 /why-did-the-cdc-develop-a-plan-for-a-zombie-apocalypse/239246/.

Gorski, David. "ITNJ 'Commissioner': A Woo-Full 'Honor' Bestowed upon Del Bigtree and Robert O. Young." *Respectful Insolence*, blog, July 26, 2019. https://respectfulinsolence.com/2019/07/26/itnj-commissioner/.

Graves Fitzsimmons, Emma. "Wisconsin Couple Sentenced in Death of Their Sick Child." *New York Times*, October 7, 2009. www.nytimes.com/2009/10/08 /us/08sentence.html.

Greene, Asa. *The Life and Adventures of Dr. Dodimus Duckworth, A.N.Q. to Which Is Added, the History of a Steam Doctor: In Two Volumes. Vol. I[–II].* New York: Peter Hill, 1833.

Greene, Mike. "There Is Hope: Dietary Supplement Activity in Congress in the Trump Era." *Natural Products Insider*, November 17, 2017. www.natural productsinsider.com/legal-compliance/there-hope-dietary-supplement -activity-congress-trump-era.

Grenon, Mark. "G2Voice Broadcast #188—Letter to President Trump and Response to FDA/FTC About Their Attack on Our Sacraments! 4-19-20." Video, Brighteon, April 19, 2020. www.brighteon.com/aedb4e1b-3a47 -434f-8548-7efe585a1cf1?fbclid=IwAR3iLyvkChEDLLv1_6gwu6A9ky2Z c93Ih0nBhiCPi5DoZQG2VjXarnIkmdw.

Grenon, Mark. "It has been 281 days for Joe and I in Columbian maximum prison and 316 days for Jonathan and Jordan in Florida jails!" Facebook, May 18, 2021. www.facebook.com/mark.grenon/posts/10165752248095160.

Grenon, Mark S. Imagine, a World Without DIS-EASE, Volume One. Self-published, 2018.

Gross, Elana. "Ben Carson Says He Took Oleandrin, an FDA-Rejected Supplement Touted by MyPillow Founder, as Coronavirus Treatment." Forbes, November 19, 2020. www.forbes.com/sites/elanagross/2020/11/19/ben -carson-says-he-took-oleandrin-an-fda-rejected-supplement-touted -by-mypillow-founder-as-coronavirus-treatment/?sh=461d042c1074.

Grossman, Lewis A. "The Origins of American Health Libertarianism." Yale Journal of Health Policy, Law and Ethics 8, no. 1 (2013): 79–134.

Haag, Justin. "Former Eagles Announce Gifts to Campaign." Chadron State College News, December 17, 2010. www.csc.edu/news/story.csc?article=8995.

Haelle, Tara. "This Is the Moment the Anti-Vaccine Movement Has Been Waiting For." New York Times, August 31, 2021. www.nytimes.com/2021/08/31 /opinion/anti-vaccine-movement.html.

Haller, John, Jr. Alternative/Complementary Medicine: 19th and Early 20th Century Reference Material: Colleges, Journals, Societies. Open SIUC, March 2021. https://opensiuc.lib.siu.edu/cgi/viewcontent.cgi?article=1000 &context=histcw_acm.

Hamowy, Ronald. "The Early Development of Medical Licensing Laws in the United States, 1875–1900." Journal of Libertarian Studies (1978): 73–119. https://cdn.mises.org/3_1_5_0.pdf.

Hananoki, Eric. "Trump VP Contender Newt Gingrich Profited from Sending Cancer 'Cure' Emails." Media Matters, July 6, 2016. www.mediamatters .org/newt-gingrich/trump-vp-contender-newt-gingrich-profited-sending -cancer-cure-emails.

Hancock, Jay. "The Stealth Campaign to Kill Off Obamacare." New York Times, July 27, 2018. www.nytimes.com/2018/07/27/business/the-stealth -campaign-to-kill-off-obamacare.html.

Harden, Blaine. "Old Remedy Gets New Leech on Life." Washington Post, February 24, 1995. www.washingtonpost.com/archive/politics/1995/02/24/old -remedy-gets-new-leech-on-life/7a3d2204-674d-4394-99b5-5160cf173816/.

Harris, Lasana T., and Susan T. Fiske. "Dehumanizing the Lowest of the Low: Neuroimaging Responses to Extreme Out-Groups." Psychological Science 17, no. 10 (October 2006): 847–853. https://doi.org/10.1111 /j.1467-9280.2006.01793.x.

Harris, Lasana T., and Susan T. Fiske. "Social Groups That Elicit Disgust Are Differentially Processed in mPFC." *Social Cognitive and Affective Neuroscience* 2, no. 1 (March 2007): 45–51. https://doi.org/10.1093/scan/nsl037.

Harris, Lasana T., et al. "Regions of the MPFC Differentially Tuned to Social and Nonsocial Affective Evaluation." *Cognitive, Affective, and Behavioral Neuroscience* 7 (2007): 309–316. https://doi.org/10.3758/CABN.7.4.309.

Hayward, Oliver S. "A Search for the Real Nathan Smith." *Journal of the History of Medicine and Allied Sciences* 15, no. 3 (1960): 268–281. www.jstor.org /stable/24620795.

Health Systems Governance and Financing Team. *Global Spending on Health: Weathering the Storm.* World Health Organization, 2020. www.who.int /publications/i/item/9789240017788.

Healthcare Triage. "How Does the FDA Approve a Drug?" Video, YouTube, July 20, 2015. www.youtube.com/watch?v=WUsO6PH_O54.

HealthKeepers Online. February 14, 2005. Archived at Wayback Machine. https://web.archive.org/web/20050214044329/https://healthkeepers.net/.

Heffernan, Conor. "The Long and Strange History of America's $36 Billion Supplement Industry." *Flux*, August 17, 2021. https://flux.community /conor-heffernan/2021/08/long-and-strange-history-americas-36-billion -supplement-industry.

Hein, Alexandra. "'QLaser' TV Infomercial Doc Gets 12 Years in Prison for Selling Scam Device." Fox News, December 27, 2021. www.foxnews.com/health /qlaser-tv-infomercial-doc-gets-12-years-in-prison-for-selling-scam-device.

Heinerman, John. *Joseph Smith and Herbal Medicine.* Monrovia, CA: Majority of One Press, 1975.

Help the Neumanns. "Help the Neumanns and Help Yourself." July 6, 2008. Archived at Wayback Machine. https://web.archive.org/web/20080706111755 /https://www.helptheneumanns.com/.

Henney, Jane E. "Cyberpharmacies and the Role of the US Food and Drug Administration." *Journal of Medical Internet Research* 3, no. 1 (2001): E3. https://doi.org/10.2196/jmir.3.1.e3.

"Herbalist in Alpine Pleads Guilty to Reduced Charge." *Deseret News*, February 5, 1996. www.deseret.com/1996/2/5/19223271/herbalist-in-alpine-pleads -guilty-to-reduced-charge.

Herwig, Miriam. "Cure Worse than Ailment: Boiled Alive." *The Herald*, February 3, 2006. www.ourherald.com/articles/cure-worse-than-ailment-boiled-alive/.

Herwig, Wesley. "A Patient Boiled Alive (Or: Why Jehiel Smith, a Thomsonian Physician, Left East Randolph, Vermont in a Hurry)." *Vermont History* 44, no. 4 (1976): 224–227. https://vermonthistory.org/journal/misc/Thomsonian Cure.pdf.

Hogan, Ron. "The Walking Dead vs. Real-Life Survivalists: How to Prep for the Zombie Apocalypse." *Den of Geek*, October 2, 2020. www.denofgeek.com /tv/the-walking-dead-how-to-survive-zombie-apocalypse/.

Holland, Byron. "Stopping Illegal Activity Online—It's More Complicated Than It Seems." CircleID, October 30, 2014. https://circleid.com/posts/20141030_stopping_illegal_activity_online_more_complicated_than_it_seems.

Holmes, Oliver Wendell. "The Medical Profession in Massachusetts." In *Medical Essays, 1842–1882.* www.gutenberg.org/files/2700/2700-h/2700-h.htm#link2H_4_0010.

Holmes, Simon. "Blind Woman Regains Her Sight in 'Miraculous Recovery' After Praying to the Relics of a Lebanese Saint in a Phoenix Church." *Daily Mail*, February 6, 2017. www.dailymail.co.uk/news/article-4195284/Blind-woman-regains-sight-praying-saint.html.

Hong, Nicole. "Inside One Company's Struggle to Get All Its Employees Vaccinated." *New York Times*, August 6, 2021. www.nytimes.com/2021/08/06/nyregion/employee-vaccination-business-ny.html.

Hospital Stats. "ER Wait Time in New York Hospitals." Accessed June 8, 2022. www.hospitalstats.org/ER-Wait-Time/New-York-NY-Metro.htm.

Hotez, Peter J. "America's Deadly Flirtation with Antiscience and the Medical Freedom Movement." *Journal of Clinical Investigation* 131, no. 7 (2021): e149072. https://doi.org/10.1172/JCI149072.

Hubbard, Amy. "Florida Senate Bill Amended to Include Zombie Apocalypse." *Los Angeles Times*, April 30, 2014. www.latimes.com/nation/nationnow/la-na-nn-zombie-apocalypse-florida-bill-20140430-htmlstory.html.

Humble, Jim. *The Miracle Mineral Supplement of the 21st Century, 3rd Edition.* Charleston, SC: Booksurge, 2006.

Huntington, Stewart. "Lytle Faces $12 Million Restitution Burden in Medical Fraud Case." Kota Territory ABC, September 21, 2018. www.kotatv.com/content/news/Lytle-faces-12-million-restitution-burden-in-medical-fraud-case-493979241.html.

Huntington, Stewart. "Lytle Sentenced to 12 Years for Laser Device Fraud." Kota Territory ABC, April 20, 2018. www.kotatv.com/content/news/Lytle-sentenced-to-12-years-for-laser-device-fraud-480437443.html.

Ideal Health and Trump Network. "AllerTest." September 2, 2011. Archived at Wayback Machine. http://web.archive.org/web/20110902080450/http://www.idealhealth.com/Custom-Test/AllerTest.aspx.

Ideal Health and Trump Network. "OsteoTest." September 2, 2011. Archived at Wayback Machine. http://web.archive.org/web/20110902080837/http://www.idealhealth.com/Custom-Test/OsteoTest.aspx.

Imrie, Robert. "Wis. Dad of Dead Girl Says He Trusted God to Heal." *The Eagle*, July 29, 2009. https://theeagle.com/news/national/wis-dad-of-dead-girl-says-he-trusted-god-to/article_f417b13f-59a1-5d82-8dd7-640d16d8cd96.html.

Institute of Medicine (US) and National Research Council (US) Committee on the Framework for Evaluating the Safety of Dietary Supplements. *Dietary Supplements: A Framework for Evaluating Safety.* Washington, DC: National Academies Press, 2005.

International Tribunal for Natural Justice. "Dr. Robert O. Young ITNJ Testimony." Video, YouTube, November 2, 2019. www.youtube.com/watch?v =gKjnEz5s37o\ (this video has been removed for violating YouTube's Community Guidelines).

International Tribunal for Natural Justice. "Jim Humble—ITNJ Witness Testimony." Video, YouTube, October 3, 2019. www.youtube.com/watch?v=9H4 DxZ6pQZ0 (this video has been removed for violating YouTube's Community Guidelines).

Jain, Minoj. "Medical Tourism Draws Growing Numbers of Americans to Seek Health Care Abroad." *Washington Post*, April 4, 2011. www.washingtonpost .com/national/health/medical-tourism-draws-growing-numbers-of-americans -to-seek-health-care-abroad/2011/02/09/AFkbobeC_story.html.

Jeukendrup, Asker. "Contamination of Nutrition Supplements." *My Sport Science*, accessed June 7, 2022. www.mysportscience.com/post/contamination -of-nutrition-supplements.

Jim Humble Live. "The Story of Earth as Recalled by Archbishop Jim Humble." Video, YouTube, December 3, 2012. Archived at Wayback Machine. https://web.archive.org/web/20130810164221/https://www.youtube.com /watch?v=Uf3uI73G2ZE.

J. M. Bullion. "1/10 Oz Australian Battle of the Coral Sea Gold Coin." Accessed March 19, 2022. www.jmbullion.com/2014-1-10-oz-battle-of-the-coral -sea-gold-coin/.

JohnDennis2010. "Night of the Living Pelosi." Video, YouTube, October 1, 2012. www.youtube.com/watch?v=FEdKqbqCGnc.

Johnson, Dirk. "Trials for Parents Who Chose Faith over Medicine." *New York Times*, January 20, 2009. www.nytimes.com/2009/01/21/us/21faith .html.

joshongs. "z PH Miracle Dr Robert Young TV show xvid." Video, YouTube, May 1, 2009. www.youtube.com/watch?v=8P4iBpmjIeo.

Jotatay 2K4. "Tom Horn and Steve Quayle—The Coming Zombie Apocalypse—Part 6." Video, Bitchute, May 12, 2021. www.bitchute.com/video /D0TuDRMioTf3/.

"Judge Orders Parents to Stand Trial in Prayer Death Case." *Pioneer Press*, updated November 13, 2015. www.twincities.com/2008/06/10/judge -orders-parents-to-stand-trial-in-prayer-death-case/amp/.

Kambhampaty, Anna P. "Many Americans Say They Believe in Ghosts. Do You?" *New York Times*, October 28, 2021. www.nytimes.com/2021/10/28 /style/do-you-believe-in-ghosts.html.

Kaye, David H. "International Journal of Engineering Research and Development (IJERD)." *Flaky Academic Journals*, blog, February 20, 2019. http:// flakyj.blogspot.com/2019/02/international-journal-of-engineering.html.

Kemper, Vicki. "FDA Easing Rules for Food Health Claims." *Los Angeles Times*, December 19, 2002. www.latimes.com/archives/la-xpm-2002-dec-19-na -fda19-story.html.

Khazan, Olga. "The Baffling Rise of Goop." *The Atlantic*, September, 2017. www.theatlantic.com/health/archive/2017/09/goop-popularity/539064/.

Khederian, Henry. "States with the Most and Least Doctors per Capita in 2020." *Yahoo! news*, April 22, 2020. www.yahoo.com/now/states-most-least -doctors-per-195041489.html.

Kirkpatrick, David D., and Stuart A. Thompson. "QAnon Cheers Republican Attacks on Jackson. Democrats See a Signal." *New York Times*, March 24, 2022. www.nytimes.com/2022/03/24/us/qanon-supreme-court-ketanji -brown-jackson.html.

Klaw, Spencer. "Belly-My-Grizzle." *American Heritage* 28, no. 4, (1977). www .americanheritage.com/belly-my-grizzle.

Klein, Kami. "Morningside Disaster Team in Florida—Lives Can Change in Only a Day." *Jim Bakker Show*, September 27, 2017. https://jimbakkershow .com/news/morningside-disaster-team-florida-lives-can-change-day/.

Kneeland, Douglas E. "The 1972 Campaign." *New York Times*, July 19, 1972. www.nytimes.com/1972/07/19/archives/mcgovern-helps-out-the-dakota -tourist-industry.html.

Knowles, David. "Carson Took Oleander Extract, Promoted by My Pillow CEO, to Treat COVID Infection." *Yahoo! news*, November 19, 2020. https://news .yahoo.com/ben-carson-took-oleander-extract-promoted-by-the-my-pillow -ceo-to-treat-his-covid-19-201219623.html.

Knowles, Eric, and Sarah DiMuccio. "How Donald Trump Appeals to Men Secretly Insecure About Their Manhood." *Washington Post*, November 29, 2018. www.washingtonpost.com/news/monkey-cage/wp/2018/11 /29/how-donald-trump-appeals-to-men-secretly-insecure-about-their -manhood/.

Kolyszko, Alicja. "I went to sleep for a while (doesn't happen lately!)." Facebook, January 22, 2021. www.facebook.com/leechesusa/posts/38519334 24870287.

Kolyszko, Edward V. "Preserving the Polish Heritage in America: The Polish Microfilm Project." *Polish American Studies* 32, no. 1 (1975): 59–63. www .jstor.org/stable/20147917.

Kolyszko, Edward V., and David J. O'Neill. *Entry into the United States*. Springfield: State Board of Education, Illinois Office of Education, 1977. https:// catalog.hathitrust.org/Record/101850532.

Kossovskaia, Irina. "Dr. Irina Kossovskaia Writer Bio." *Science to Sage Magazine*, September 6, 2013. https://sciencetosagemagazine.com/dr-irina-kossovskaia/.

Kossovskaia, Irina. "Q Laser Update." *Health Boss*, accessed March 17, 2022. https://myemail.constantcontact.com/QLaser-Update.html?soid=11052 68807269&aid=4uCD7lARITM.

Kotick, James D., and Amir Taghinia. "Prolonged Bleeding After a Single Leech Application in Pediatric Hand Surgery." *Journal of Hand and Microsurgery* 9, no. 2 (August 2017): 98–100. https://doi.org/10.1055/s-0037-1604348.

Kovar, Vincent. "What Our Favorite Monsters Tell Us About America: Vampires, Politics, and Zombies." *AtmosFX*, blog, October 12, 2017. https://atmosfx.com /blogs/community/celebration-census-four-monsters-politics-halloween.

Langlois, Shawn. "'QAnon' Book Claiming Democrats Eat Children Is Climbing the Amazon Charts." *MarketWatch*, March 5, 2019. www.marketwatch .com/story/qanon-book-claiming-democrats-eat-children-is-climbing-the -amazon-charts-2019-03-05.

Laser Light Institute. "Healing Light by Dr. Larry Lytle: A Compilation of Dr. Lytle's 'Healing Light' Articles Through January 2006." September 3, 2013. Archived at Wayback Machine. https://web.archive.org /web/20130903122103/http://www.laserlightinstitute.info/healinglight.pdf.

Last Reformation. "Received the Holy Spirit in His Bed!—Powerful Night in Florida!" Video, YouTube, June 25, 2021. www.youtube.com/watch?v =X50dUML8HtA.

Last Reformation. "Saw the Blue House in a Vision—Jesus Is Still Building His Church!—Amazing Testimony Like The. . . ." Video, YouTube, October 5, 2020. www.youtube.com/watch?v=xsf9BkGGU5A.

Leeches BG—Hirudotherapy. "World Hirudologists on TV in Sofia [Bulgaria] 2013" (translation from Bulgarian). Video, YouTube, January 24, 2014. www.youtube.com/watch?v=tIZtIc-hA78.

Legacy Healing Center. "Legacy Healing Center Now Accepts Bitcoin and Ethereum as Payment for Addiction Treatment Services." News release, Cision PRNewswire, July 15, 2021. www.prnewswire.com/news-releases /legacy-healing-center-now-accepts-bitcoin-and-ethereum-as-payment -for-addiction-treatment-services-301333772.html.

Legacy.com. "William 'Peanuts' Neumann." Obituary, August 16, 2015. www .legacy.com/us/obituaries/wausaudailyherald/name/william-neumann-obituary ?pid=175527856.

Lemke, Sarah, et al. "May Salivary Gland Secretory Proteins from Hematophagous Leeches (*Hirudo verbana*) Reach Pharmacologically Relevant Concentrations in the Vertebrate Host?" *PLoS ONE* 8, no. 9 (September 18, 2013): e73809. https://doi.org/10.1371/journal.pone.0073809.

Lennard, Natasha. "Kansas Militia Prepares for Zombies." *Salon*, January 4, 2013. www.salon.com/2013/01/04/kansas_militia_prepares_for_zombies/.

Leo, Giles, and Tristan Quinn. "The Dying Officer Treated for Cancer with Baking Soda." BBC, January 19, 2017. www.bbc.com/news/magazine -38650739.

Lerner, Sharon. "Doctor Who Joined Capitol Attacks Leads a Far-Right Campaign Against Covid-19 Vaccine." *The Intercept*, January 14, 2021. https:// theintercept.com/2021/01/14/capitol-riot-covid-vaccine-doctor/.

Levine, Jon. "Alex Jones Sounds the Alarm on Liberal Brain-Eating Lesbians (Video)." *The Wrap*, December 4, 2017. www.thewrap.com/alex-jones -sounds-the-alarm-on-liberal-brain-eating-lesbians-video/.

Levitan, Dave. "Fact Check: Rand Paul Repeats Baseless Vaccine Claims." *USA Today*, February 4, 2015. www.usatoday.com/story/news/politics/2015/02/04/fact-check-rand-paul-vaccines/22821023/.

Lewis, Nicole, Christina Cauterucci, and Anna Flagg. "Trump's Surprising Popularity in Prison." Marshall Project, March 12, 2020. www.themarshallproject.org/2020/03/12/trump-s-surprising-popularity-in-prison.

Lewis, Nicole, Aviva Shen, and Anna Flagg. "What Do We Really Know About the Politics of People Behind Bars?" Marshall Project, March 11, 2020. www.themarshallproject.org/2020/03/11/what-do-we-really-know-about-the-politics-of-people-behind-bars.

Li, Wen-Qing, et al. "Sildenafil Use and Increased Risk of Incident Melanoma in US Men: A Prospective Cohort Study." *JAMA Internal Medicine* 174, no. 6 (2014): 964–970. https://doi.org/10.1001/jamainternmed.2014.594.

Lipka, Michael, and Benjamin Wormald. "How Religious Is Your State?" Pew Research Center, February 29, 2016. www.pewresearch.org/fact-tank/2016/02/29/how-religious-is-your-state/?state=alabama.

Lonas, Lexi. "Man Claimed QAnon Made Him Kill His Children, FBI Says." MSN, August 12, 2021. www.msn.com/en-us/news/politics/man-claimed-qanon-made-him-kill-his-children-fbi-says/ar-AANf8vr?ocid=wispr&li=BBnbfcL.

London, Sharon. "The 8th Annual Health Freedom Expo Returns to the Renaissance Schaumburg Hotel and Convention Center." News release, Newswire, June 14, 2012. https://newswire.net/newsroom/financial/00069497-the-8th-annual-health-freedom-expo-returns-to-the-renaissance-schaumburg-hotel-and-convention-center.html.

Long, Josh. "Kabco Pharmaceuticals: Story of Redemption in Dietary Supplement Sector." Natural Products Insider, October 2, 2015. www.naturalproductsinsider.com/manufacturing/kabco-pharmaceuticals-story-redemption-dietary-supplement-sector.

Lopez, German. "How Americans Think the World Will End, in Charts." *Vox*, March 12, 2015. www.vox.com/2015/3/12/8194903/apocalypse-causes-poll.

Lugo, Manuel. "Are Margate Seawalls Sturdy Enough to Withstand Another Hurricane Season?" MargateNews.net, May 10, 2020. https://margatenews.net/are-margate-seawalls-sturdy-enough-to-withstand-another-hurricane-season-p1580-195.htm.

Lupkin, Sydney. "A Look at How the Revolving Door Spins from FDA to Industry." NPR, September 28, 2016. www.npr.org/sections/health-shots/2016/09/28/495694559/a-look-at-how-the-revolving-door-spins-from-fda-to-industry.

"Lytle, Kip." Obituary, *Rapid City Journal*, December 7, 2014. https://rapidcityjournal.com/obits/lytle-kip/article_2009c689-1469-514c-8019-6f8eb16161c1.html.

Lytle, Larry. Citizen Petition to the Division of Dockets Management of the Food and Drug Administration. Doc ID: FDA-2014-P-0445-0001. April

11, 2014. https://downloads.regulations.gov/FDA-2014-P-0445-0001 /attachment_2.pdf.

Lytle, Larry. *Healing Light: Energy Medicine of the Future*. Bloomington, IN: Authorhouse, 2004.

Lytle, Larry. Letter to Susan Atcher, Consumer Safety Officer of the Food and Drug Administration. "Request for Permission to Manufacture and Market Products to Private Members Only in the Private Domain." June 25, 2010. https://downloads.regulations.gov/FDA-2014-P-0445-0001/attachment_3 .pdf.

Lytle, Larry. Letter to Susan Atcher, Consumer Safety Officer of the Food and Drug Administration. "Rescission of Activities and Practices Involving Low Level Laser Devices." June 5, 2010. https://downloads.regulations.gov/FDA -2014-P-0445-0001/attachment_3.pdf.

Lytle, Larry. "Therapeutic Low Level Laser Apparatus and Method." Application for patent with the United States Patent and Trademark Office. March 29, 2005. https://patft.uspto.gov/netacgi/nph-Parser?Sect2=PTO1 &Sect2=HITOFF&p=1&u=%2Fnetahtml%2FPTO%2Fsearch-bool.html &r=1&f=G&l=50&d=PALL&RefSrch=yes&Query=PN%2F6872221.

Lytle, Larry. *Universal Healer: Book I: Osteoarthritis*. Bloomington, IN: Authorhouse, 2008.

Manella, Morgan. "90% of Americans Have Prayed for Healing, Study Finds." CNN, April 25, 2016. www.cnn.com/2016/04/25/health/healing-power-of -prayer-study/index.html.

Mantyla, Kyle. "Lance Wallnau: The Media Is Using 'Mind Control and Witchcraft' to Whip Up Opposition to Trump." Right Wing Watch, February 23, 2017. www.rightwingwatch.org/post/lance-wallnau-the-media-is-using-mind -control-and-witchcraft-to-whip-up-opposition-to-trump/.

Mantyla, Kyle. "Scott Lively Says Christians Must Prepare to Wage Violent Revolution." Right Wing Watch, May 4, 2020. www.rightwingwatch.org /post/scott-lively-says-christians-must-prepare-to-wage-violent-revolution/.

Maremont, Mark. "Ben Carson Has Had Ties to Dietary Supplement Firm That Faced Legal Challenge." *Wall Street Journal*, October 5, 2015. www .wsj.com/articles/ben-carson-has-had-ties-to-dietary-supplement-firm-that -faced-legal-challenge-1444057743.

Maremont, Mark. "A Mystery in Ben Carson's Ties With Supplement Maker Mannatech." *Wall Street Journal*, October 8, 2015. www.wsj.com/articles /BL-WB-58394.

Martial (Marcus Valerius Martialis). "Patient and Doctor." In *The World's Greatest Books: Vol. 17: Poetry and Drama*, translated by Wight Duff, edited by Arthur Mee and J. A. Hammerton. New York: W. H. Wise, 1910.

MassKids. "Civil Religious Exemptions Forced on States in 1974 by Department of Health, Education & Welfare (HEW)." Accessed March 19, 2022. www.masskids.org/index.php/religious-medical-neglect/jeopardizing -childrens-lives/hhs-policy-on-state-religious-exemptions.

Mayo Clinic. "Diabetic Ketoacidosis." Accessed March 15, 2022. www
.mayoclinic.org/diseases-conditions/diabetic-ketoacidosis/symptoms
-causes/syc-20371551.

Mazer, Benjamin. "How the 'Alt' Is Polarizing, and Harming, Medicine." *Stat*,
December 29, 2016. www.statnews.com/2016/12/29/alternative-medicine/.

McBreen, Darrin. "Rabid." Video, Banned Video, December 30, 2019. https://
banned.video/watch?id=5e0a9480cf8ec4002581e7a6.

McCall, Becky. "Risk for Erectile Dysfunction Sixfold Higher in Men
with COVID-19." Medscape, April 6, 2021. www.medscape.com
/viewarticle/948788#vp_2.

McCormick, Theodora. "The Dietary Supplement Industry in the Time of
Trump: Potential Opportunities and Pitfalls." Food and Drug Law Institute, December 2017. www.fdli.org/2017/12/dietary-supplement-industry
-time-trump-potential-opportunities-pitfalls/.

Mechanic, A. "Notice." *Botanic Watchman* 1, no. 1 (1834): 7–8. www.google
.com/books/edition/Thomsonian_Botanic_Watchman/ycIhAQAAMAAJ
?hl=en&gbpv=1&bsq=riots.

MedCrave. "Information on MedCrave Article Processing Charges." Accessed
March 20, 2022. https://medcraveonline.com/processing-fee.php.

Medical Dictionary. "Calendar." October 1, 2005. http://the-medical-dictionary
.com/progressive_supranuclear_palsy_article_7.htm.

MedZed LLC. "MedZed Names Neil A. Solomon, M.D., as Co-founder, Chief
Strategist & Chief Medical Officer." News release, Cision PRNewswire,
September 9, 2015. www.prnewswire.com/news-releases/medzed-names
-neil-a-solomon-md-as-co-founder-chief-strategist—chief-medical-officer
-300139894.html.

Mercola.com. "Horny Goat Weed." May 5, 2017. https://articles.mercola.com
/sites/articles/archive/2017/05/01/horny-goat-weed.aspx (article is no longer available).

Mercola.com. "Misleading Sunscreen Propaganda." December 26, 2012.
https://articles.mercola.com/sites/articles/archive/2012/12/26/misleading
-sunscreen-propaganda.aspx (article is no longer available).

Metro. "Leech Therapy: Bloodsuckers in Brooklyn." April 18, 2014. www
.metro.us/leech-therapy-bloodsuckers-in-brooklyn/.

Mikkelson, David. "LQP-79 Zombie Virus." Snopes, July 12, 2012. www
.snopes.com/fact-check/lqp-79-zombie-virus/.

Miller, Emily. *Emily Gets Her Gun: But Obama Wants to Take Yours*. Washington, DC: Regnery Publishing, 2013.

Miller, Robert D. *Legal and Professional Actions Involving Medical Consent
and Refusal in the Nineteenth Century*. 2020. https://minds.wisconsin.edu
/bitstream/handle/1793/80712/LEGAL%20AND%20PROFESSIONAL
%20ACTIONS%20INVOLVING%20MEDICAL%20CONSENT%20AND
%20REFUSAL%20IN%20THE%20NINETEENTH%20CENTURY%20
-%20final%20.pdf?sequence=1&isAllowed=y.

Miller, Ronald V., Jr. "Average Injury Verdicts in California," *Lawsuit Information Center Blog*, December 12, 2021. www.lawsuit-information-center .com/average_injury_verdicts_in_cal.html.

Mirkin, Gabe. "Acid/Alkaline Theory of Disease Is Nonsense." Quackwatch, January 11, 2009. https://quackwatch.org/related/DSH/coral2/.

Mishra, Suruchi, et al. "Dietary Supplement Use Among Adults: United States, 2017–2018." National Center for Health Statistics Data Brief No. 399, February 2021. www.cdc.gov/nchs/products/databriefs/db399.htm.

Momintheworks. "Jim Bakker Show (Aired on April 6th 2021): The Supernatural: More Natural than You Might Think Day 2." Video, YouTube, April 6, 2021. www.youtube.com/watch?v=Wy6JLS5dmeU.

Morgan, John. *A Bitter Pill: How Big Pharma Lobbies to Keep Prescription Drug Prices High*. Citizens for Responsibility and Ethics in Washington, June 18, 2018. www.citizensforethics.org/reports-investigations/crew-reports/a -bitter-pill-how-big-pharma-lobbies-to-keep-prescription-drug-prices-high/.

Morrissey, Charles T. "Inspiration and Perspiration: Vermont and the Thomsonian Cure for Illness." *Vermont History* 44, no. 4 (1976): 222–224. https:// vermonthistory.org/journal/misc/ThomsonianCure.pdf.

Moya, Alfred (@BlogOcala). "Ask your friends if they have tried BioSynergy supplements like L-theanine &GABA to reduce stress & improve mood #ad http://spn.tw/tXVam." Twitter, March 7, 2011. https://twitter.com /BlogOcala/status/44842634249912320.

Moya, Alfred. "Chief Investment Officer and Bitcoin Evangelist at Bitcoins-Vendor.com." LinkedIn profile, accessed March 20, 2022. www.linkedin .com/in/alfredmoya.

Mullen O'Keefe, Shannon. "Gallup Vault: New Vaccines Not Wildly Popular in U.S." *Gallup News*, September 10, 2020. https://news.gallup.com /vault/319976/gallup-vault-new-vaccines-not-wildly-popular.aspx.

Murphy, Tim. "Opening Statement: Hearing on 'Counterfeit Drugs: Fighting Illegal Supply Chains.'" Homeland Security Digital Library, February 27, 2014. www.hsdl.org/?view&did=750762.

Musk, Elon (@elonmusk). "Based on current trends, probably close to zero new cases in US too by end of April." Twitter, March 19, 2020. https://t witter.com/elonmusk/status/1240754657263144960?ref_src=twsrc%5Etfw %7Ctwcamp%5Etweetembed%7Ctwterm%5E1240754657263144960 %7Ctwgr%5E%7Ctwcon%5Es1_&ref_url=https%3A%2F%2Fwww .insidehook.com%2Farticle%2Ftech%2Felon-musk-worst-tweets.

Myers, Steve, and Josh Long. "Trump Effect: Big FDA Changes Afoot?" *Natural Product Insider*, March 8, 2017. www.naturalproductsinsider.com /regulatory/trump-effect-big-fda-changes-afoot.

Nakamoto,Tetsuo. "Science." *Theodent*, blog, accessed June 8, 2022. https:// theodent.com/blogs/science.

Nasiruddin, Melissa, Monique Halabi, and Alexander Dao. "Zombies: A Pop Culture Resource for Public Health Awareness." *Emerging Infectious*

Diseases 19, no. 5 (2013): 809–813. https://doi.org/10.3201/eid1905
.ad1905.

Natures Sunshine. "Goodbye to Clinton Ray Miller, the Father of Health
Freedom; 1921–2013." July 25, 2013. www.naturessunshine.com/blog/en
/goodbye-to-clinton-ray-miller-the-father-of-health-freedom-1921-2013/.

NBC Miami. "Margate Man Found Not Guilty in Oral Sex Murder Trial." May
22, 2017. www.nbcmiami.com/news/local/closing-arguments-underway-in
-oral-sex-defense-trial/96994/.

Neergaardd, Lauran. "FDA Warns Dietary Supplement Industry." Associated
Press, December 18, 2002. https://apnews.com/article/61e16a6d34a2e78
160247831ba155363.

Neumann, Leilani. "Bless your husband or the father of your child/children
today, no matter what, in both words and actions." Facebook, June 17,
2018. www.facebook.com/photo.php?fbid=1713247015438220&set=pb
.100002588152723.-2207520000..&type=3.

Neumann, Leilani. "Happy 34 years to us." Facebook, June 6, 2021. www
.facebook.com/photo/?fbid=4000428346720064&set=ecnf.10000
2588152723.

"New Medicine Based on an 88 Year Old Theory by Albert Einstein Can Help
Almost Everyone Who Is Sick or Injured." Paid advertisement, *Sarasota
Herald Tribune*, September 11, 2008. https://news.google.com/newspapers
?nid=1774&dat=20080911&id=alMhAAAAIBAJ&sjid=dIUFAAAAIBAJ
&pg=6605,35299.

Nielsen, Tor. "The COVID-19 Pandemic Is Changing Our Dreams." *Scientific
American*, October 1, 2020. www.scientificamerican.com/article/the-covid
-19-pandemic-is-changing-our-dreams/.

Nimmo, Jamie. "Exposed: The Conspiracy Theorists Who Claim Coronavirus
Is Linked to 5G, Including the Cousin of a Cabinet Minister and a Former
CIA Spy." *Daily Mail*, April 11, 2020. www.dailymail.co.uk/news/article
-8211171/Exposed-conspiracy-theorists-claim-coronavirus-linked-5G
.html.

NovaCare, LLC. "About Us." LinkedIn, accessed March 20, 2022. www.linkedin
.com/company/novacare-llc.

Novack, Sophie. "How Anti-Vaxxers Are Injecting Themselves into the Texas Republican Primaries." *Texas Observer*, February 28, 2018. www.texasobserver
.org/anti-vaxxers-injecting-texas-republican-primaries/.

Novick, Ilana. "Trump Appeals to Men's Deepest Insecurities, Research Finds."
Truthdig, November 29, 2019. www.truthdig.com/articles/researchers
-explain-how-trump-wins-men-over-by-appealing-to-their-insecurities/.

NPR Illinois. "Calendar: Trinity Health Freedom Expo." October 1, 2021. www
.nprillinois.org/community-calendar/event/trinity-health-freedom-expo.

Office of the District Attorney County of San Diego. "DA Charges Two with
Conspiracy to Practice Medicine Without a License: Defendants Using
I-V Treatments on Patients at Avocado Ranch." News release, January 24,

2014. https://quackwatch.org/wp-content/uploads/sites/33/quackwatch/casewatch/crim/ro_young/news_release.pdf.

"Officials in Dakota Ask Nation to Give Cash as Flood Aid." *New York Times*, June 16, 1972. www.nytimes.com/1972/06/13/archives/survivors-of-dakota-flood-vow-to-get-on-with-it.html.

Ofgang, Erik. "When Yale Medical Students Robbed a Grave for Science, New Haven Erupted in Fury." *Connecticut Magazine*, March 19, 2018. www.connecticutmag.com/the-connecticut-story/when-yale-medical-students-robbed-a-grave-for-science-new-haven-erupted-in-fury/article_94312fde-27c5-11e8-a23d-cf5e1f70160e.html.

Ojewole, J. A. "African Traditional Medicines for Erectile Dysfunction: Elusive Dream or Imminent Reality?" *Cardiovascular Journal of Africa* 18, no. 4 (2007): 213–215. www.ncbi.nlm.nih.gov/pmc/articles/PMC4170225/.

Olson, DaiWai M., and John C. Bazil. "Of Zombies and Evidence." *Journal of Neuroscience Nursing* 51, no. 1 (February 2019): 7. https://doi.org/10.1097/JNN.0000000000000421.

On the Issues. "Libertarian Party on Health Care." Accessed March 19, 2022. www.ontheissues.org/celeb/Libertarian_Party_Health_Care.htm.

Open Secrets. "Summary: Nutritional and Dietary Supplements Interest Groups." Accessed March 19, 2022. www.opensecrets.org/industries/indus.php?cycle=2016&ind=H4600.

The Original Skeptical Raptor. "Another Anti-Vaccine Article: Bad Journal, Bad Data." *Skeptical Raptor*, blog, February 1, 2017. www.skepticalraptor.com/skepticalraptorblog.php/another-anti-vaccine-article-bad-journal-bad-data/.

Osteopathic Medical Board of California. "In the Matter of the Accusation Against: Bennie S. Johnson, D.O." Case No. 00-2013-003759. April 3, 2017. https://quackwatch.org/wp-content/uploads/sites/33/quackwatch/casewatch/board/med/johnson_b/revocation.pdf.

Our World in Data. "Daily New Confirmed COVID-19 Deaths per Million People." Accessed June 8, 2022. https://ourworldindata.org/explorers/coronavirus-data-explorer.

Pandey, Renu, Larry Lytle, and Alok Mishra. "Low Level Laser Therapy (Lllt) for the Treatment of Hypertension." *International Journal of Engineering Research and Development* 6, no. 3 (March 2013): 35–38. http://ijerd.com/paper/vol6-issue3/S%20pdf/F06033538.pdf.

Parker Bowles, Emma. "Gruesome, Medieval and Utterly Bizarre . . . but Leeches Freed Me from Awful Migraines." *Daily Mail*, June 3, 2013. www.dailymail.co.uk/health/article-2334337/Gruesome-medieval-utterly-bizarre—leeches-freed-awful-migraines.html.

"A Parody on 'Mary's Ghost'; or, The Doctors and Body-Snatchers. A Pathetic Tale, with Numerous Additions." Norwich, UK: Christopher Berry, 1829. Accessed June 24, 2022. https://archive.org/details/b30375198/page/6/mode/2up.

People v. Robert O. Young. Plea of Guilty/No Contest—Felony. Case no. SCD 253359. Filed April 12, 2017. https://centerforinquiry.org/wp-content/uploads/sites/33/quackwatch/young_plea.pdf.

Perlman, Melissa. "What Started as Group of Anti-Vax Moms Led by Stockton Woman Is Now 'Mamalitia.'" CBS Sacramento, April 29, 2021. https://sacramento.cbslocal.com/2021/04/29/what-started-as-group-of-anti-vax-moms-is-now-mamalitia/.

Perlstein, Rick. "Eye on the Pyramids (Part 4: The Incredible Bread Machine)." *The Nation*, October 30, 2013. www.thenation.com/article/archive/eye-pyramids-part-4-incredible-bread-machine/.

Perlstein, Rick. "The Long Con." *The Baffler*, November 2012. https://thebaffler.com/salvos/the-long-con.

Perry, Susan. "How Sen. Hatch Has Held Back the Regulation of Dietary Supplements." *MinnPost*, June 21, 2011. www.minnpost.com/second-opinion/2011/06/how-sen-hatch-has-held-back-regulation-dietary-supplements/.

Perry, Susan. "Trump's Short, Failed Venture into Vitamin Supplement Hucksterism." *MinnPost*, March 4, 2016. www.minnpost.com/second-opinion/2016/03/trumps-short-failed-venture-vitamin-supplement-hucksterism/.

Pew Research Center. "Vast Majority of Americans Say Benefits of Childhood Vaccines Outweigh Risks: Americans' Health Care Behaviors and Use of Conventional and Alternative Medicine." Pew Research Center, February 2, 2017. www.pewresearch.org/science/2017/02/02/americans-health-care-behaviors-and-use-of-conventional-and-alternative-medicine/.

pH Miracle Products. "Disclaimer." Accessed March 15, 2022. https://phmiracleproducts.com/pages/disclaimer.

Phadke, Varun K. "Association Between Vaccine Refusal and Vaccine-Preventable Diseases in the United States: A Review of Measles and Pertussis." *JAMA* 315, no. 11 (2016): 1149–1158. https://doi.org/10.1001/jama.2016.1353.

Phend, Rachel. "Anticoagulation Guidance Emerging for Severe COVID-19." *MedPage Today*, January 20, 2021. www.medpagetoday.com/infectiousdisease/covid19/85865?fbclid=IwAR2RZCTQE4OdwJk51_9nbYu-YyTj8FCNZcE-LbnUP9R_luEl_OKX_JMmw-Y.

Piller, Charles. "Exclusive: FDA Enforcement Actions Plummet Under Trump." *Science*, July 2, 2019. www.science.org/content/article/exclusive-fda-enforcement-actions-plummet-under-trump.

Piller, Charles, and Jia You. "Hidden Conflicts? Pharma Payments to FDA Advisers After Drug Approvals Spark Ethical Concerns." *Science*, July 5, 2018. www.sciencemag.org/news/2018/07/hidden-conflicts-pharma-payments-fda-advisers-after-drug-approvals-spark-ethical.

Piña, Tinabeth. "Take Bugs Instead of Drugs!" Video, YouTube, October 31, 2014. www.youtube.com/watch?v=otDhdlL79H0&list=PL3unzgrm2ZXHQjWxeexz9dzUmQL2D1a-8.

Prevennia. "Dr. Alan Keyes Joins Prevennia in Its Fight Against Life Altering Disease." News release, August 18, 2011. www.benzinga.com/pressreleases /11/08/p1865669/dr-alan-keyes-joins-prevennia-in-its-fight-against-life -altering-diseas.

Prominski, Patrick. "Samuel Thomson's Crusade: Populism, Folk Remedy, and Tradition in Timothy Flint and Catharine Maria Sedgwick." *Literature and Medicine* 38, no. 1 (2020): 189–210. https://doi.org/10.1353/lm.2020 .0008.

QLasers PMA. "2014 08 28 13 37 QTalk with Dr Larry Lytle Healing Light An Introduction to Energy Medicine." Video, YouTube, August 29, 2014. www .youtube.com/watch?v=SOP0tLkaPNs&t=youtube.com/watch ?v=SOP0tLkaPNs&t=256s.

QLasers PMA. "Addressing the Symptoms of Dental Distress Syndrome." Video, YouTube, January 31, 2014. www.youtube.com/watch?v=rOjOVty K5Gw.

QLasers PMA. "Healing Light Saves the Little Bear." Video, YouTube, September 24, 2014. www.youtube.com/watch?v=f2kYRjXwUAk.

QLasers PMA. "This account has been suspended." April 18, 2015. Archived at Wayback Machine. https://web.archive.org/web/20150418214644/http:// www.qlaserspma.com/cgi-sys/suspendedpage.cgi.

QLasers PMA. "Welcome to QLasers Private Membership Association." September 27, 2010. Archived at Wayback Machine. https://web.arc hive.org/web/20100927220108/http://www.qlaserspma.com/.

Quayle, Steve. "Zombies: The Calling Forth of the Damned: The Zombie Resurrection and the Day of the Lord." Accessed March 20, 2022. www .stevequayle.com/index.php?s=285.

Raman, Ryan. "What Is the Gerson Therapy, and Does It Fight Cancer?" *Healthline*, March 18, 2019. www.healthline.com/nutrition/gerson-therapy #what-it-is.

Rambajan, I. "Highly Prevalent Falciparum Malaria in North West Guyana: Its Development History and Control Problems." *Bulletin of the Pan American Health Organization* 28, no. 3 (1994): 193–201. https://pubmed.ncbi.nlm .nih.gov/7951362/.

Rapid City Public Library. "Rapid City 1972 Flood Oral History—Larry Lytle." Video, Vimeo, September 5, 2012. https://vimeo.com/48920247.

Rapid City Public Library Digital Collection. "1972 Flood Victims." Accessed June 26, 2022. http://ppolinks.com/rcplib/SID-0000000176411.pdf.

Ratini, Melinda. "What to Expect in Your 70s." WebMD, August 4, 2021. www .webmd.com/healthy-aging/ss/slideshow-what-to-expect-in-your-70s.

Realtor.com. "Ronnie Weir." Accessed March 19, 2022. www.realtor.com /realestateagents/ronnie-weir_rapid-city_sd_2789815.

Redpath-Fruth Funeral Home. "Wendell W. Whitman." Obituary, May 21, 2008. www.redpathfruthfuneralhome.com/obituary/Wendell-Whitman.

Reese, David Meredith. *Humbugs of New-York: Being a Remonstrance Against Popular Delusion; Whether in Science, Philosophy, or Religion*. New York: John S. Taylor, Brick-Church Chapel, 1838.

Reinhart, R. J. "Fewer in U.S. Continue to See Vaccines as Important." Gallup News, January 14, 2020. https://news.gallup.com/poll/276929/fewer-continue-vaccines-important.aspx.

Religion News Blog. "Jury Convicts Mother Who Prayed for Daughter Instead of Treating Her Fatal Diabetes." May 23, 2009. www.religionnewsblog.com/23480/madeline-neumann-mother-convicted.

Religion News Blog. "Mom on Trial for Daughter's Faith Healing Death Falls Ill." May 18, 2009. www.religionnewsblog.com/23475/madeline-neumann-15.

Religion News Blog. "Mother Thought Sickness Was Sin; 911 Called Twelve Hours After Daughter Went into Coma." May 20, 2009. www.religionnewsblog.com/23478/madeline-neumann-faith-healing-3.

Religion News Blog. "Police: Girl Died as Parents Prayed Instead of Seeking Help." March 26, 2008. www.religionnewsblog.com/20958/madeline-neumann.

Reuters. "Fact Check: No Evidence Bill Gates Said 'At Least 3 Billion People Need to Die.'" January 29, 2021. www.reuters.com/article/uk-factcheck-bill-gates-fake-3-billion-q-idUSKBN29Y20D.

Rice, Charles, and Frederick Albert Castle. "The Leech Trade." In *New Remedies: A Quarterly Retrospect of Therapeutics, Pharmacy and Allied Subjects*, vol. 2. New York: William Wood and Company, 1873.

Right Wing Watch (@RightWingWatch). "Jo Rae Perkins, the GOP's Senate nominee in Oregon and a full-blown QAnon supporter, says mask mandates and social distancing guidelines are part of a plot to turn us into zombies." Twitter, August 14, 2020. https://twitter.com/RightWingWatch/status/1294275689319936002.

Ripley, Anthony. "Deaths Pass 200 in Dakota Flood; Search Goes On." *New York Times*, June 12, 1972. www.nytimes.com/1972/06/12/archives/deaths-pass-200-in-dakota-flood-search-goes-on-87-bodies-are.html.

Robert L. Lytle v. Gerald Berg. No. 12-3321 (8th Cir. 2013). https://law.justia.com/cases/federal/appellate-courts/ca8/12-3321/12-3321-2013-04-01.html.

Robert Larry Lytle v. Charles Hendrix. No. 4:19-cv-00270-KGB (USDC, E.D. Ark., Cent. Div., March 9, 2020). www.leagle.com/decision/infdco202003 10921.

Roberts, Brooklyn. "Health Care Freedom: Easier Access to Quality Care." *American Legislative Exchange Council News*, October 1, 2020. www.alec.org/article/health-care-freedom-easier-access-to-quality-care/.

Rodrick, Stephen. "Robert Redford's Restless Solitude." *Men's Journal*, October 15. 2013. www.mensjournal.com/entertainment/robert-redfords-restless-solitude-20131015/.

Rodriguez, Laura. "Leech Therapy Gaining Popularity in South Florida." NBC Miami, May 24, 2016. www.nbcmiami.com/news/local/leech-therapy-gaining-popularity-in-south-florida/55659/.

Rogers, Phil. "Letters Reveal What Inmates Had to Say About Blagojevich Amid Renewed Plea for Freedom." NBC Chicago, July 12, 2016. www.nbcchicago.com/news/local/prosecutors-want-blagojevich-to-serve-full-original-sentence/2008995/.

Romez, Clarissa, et al. "Case Report of Instantaneous Resolution of Juvenile Macular Degeneration Blindness After Proximal Intercessory Prayer." *Explore* 17, no. 1 (2021): 79–83. https://doi.org/10.1016/j.explore.2020.02.011.

Roopnarine, Lomarsh. "Wounding Guyana: Gold Mining and Environmental Degradation." *Revista Europea de Estudios Latinoamericanos y Del Caribe / European Review of Latin American and Caribbean Studies*, no. 73 (2002): 83–91. www.jstor.org/stable/25675989.

Roose, Kevin. "Yoga Teachers Take on QAnon." *New York Times*, September 15, 2020. www.nytimes.com/2020/09/15/technology/yoga-teachers-take-on-qanon.html.

Ross, Casey, Max Blau, and Kate Sheridan. "Medicine with a Side of Mysticism: Top Hospitals Promote Unproven Therapies." *Stat*, March 7, 2017. www.statnews.com/2017/03/07/alternative-medicine-hospitals-promote/.

Ross, Jaimie. "Suspected U.K. Mass Shooter Said He Was American, Trump-Supporting Virgin." *Daily Beast*, August 13, 2021. www.thedailybeast.com/jake-davison-suspected-mass-shooter-said-he-was-an-american-trump-supporting-virgin.

Rothstein, William G. "Review of *The People's Doctors: Samuel Thomson and the American Botanical Movement, 1790–1860*." *Bulletin of the History of Medicine* 76, no. 1 (2002): 147–148. https://doi.org/10.1353/bhm.2002.0044.

Rough, Ginger, and Robert Anglen. "Jared Fogle Attacked in Prison by Arizona Criminal: 'He Could Have Killed Him If He Wanted To.'" *AZCentral.com*, March 16, 2016. www.azcentral.com/story/entertainment/people/2016/03/16/jared-fogle-prison-attack-steven-niggs-arizona/81863940/.

Rubik, B. "Sympathetic Resonance Technology: Scientific Foundation and Summary of Biologic and Clinical Studies." *Journal of Alternative and Complementary Medicine* 8, no. 6 (2002): 823–856. https://doi.org/10.1089/10755530260511838.

Rural Health Information Hub. "Healthcare Access in Rural Communities." August 18, 2021. www.ruralhealthinfo.org/topics/healthcare-access.

Russon, Jen. "Rescue Dog Warns Family About Alligator Lurking at Front Door." *Coral Springs Talk*, May 30, 2019. https://coralspringstalk.com/rescue-dog-warns-family-about-alligator-lurking-at-front-door-23312.

Sackett, David L. "Evidence Based Medicine: What It Is and What It Isn't." *British Medical Journal* 312 (1996): 71–72. www.ncbi.nlm.nih.gov/pmc/articles/PMC2349778/pdf/bmj00524-0009.pdf.

Safe Information. "Jim Humble über Aliens deutsch Bewusst TV 4 11 2015 Reupload 2020" [Jim Humble on Aliens German Bewusst TV]. Video, You-Tube, May 2, 2020. www.youtube.com/watch?v=_HfSkC6pDnc.

Safe Trek. "Products." Accessed March 19, 2022. www.safetrek.com/.

Sanders, Linley. "14% of Americans Have a Zombie Apocalypse Plan." You GovAmerica, October 1, 2019. https://today.yougov.com/topics/entertainment /articles-reports/2019/10/01/zombie-apocalypse-plan.

Sandler, Rachel. "FDA Rejects Oleandrin, Extract Pushed by MyPillow CEO, as a Dietary Supplement." *Forbes*, September 4, 2020. www.forbes.com /sites/rachelsandler/2020/09/04/fda-rejects-oleandrin-extract-pushed-by -mypillow-ceo-as-a-dietary-supplement/?sh=5abdb6853afe.

Sandstrom, Aleksandra. "Most States Allow Religious Exemptions from Child Abuse and Neglect Laws." Pew Research Center, August 12, 2016. www .pewresearch.org/fact-tank/2016/08/12/most-states-allow-religious-exemptions -from-child-abuse-and-neglect-laws/.

Saper, Robert B. "Overview of Herbal Medicine and Dietary Supplements." UpToDate, October 26, 2021. www.uptodate.com/contents/overview-of -herbal-medicine-and-dietary-supplements.

Schlenoff, Dan. "50, 100 & 150 Years Ago: March 2021." *Scientific American*, March 1, 2021. www.scientificamerican.com/article/50-100-150-years-ago -march-2021/.

Schlozman, Steven. "The Harvard Doctor Who Accidentally Unleashed a Zombie Invasion." *New York Times Magazine*, October 25, 2013. www .nytimes.com/2013/10/27/magazine/the-harvard-doctor-who-accidentally -unleashed-a-zombie-invasion.html.

Schontzler, Gail. "Fallout Fears Hit Bozeman, Spark Run on Pills." *Bozeman Daily Chronicle*, March 17, 2011. www.bozemandailychronicle.com/news /fallout-fears-hit-bozeman-spark-run-on-pills/article_634cabbe-5031-11e0 -8d52-001cc4c002e0.html.

Schwalfenberg, Gerry K. "The Alkaline Diet: Is There Evidence That an Alka-line pH Diet Benefits Health?" *Journal of Environmental and Public Health* (2012). https://doi.org/10.1155/2012/727630.

Schwartz, Matthew S. "Missouri Sues Televangelist Jim Bakker for Selling Fake Coronavirus Cure." NPR, March 11, 2020. www.npr.org/2020/03 /11/814550474/missouri-sues-televangelist-jim-bakker-for-selling-fake -coronavirus-cure.

Scutti, Susan. "Choosing Alternative Cancer Therapy Doubles Risk of Death, Study Says." CNN, August 17, 2017. www.cnn.com/2017/08/17/health /alternative-vs-conventional-cancer-treatment-study/index.html.

Siegler, Kirk. "The Struggle to Hire and Keep Doctors in Rural Areas Means Patients Go Without Care." NPR, May 21, 2019. www.npr.org/sections /health-shots/2019/05/21/725118232/the-struggle-to-hire-and-keep-doctors -in-rural-areas-means-patients-go-without-c.

Slawson, Robert G. "Medical Training in the United States Prior to the Civil War." *Journal of Evidence-Based Complementary and Alternative Medicine* 17, no. 1 (2012): 11–27. https://doi.org/10.1177/2156587211427404.

Slisco, Aila. "Radio Host Steve Quayle Claims Zombies Could Attack Earth on Televangelist Jim Bakker's Show." *Newsweek*, April 6, 2021. www .newsweek.com/radio-host-steve-quayle-claims-zombies-could-attack -earth-televangelist-jim-bakkers-show-1581483.

Smith, R. Jeffrey, and Jeffrey H. Birnbaum. "Drug Bill Demonstrates Lobby's Pull." *Washington Post*, January 11, 2007. www.washingtonpost.com /wp-dyn/content/article/2007/01/11/AR2007011102081.html.

Smith Weinstock, Joanna. "Samuel Thomson's Botanic System: Alternative Medicine in Early Nineteenth Century Vermont." *Vermont History* 56, no. 1 (1988): 5–20. https://vermonthistory.org/journal/misc/SamuelThomsons BotanicSystem.pdf.

SnyderHealth. "Dr. Robert Young on CNN Discussing His Alkaline Diet, the pH Miracle Program." Video, YouTube, January 31, 2007. www.youtube .com/watch?v=T0nwZPqbCbo&t=4s.

Solender, Andrew. "U.S. Army Halted Tests on Oleandrin, a Drug Touted to Trump as Covid-19 Cure by MyPillow CEO Lindell." *Forbes*, September 4, 2020. www.forbes.com/sites/andrewsolender/2020/08/19/us-army-halted -tests-on-oleandrin-a-drug-touted-to-trump-as-covid-19-cure-by-mypillow -ceo-lindell/?sh=699dd6513bb6.

Speigel, Lee. "Morgan Freeman: 'We May Already Be in the Midst of a Growing Zombie Apocalypse.'" *HuffPost*, June 25, 2014. www.huffpost.com /entry/morgan-freeman-zombie-apocalypse_n_5531252?utm_hp_ref =zombie-apocalypse.

Spencer, Samuel. "QAnon Believers Tell Borat That Hillary and Bill Clinton Drink Blood in Movie Sequel." *Newsweek*, October 23, 2020. www .newsweek.com/borat-2-movie-qanon-bill-clinton-hillary-clinton-blood -1541366.

"Startling Theories as to Odors." *New York Times*, December 23, 1884. https:// timesmachine.nytimes.com/timesmachine/1884/12/23/106290806.html.

State of Wisconsin v. Dale R. Neumann. 348 Wis. 2d 455, 832 N.W.2d 560, 2013 WI 58 (Wis. 2013). https://casetext.com/case/state-v-neumann-10.

State of Wisconsin v. Dale R. Neumann. "Appeal No. 11 AP 1044- CR" (Wis. Ct. App. D3 July 19, 2011). https://acefiling.wicourts.gov/document/eFiled /2011AP001105/68426.

State of Wisconsin v. Dale R. Neumann and Leilani E. Neumann. "Certification." 2011AP1044-CR, 2011AP1105-CR, Cir. Ct. Nos. 2008CF324, 2008CF323 (Wis. Ct. App. D3 May 1, 2012). www.wicourts.gov/ca/cert /DisplayDocument.pdf?content=pdf&seqNo=81830.

State of Wisconsin v. Dale R. Neumann and Leilani E. Neumann. "Certification from the Court of Appeals." Case No.: 2011AP1044-CR & 2011AP1105-CR

(Wis. Sup. Ct. July 3, 2013). www.wicourts.gov/sc/opinion/DisplayDocument
.html?content=html&seqNo=98993.

State of Wisconsin v. Leilani E. Neumann. "Appeal No. 2011AP001105—CR"
(Wis. Ct. App. D3 July 19, 2011). https://acefiling.wicourts.gov/document
/eFiled/2011AP001105/68426.

Sunshine Health Freedom Organization. "Board of Directors." Accessed March
19, 2022. https://sunshinehealthfreedom.org/?page_id=103.

Swan, Rita. "Children's Healthcare Is a Legal Duty, Inc." *Child, Inc.*, 2008.
http://childrenshealthcare.org/wp-content/uploads/2010/10/2008-01-fnl
.pdf.

Swann, John P. "The History of Efforts to Regulate Dietary Supplements in the
USA." *Drug Testing and Analysis* 8 (2016): 271–282. https://doi.org/10.1002
/dta.1919.

Swanson, Ana. "The Trump Network Sought to Make People Rich but Left Behind Disappointment." *Washington Post*, March 23, 2016. www.washington
post.com/news/wonk/wp/2016/03/23/the-trump-network-sought-to-make
-people-rich-but-left-behind-disappointment/.

Swarthmore College Linguistics Department. "Zombies Reimagined: A Critical
Discourse Analysis of Popular Culture." Accessed March 20, 2022. https://
ds-pages.swarthmore.edu/zombies-reimagined/.

Swetlitz, Ike. "Donald Trump, Bad Science, and the Vitamin Company That Went
Bust." *Stat*, March 2, 2016. www.statnews.com/2016/03/02/donald-trump
-vitamin-company/.

Taboada, Luis De. "Light-Emitting Device and Method for Providing Photo-
therapy to the Brain." Application for patent with the United States Patent
and Trademark Office, November 23, 2021. https://patft.uspto.gov/netacgi
/nph-Parser?Sect1=PTO2&Sect2=HITOFF&p=1&u=%2Fnetahtml
%2FPTO%2Fsearch-bool.html&r=1&f=G&l=50&col=AND&d=PTXT&s1
=%22Larry+Lytle%22&OS=%22Larry+Lytle%22&RS=%22Larry+Lytle
%22.

Tallman, Deanna. "Goldline Announces New Exclusive Gold and Silver Bullion Coins." News release, Business Wire, May 5, 2014. www.businesswire
.com/news/home/20140505005134/en/Goldline-Announces-New-Exclusive
-Gold-and-Silver-Bullion-Coins.

Tatro, Samantha. "'pH Miracle' Author Robert O. Young Sentenced." NBC
San Diego, June 29, 2017. www.nbcsandiego.com/news/local/ph-miracle
-author-robert-o-young-sentenced/19346/.

Thomas, Liji. "Big Pharma More Profitable than Most Other Large Public Firms." News Medical, March 3, 2020. www.news-medical.net/news
/20200303/Big-Pharma-more-profitable-than-most-other-large-public
-firms.aspx.

Tillman, Zoe. "A Capitol Rioter Says He's Working on a Video Game Featuring
Donald Trump Shooting 'Dem Zombies' and 'Antifa.'" *BuzzFeed News*, July

29, 2021. www.buzzfeednews.com/article/zoetillman/jan-6-capitol-rioter-donald-trump-shooter-video-game.

Tilton, George Henry. *A History of Rehoboth, Massachusetts; Its History for 275 Years, 1643–1918, in Which Is Incorporated the Vital Parts of the Original History of the Town.* Boston: George Henry Tilton, 1918.

Trinity Health Freedom Expo. "About." Accessed March 20, 2022. https://trinityhealthfreedomexpo.com/about/.

Trinity School of Natural Health. "About." Accessed March 20, 2022. www.trinityschool.org/about.

Trinity School of Natural Health. "Master Iridologist." Accessed March 19, 2022. www.trinityschool.org/program/mi.

TrumpNetwork411. "The Trump Network—Donald Trump and Ideal Health Team Up." Video, YouTube, 2010. www.youtube.com/watch?v=fK9AhOo3Fj0.

Tupper, Seth. "Laser Man, Part 1." *Rapid City Journal*, March 19, 2017. https://rapidcityjournal.com/news/local/laser-man-part-1-investigation-of-lytle-is-16-year-saga/article_ba54eb5d-d3fa-52ba-b98d-8ecf060e2886.html#tracking-source=in-article.

TV Series Finale. "The Bachelor: Season 21 Ratings." May 12, 2017. https://tvseriesfinale.com/tv-show/bachelor-season-21-ratings/.

Twohey, Megan. "Ted Cruz's Father Worked with Supplements Maker Sued by Investors." *New York Times*, April 29, 2016. www.nytimes.com/2016/04/30/us/politics/rafael-cruz-mannatech.html.

Uhlig, Keith. "Couple Convicted in Prayer Death Case Hope for New Start with Coffee Shop in Stratford." *Wausau Daily Herald*, June 15, 2018. www.wausaudailyherald.com/story/news/2018/06/15/leilani-dale-neumann-prayer-death-couple-hope-new-start-stratford-coffee-shop/699773002/.

United States of America v. 2035, Inc. and Robert L. Lytle. CA no. 14-5075 (US Dis. Ct. D.S.D. October 21, 2014). www.justice.gov/sites/default/files/opa/press-releases/attachments/2014/11/04/qlasers_complaint.pdf.

United States of America v. 2035, Inc. and Robert L. Lytle. "Order of Permanent Injunction." Case 5:14-cv-05075-JLV Document 138 (US Dis. Ct. D.S.D. Western Div., October 6, 2015). www.justice.gov/opa/page/file/1356546/download.

United States of America v. 2035 Inc. et al. No. 5:2014cv05075—Document 47 (D.S.D. 2015). https://law.justia.com/cases/federal/district-courts/south-dakota/sddce/5:2014cv05075/55548/47/.

United States of America v. Genesis II Church of Health and Healing et al. No. 1:2020cv21601—Docket (USDC District of Southern Fla., April 16, 2020). https://dockets.justia.com/docket/florida/flsdce/1:2020cv21601/569990.

United States of America v. Grenon et al. No. 1:21-cr-20242—Docket (USDC District of Southern Fla., April 22, 2021). www.pacermonitor.com/public/case/40347064/USA_v_Grenon_et_al.

United States of America v. Lytle et al. No. 5:2021cv05011—Docket (D.S.D. February 19, 2021). https://dockets.justia.com/docket/south-dakota/sddce /5:2021cv05011/70594.

United States of America v. Mark Scott Grenon, Jonathan David Grenon, Jordan Paul Grenon, and Joseph Timothy Grenon. Case no. 21-20242-CR-ALTONAGA/ TORRES (USDC Southern District of Florida, April 22, 2021). https:// cdn.centerforinquiry.org/wp-content/uploads/sites/33/2016/10/24194401 /indictment.pdf.

United States of America v. Mark Scott Grenon, Jonathan David Grenon, Jordan Paul Grenon, and Joseph Timothy Grenon. No. 20-3050-MJ-Otazo-Reyes: Government's Memorandum in Support of Detention (USDC District of Southern Fla., July 8, 2020). www.docketbird.com/court-cases/USA-v -Grenon-et-al/flsd-1:2020-mj-03050.

United States v. Robert L. Lytle. No. 17-2421 (8th Cir. 2018). https://law.justia .com/cases/federal/appellate-courts/ca8/17-2421/17-2421-2018-08-31.html.

United States of America v. Robert Larry Lytle. 5:17-CR-50020-01-RAL (D.S.D. August 12, 2020). https://casetext.com/case/united-states-v-lytle-22.

United States of America v. Robert Larry Lytle, Irina Kossovskaia and Fredretta Eason. CR: 17-50020 (US Dis. Ct. D.S.D. January 26, 2017). www.justice .gov/opa/press-release/file/934111/download.

United States of America v. Ronald D. Weir, Jr. Charges. CR: 17-50020 (US Dis. Ct. D.S.D. Western Div., January 30, 2017). www.justice.gov/opa /press-release/file/934116/download.

United States of America v. Ronald D. Weir, Jr. "Factual Basis Statement." CR: 17-50020 (US Dis. Ct. D.S.D. Western Div., January 30, 2017). www.justice .gov/opa/press-release/file/934126/download.

United States of America v. Ronald D. Weir, Jr. "Opinion and Order Denying Motion for Furlough." No. 5:17-CR-50022-RAL (US Dis. Ct. D.S.D. Western Div., August 3, 2018). www.leagle.com/decision/infdco20180806b84.

Unleavened Bread Ministries. "Could Hillary Be President When the U.S. Falls?" Accessed March 15, 2022. www.ubm1.org/?page=presidenthillary.

Unleavened Bread Ministries. "Drugs Cause Murderous Rampages." Accessed March 15, 2022. www.ubm1.org/?page=drugsrampages.

Unleavened Bread Ministries. "Immunized from Christianity." Accessed March 15, 2022. www.ubm1.org/?page=immunized.

Unleavened Bread Ministries. "Preserved from the Beast." Podcast Addict, December 8, 2021. www.podcastaddict.com/episode/132451223.

Unleavened Bread Ministries. "Preserved from the Beast (1)." Accessed March 15, 2022. www.ubm1.org/?page=preserved-from-the-beast.

UPI. "Aid for Victims of Flood." *New York Times,* June 25, 1972. www.nytimes .com/1972/06/25/archives/aid-for-victims-of-flood.html.

UPI. "Flood Kills 155 in South Dakota; 5,000 Homeless." *New York Times,* June 14, 1982. www.nytimes.com/1972/06/11/archives/flood-kills-155-in -south-dakota-5000-homeless-rapid-city-area.html.

UPI. "Quick Tax Relief on Floods Backed." *New York Times*, July 1, 1972. www
.nytimes.com/1972/07/01/archives/quick-tax-relief-on-floods-backed-senate
-favors-immediate.html.

UPI. "Rapid City Recalls Devastating Flood of 1972." *New York Times*, June 14,
1982. www.nytimes.com/1982/06/14/us/rapid-city-recalls-devastating-flood
-of-1972.html.

US Department of Health and Human Services. "Federal Judge Issues Permanent Injunction Against South Dakota Laser Manufacturer." News release,
October 7, 2015. Archived at Wayback Machine. https://wayback.archive
-it.org/7993/20170111092353/http://www.fda.gov/NewsEvents/Newsroom
/PressAnnouncements/ucm466044.htm.

US Department of Justice. "Medical Device Manufacturer Permanently En-
joined." News release, October 7, 2015. www.justice.gov/opa/pr/medical
-device-manufacturer-permanently-enjoined.

US Department of Justice. "Three Conspirators Sentenced in $16.6m Fraud-
ulent Medical Device Scheme." News release, April 23, 2018. www.justice
.gov/opa/pr/three-conspirators-sentenced-166m-fraudulent-medical-device
-scheme.

US Department of Justice. "Three Individuals Arrested and Charged in South
Dakota Fraudulent Medical Device Scheme." News release, January 31,
2017. www.justice.gov/usao-sd/pr/three-individuals-arrested-and-charged
-south-dakota-fraudulent-medical-device-scheme.

US Federal Trade Commission. Warning Letter to Robert O. Young, September 22, 2020. www.ftc.gov/system/files/warning-letters/ftc-covid-19-letter
-robert_o_young.pdf.

US Food and Drug Administration. "BeSafeRx: Frequently Asked Questions
(FAQs)." Accessed June 7, 2022. www.fda.gov/drugs/besaferx-your-source
-online-pharmacy-information/besaferx-frequently-asked-questions
-faqs.

US Food and Drug Administration. "Contact Lens Care Products—Premarket
Notification 510(k) Guidance." May 1, 1997. www.fda.gov/medical-devices
/guidance-documents-medical-devices-and-radiation-emitting-products
/contact-lens-care-products-premarket-notification-510k-guidance.

US Food and Drug Administration. "Fact Sheet: FDA at a Glance." November
2021. www.fda.gov/about-fda/fda-basics/fact-sheet-fda-glance.

US Food and Drug Administration. "FDA and the Work/Life Balance." Video,
YouTube, July 28, 2014. www.youtube.com/watch?v=yh9mqzrgjks.

US Food and Drug Administration. "FDA Warns Consumers of Serious
Harm from Drinking Miracle Mineral Solution (MMS)." News release,
July 30, 2010. Archived at Wayback Machine. https://wayback.archive-it
.org/7993/20170112005302/http://www.fda.gov/NewsEvents/Newsroom
/PressAnnouncements/2010/ucm220747.htm.

US Food and Drug Administration. "Guidance for Industry: Qualified Health
Claims in the Labeling of Conventional Foods and Dietary Supplements;

Availability." *Federal Register*, December 20, 2002. www.federalregister.gov /documents/2002/12/20/02-32194/guidance-for-industry-qualified-health -claims-in-the-labeling-of-conventional-foods-and-dietary.

US Food and Drug Administration. "Health Fraud Product Database." Accessed June 7, 2022. www.fda.gov/consumers/health-fraud-scams/health -fraud-product-database.

US Food and Drug Administration. *Investigations Operations Manual 2021*. Updated November 3, 2020. www.fda.gov/downloads/iceci/inspections/iom /ucm607759.pdf.

US Food and Drug Administration. "Questions and Answers on Dietary Supplements." Accessed June 7, 2022. www.fda.gov/food/information -consumers-using-dietary-supplements/questions-and-answers-dietary -supplements..

US Food and Drug Administration. "Remarks by Lowell Schiller, JD at the Council for Responsible Nutrition Conference—11/7/2019." November 6, 2019. www.fda.gov/medical-devices/guidance-documents-medical -devices-and-radiation-emitting-products/contact-lens-care-products -premarket-notification-510k-guidance.

US Food and Drug Administration. Warning Letter to Genesis II Church of Health and Healing, Mark Grenon, Joseph Grenon, Jordan Grenon, and Jim Humble. November 6, 2019. www.ftc.gov/system/files/warning-letters /fda-covid-19-letter-genesis_ii_church_of_health_and_healing.pdf.

US Food and Drug Administration. Warning Letter to Phoenix Biotechnology, Inc. December 15, 2020. www.fda.gov/inspections-compliance -enforcement-and-criminal-investigations/warning-letters/phoenix -biotechnology-inc-612178-12152020.

US Food and Drug Administration. Warning Letter to Robert L. Lytle. March 3, 2011. Archived at Wayback Machine. https://wayback.archive-it.org /7993/20170112094002/http://www.fda.gov/ICECI/EnforcementActions /WarningLetters/ucm246619.htm.

US Food and Drug Administration. "Welcome to FDA's White Oak Campus." Video, YouTube, April 19, 2017. www.youtube.com/watch?v=DqimZYtaqHw.

US Patent and Trademark Office. "Results of Search in US Patent Collection db for: ('laser' and 'lytle'): 1209 patents." Accessed March 19, 2022. https://patft .uspto.gov/netacgi/nph-Parser?Sect1=PTO2&Sect2=HITOFF&u =%2Fnetahtml%2FPTO%2Fsearch-adv.htm&r=0&f=S&l=50&d=PTXT&RS =laser&Refine=Refine+Search&Query=%22laser%22+AND+%22lytle%22.

US Zombie Outbreak Response Team. "About Us." Accessed March 20, 2022. https://uszort.com/.

Vaes, Jeroen, et al. "On the Behavioral Consequences of Infrahumanization: The Implicit Role of Uniquely Human Emotions in Intergroup Relations." *Journal of Personality and Social Psychology* 85, no. 6 (2004): 1016–1034. https://doi.org/10.1037/0022-3514.85.6.1016.

Van Vleck, Richard. "The Electronic Reactions of Albert Abrams." *American Artifacts*, accessed June 26, 2022. www.americanartifacts.com/smma/abrams/abrams.htm.

Vance, Lawrence M. "Conservatives and Medical Freedom," Future of Freedom Foundation, October 30, 2012. www.fff.org/explore-freedom/article/conservatives-and-medical-freedom/.

Vanegeren, Jessica. "Dueling Bills Take Aim at Religious Exemption." *Cap Times*, November 17, 2009. https://madison.com/ct/news/local/govt_and_politics/dueling-bills-take-aim-at-religious-exemption/article_ba6f00b4-d38b-11de-871b-001cc4c03286.html.

Vanegeren, Jessica. "Prayer Death Case Headed to State Supreme Court, Experts Say." *Cap Times*, March 19, 2010. https://madison.com/ct/news/local/crime_and_courts/prayer-death-case-headed-to-state-supreme-court-experts-say/article_85c9b9e0-b195-5b08-bd76-6df955e64adf.html.

Vervaeke, John, Christopher Mastropietro, and Filip Miscevic. *Zombies in Western Culture: A 21st Century Crisis*. Open Book Publishers, 2017. https://books.openedition.org/obp/4271?lang=en.

Vintage King. "You Can't Say I Didn't Tell You." Video, Facebook, March 31, 2021. www.facebook.com/vintageking2020/videos/136240745104365/.

Volckhausen, Taran. "Amazon Gold Mining Wipes out Rainforest Regeneration for Years: Study." *Mongabay*, August 4, 2020. https://news.mongabay.com/2020/08/amazon-gold-mining-wipes-out-rainforest-regeneration-for-years-study/.

Voytko, Lisette. "Maye Musk—Elon's Mom—Plugs $100 Anti-Aging Supplement, but Says She Hasn't 'Noticed' if It's Working." *Forbes*, September 28, 2021. www.forbes.com/sites/lisettevoytko/2021/09/28/maye-musk-elons-mom-plugs-100-anti-aging-supplement-but-says-i-havent-noticed-if-its-working/?sh=55f0af6e50cf.

Walton, Geri. " A Rat Problem in France in the Early 1800s." *Geri Walton Blog*, March 18, 2016. www.geriwalton.com/a-rat-problem-in-france-in-1800s/.

Watson, Steve. "Video: Trump Runs 'Zombie Biden' Ad During *Fear the Walking Dead* Broadcast." Infowars, October 26, 2020. www.infowars.com/posts/video-trump-runs-zombie-biden-ad-during-fear-the-walking-dead-broadcast/.

WCG-FDAnews Video Library. "A Day in the Life of an FDA Investigator." Video, YouTube, February 10, 2015. www.youtube.com/watch?v=qFlrD3kJfq4.

WCG-FDAnews Video Library. "A Day in the Life of FDA's Field Investigators." Video, YouTube, February 10, 2015. www.youtube.com/watch?v=jF_5MFZ08LA.

Weather Underground. "Livingston, MT Weather History." Accessed March 19, 2022. www.wunderground.com/history/daily/us/mt/livingston/KLVM/date/2004-2-19.

WebMD. "The Online Pharmacy Phenomenon." April 1999. www.webmd.com/a-to-z-guides/features/online-pharmacy-phenomenon.

Weisz, George. "From Clinical Counting to Evidence-Based Medicine." In *Body Counts: Medical Quantification in Historical and Sociological Perspective.* Montreal: McGill-Queen's University Press, 2005.

West, Marc. "Correlation of the Week: Zombies, Vampires, Democrats and Republicans." *Where Science Meets Pop Culture*, May 23, 2009. www.mrscienceshow.com/2009/05/correlation-of-week-zombies-vampires.html.

White, Jamie. "Mind Control: Scientists Engineer 'Magneto' Protein Capable of Remotely Controlling Brain and Behavior." Infowars, May 17, 2021. www.infowars.com/posts/mind-control-scientists-engineer-magneto-protein-capable-of-remotely-controlling-brain-behavior/.

Wilcox, Lindsay. "Physician Salary Report 2021: Compensation Steady Despite COVID-19." *Weatherby Healthcare* (blog), May 26, 2021. https://weatherbyhealthcare.com/blog/annual-physician-salary-report.

Wilson, John L. *Stanford University School of Medicine and the Predecessor Schools: An Historical Perspective.* 1998, accessed June 26, 2022. https://lane.stanford.edu/med-history/wilson/chap06.html.

WLUK-TV Fox 11. "Neumann Testifies." Video, YouTube, July 31, 2009. www.youtube.com/watch?v=z8EgKmMwff8.

Wolfe, Jan. "Four Officers Who Responded to U.S. Capitol Attack Have Died by Suicide." Reuters, August 2, 2021. www.reuters.com/world/us/officer-who-responded-us-capitol-attack-is-third-die-by-suicide-2021-08-02/.

Wong, Venessa. "Disgraced Dentist Zapped by Feds over Phony AIDS Laser." *BuzzFeed News*, October 11, 2015. www.buzzfeednews.com/article/venessawong/home-lasers-claiming-to-treat-cancer.

World Bank. "Physicians (per 1,000 People)—United States." Accessed March 19, 2022. https://data.worldbank.org/indicator/SH.MED.PHYS.ZS?locations=US.

Wouters, Olivier J. "Lobbying Expenditures and Campaign Contributions by the Pharmaceutical and Health Product Industry in the United States, 1999–2018." *JAMA Internal Medicine* 180, no. 5 (2020): 688–697. https://doi.org/10.1001/jamainternmed.2020.0146.

Yolin, Herbert S. "The Oral Cavity as a Guide for the Application of Low Level Laser Energy and Its Direct Effect on the Autonomic Nervous System Providing True Energy Healing for All Health Practitioners." *Proceedings of SPIE* 6846 (February 21, 2008). https://doi.org/10.1117/12.764195.

YouGov America. "The Most Popular All-Time Writers (Q2 2022)." Accessed March 31, 2022. https://today.yougov.com/ratings/arts/popularity/all-time%20writers/all.

Young, James Harvey. "The Todstool Millionaires: Chapter 4." Quackwatch, June 1, 2002. https://quackwatch.org/hx/tm/4-2/.

Young, Molly. "How Disgust Explains Everything." *New York Times Magazine*, December 27, 2021. www.nytimes.com/2021/12/27/magazine/disgust-science.html.

Young, Robert. "About." Accessed March 15, 2022. www.drrobertyoung.com /meet-dr-young.

Young, Robert. "The Alkalizing Benefits of Chlorine Dioxide (ClO2) in Human Health." Accessed March 15, 2022. www.drrobertyoung.com/post/the -alkalizing-benefits-of-chlorine-dioxide-clo2-in-human-health.

Young, Robert. "Alkalizing Nutritional Therapy in the Prevention and Reversal of Any Cancerous Condition." *International Journal of Complementary and Alternative Medicine* 2, no. 46 (2015). https://medcraveonline.com /IJCAM/IJCAM-02-00046. (Author's note: This journal has been flagged by the blog *Skeptical Raptor* as a predatory academic publisher, in part because it charges fees for submissions and has no proven standards for publication.)

Young, Robert. "Back to the Future: Jane Clayson of *The Morning Show* Shares the pH Miracle." Video, YouTube, January 24, 2021. www.youtube.com /watch?v=IJDOREbw4gA.

Young, Robert. "Biological Transformation in Dark Field Microscopy." Video, YouTube, September 5, 2018. www.youtube.com/watch?v=kvTlUGkgQEI.

Young, Robert. "The Cause and Self-Cure for Erectile Dysfunction & Improved Sex Life!" Accessed March 15, 2022. www.drrobertyoung.com/post /the-cause-and-self-cure-for-erectile-dysfunction-improved-sex-life.

Young, Robert. "Curriculum Vitae." Accessed March 15, 2022. www.drrobert young.com/curriculim-vitae.

Young, Robert. "Dawn Shares the Truth About Her Alkaline Child Birth with Shelley Young." Video, YouTube, December 4, 2018. www.youtube.com /watch?v=yDZB5ArUoXE.

Young, Robert. "Disclaimer." Accessed March 15, 2022. www.drrobertyoung .com/disclaimer.

Young, Robert. "Dr. Ben Johnson DO Shares is [*sic*] pH Miracle." Video, YouTube, September 15, 2018. www.youtube.com/watch?v=r9tgVvgegn4.

Young, Robert. "Dr. Charlie Ward Interviews Dr. Robert O. Young on What Is Really Going On?" Video, YouTube, October 19, 2020. www.youtube.com /watch?v=eqXhklpLqMM.

Young, Robert. "Dr. Joseph Mercola Interviews Robert O Young MS, DSc, PhD (The Complete Interview)." Video, YouTube, November 22, 2019. www .youtube.com/watch?v=5NFlsWDPBRs&t=1675s.

Young, Robert. "Dr. Robert O Young's Harvard Lecture—Towards the Ethics of Healing." Video, YouTube, December 3, 2018. www.youtube.com /watch?v=c-I-FyW-qmQ.

Young, Robert. "God Has Written His Name in Every Strand of Human DNA." Accessed March 15, 2022. www.drrobertyoung.com/post/god-has-written -his-name-in-every-strand-of-your-dna.

Young, Robert. "Health Sovereignty & Truth." Video, YouTube, January 29, 2021. www.youtube.com/watch?v=SX0PVjHgtGc.

Young, Robert. "High Crimes, Treason and Misdemeanors." Accessed March 15, 2022. www.drrobertyoung.com/post/high-crimes-treason-and-misdemeanors.

Young, Robert. "Just Believe and Miracles Are Possible." Video, YouTube, October 22, 2020. www.youtube.com/watch?v=yljF-tfT6Mg.

Young, Robert. "Just Believe and Miracles Will Happen." Accessed March 15, 2022. www.drrobertyoung.com/post/just-believe-and-miracles-will-happen.

Young, Robert. "A Lecture and Interview in Roma, Italy on the pH Miracle for Cancer and Then to the Vatican and the Pope." Video, YouTube, January 4, 2021. www.youtube.com/watch?v=qOtQmKe4svk.

Young, Robert. "The Many Healthy Restorative Benefits of Innerlight Blue Light." Video, YouTube, July 20, 2018. www.youtube.com/watch?v=qWqJx1TqeI8.

Young, Robert. "Message to My Critics." Accessed March 15, 2022. www.drrobertyoung.com/message.

Young, Robert. "Part 1—A Conversation on Inflammatory Ductal Cell Carcinoma Breast Cancer." Video, YouTube, November 6, 2020. www.youtube.com/watch?v=S3tXTyIYwi4.

Young, Robert. "Peer-Reviewed Articles." Accessed March 15, 2022. www.drrobertyoung.com/peer-reviewed-articles.

Young, Robert. "Preventing and Reversing Hair Loss." *pHorever Young* (blog), May 10, 2007. https://phoreveryoung.wordpress.com/2007/05/10/preventing-and-reversing-hair-loss/.

Young, Robert. "The Ranch of the Sun." Video, YouTube, January 31, 2016. www.youtube.com/watch?v=MUymssxXDN8.

Young, Robert. "The Real Truth About Dawn Kali's Breast Cancer." Video, YouTube, December 4, 2018. www.youtube.com/watch?v=X718ndGjZos.

Young, Robert. "Sacha Stone Interviews Commissioner Dr Robert O Young of the ITNJ [Part 2]." Video, YouTube, August 21, 2020. www.youtube.com/watch?v=OzKQsF-eOLg.

Young, Robert. "Saving the Animals and Humans in Africa and in America!" Accessed March 15, 2022. www.drrobertyoung.com/post/saving-the-animals-humans-in-africa-and-in-america.

Young, Robert. "Scanning and Transmission Electron Microscopy Reveals Graphene and Parasites in CoV-19 Vaccines." Accessed March 15, 2022. www.drrobertyoung.com/post/transmission-electron-microscopy-reveals-graphene-oxide-in-cov-19-vaccines.

Young, Robert. "The True Cause of COVID-19 Revealed with Dr. Robert O. Young." Accessed March 15, 2022. www.drrobertyoung.com/post/true-cause-of-covid-19-revealed-with-dr-robert-o-young.

Young, Robert. "The Truth About Dawn Kali!" Video, YouTube, December 4, 2018. www.youtube.com/watch?v=kC4ga2eC3WM.

Young, Robert. "The Truth About Kim Tinkham and Breast Cancer." Video, YouTube, November 11, 2020. www.youtube.com/watch?v=YSBrH8cDmUM.

Young, Robert. "Wake Up Humanity! The Plandemic Is Real!" Accessed March 15, 2022. www.drrobertyoung.com/post/the-plandemic-is-real.

Young, Robert. "Who Had Their Finger on the Magic of Life—Antoine Béchamp or Louis Pasteur?" *International Journal of Vaccines and Vaccination* 2, no. 47 (2016). https://medcraveonline.com/IJVV/IJVV-02-00047. (Author's note: This journal has been flagged by the blog *Skeptical Raptor* as a predatory academic publisher, in part because it charges fees for submissions and has no proven standards for publication.)

Youngdahl, Karie. "President-Elect Donald Trump and Vaccines." History of Vaccines, November 10, 2016. https://historyofvaccines.org/blog/president-elect-donald-trump-and-vaccines.

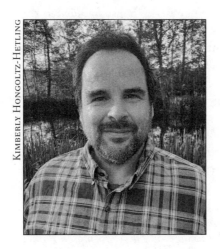

MATTHEW HONGOLTZ-HETLING is a journalist specializing in narrative features and investigative reporting. He has been named a finalist for the Pulitzer Prize, won a George Polk Award, and been voted Journalist of the Year by the Maine Press Association, among numerous other honors. He is the author of one previous book, *A Libertarian Walks into a Bear*, and he has written for the *New Republic*, *USA Today*, *Popular Science*, *Atavist Magazine*, Pulitzer Center on Crisis Reporting, the Associated Press, and elsewhere. He lives in Vermont.

PublicAffairs is a publishing house founded in 1997. It is a tribute to the standards, values, and flair of three persons who have served as mentors to countless reporters, writers, editors, and book people of all kinds, including me.

I. F. STONE, proprietor of *I. F. Stone's Weekly*, combined a commitment to the First Amendment with entrepreneurial zeal and reporting skill and became one of the great independent journalists in American history. At the age of eighty, Izzy published *The Trial of Socrates*, which was a national bestseller. He wrote the book after he taught himself ancient Greek.

BENJAMIN C. BRADLEE was for nearly thirty years the charismatic editorial leader of *The Washington Post*. It was Ben who gave the *Post* the range and courage to pursue such historic issues as Watergate. He supported his reporters with a tenacity that made them fearless and it is no accident that so many became authors of influential, best-selling books.

ROBERT L. BERNSTEIN, the chief executive of Random House for more than a quarter century, guided one of the nation's premier publishing houses. Bob was personally responsible for many books of political dissent and argument that challenged tyranny around the globe. He is also the founder and longtime chair of Human Rights Watch, one of the most respected human rights organizations in the world.

• • •

For fifty years, the banner of Public Affairs Press was carried by its owner Morris B. Schnapper, who published Gandhi, Nasser, Toynbee, Truman, and about 1,500 other authors. In 1983, Schnapper was described by *The Washington Post* as "a redoubtable gadfly." His legacy will endure in the books to come.

Peter Osnos, *Founder*